THE CHRONICALLY
DISTRESSED CLIENT

A model for intervention in the community

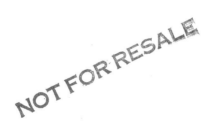

THE CHRONICALLY DISTRESSED CLIENT

A model for intervention in the community

FRANCES POWER ROWAN, R.N., M.S.

Team Leader, Day Treatment Program,
West Central Community Services Center,
Willmar, Minnesota

The C. V. Mosby Company

ST. LOUIS • TORONTO • LONDON   1980

The C. V. Mosby Company
11830 Westline Industrial Drive, St. Louis, Missouri 63141

Library of Congress Cataloging in Publication Data

Rowan, Frances Power, 1938-
   The chronically distressed client.

   Bibliography: p.
   Includes index.
   1. Mentally ill—Rehabilitation.   2. Mentally ill—
Rehabilitation—Case studies.   3. Community mental
health services.   4. Psychiatric nursing.   I. Title.
RC439.5.R68   610.73′68   79-22475
ISBN 0-8016-4204-3

C/M/M   9   8   7   6   5   4   3   2   1   05/C/606

To my mother

Theresa Foley Power

whose caring continues to unfold growth,

whose strength continues to adapt to life's demands,

and who finds fun in living for the moment.

She stands in testimony to the polarization of

true ego integrity and the flowering of wisdom.

FOREWORD

Although much has been written describing the science and art of nursing, there is little in the nursing literature illustrating how the two blend to become nursing practice. Frances Power Rowan does that in this book.

But she does more than that. In the preface and the first two chapters the reader is given a clear, understandable, explicit statement of nursing philosophy, nursing process, nursing practice, and the variables used to determine and evaluate care. The case studies in the next eight chapters illustrate the consistent application of that framework in practice.

Those who claim that psychiatric nursing is basically just process will find that position challenged. The content of practice is emphasized along with the continual evaluation and reevaluation of the client's response to explicit nursing interventions.

Those who minimize the importance of nursing process will also find that position challenged. Characteristics of the effective nurse are emphasized. The concept of a professional relationship is discussed. And a four-step nursing process is identified as the structural framework for practice.

The listing of variables and the use of the data base to determine and evaluate nursing care will stimulate considerable thought. Although additional testing is required to assure the validity and independence of the variables and to create a sound psychometric scale, a good beginning is here. The author has avoided premature claims about scaling and scoring, and this, too, is commendable.

What is most exciting to me is that as the author agonized intellectually over her own practice, doing a critical analysis and scholarly synthesis, she produced a book that is more than a contribution to the psychiatric nursing literature. Frances Power Rowan, through an inductive analysis of her practice, has helped define the very scope and nature of nursing knowledge and nursing practice.

Carol A. Lindeman, R.N., Ph.D., F.A.A.N.

PREFACE

In practice settings, nursing and nurses are in a special position. The clinician is placed by time, space, and skill most closely to the client's inner self. The pivot of any nurse's practice, especially in the psychosocial area, is to assist this inner self to cope in a healthy manner with traumatic experiences and to adapt to the living situation. All people cope in some way with life, its various predictable and unpredictable crises, the suffering and enjoyment of daily living, and all experiences, both positive and negative, that life provides. Unhealthy coping patterns are attempts to struggle with life and to protect the self from further pain. Healthy coping mechanisms are attempts to resolve conflicts and problems and to reach a relative level of equilibrium and emotional healing. Nurses willing to develop their communication skills and risk displaying a caring posture have within their grasp the ability to motivate or influence another human being's coping behaviors and coping patterns and thus affect human life.

Caring for individuals with long-term coping difficulties and chronic life disruptions can be a challenge. The attitude of the nurse within this relationship—sensitivity, empathy, flexibility, professional competency, proficiency, accountability, knowledge, care and concern, and self-investment—is crucial to help modify patterns of coping behaviors in the dilemma-filled lives of clients who receive the indelible label of "chronic." One does not readily adjust to the slow, deliberate stride called for in these situations. The fast-paced challenge of critical or crisis situations often has a more mobilizing effect on the nurse. The invitation of involvement with extended care clients lies in grappling with dilemmas and confronting the intricate entanglements of lives rooted in anxiety, dependence, and low self-concept. One perceives the confrontation as an uphill struggle and the task as toilsome. The conclusions from application of nursing process evaluation demand constant assessment with an expanded data base and increased validation. These vulnerable clients seem to live in a maze of self-defeat. The nurse must be keenly insightful and flexible if this maze is to resolve into a durable and renewed existence for the client. Often the evaluation mandates for the nurse frequent and increasingly innovative and creative use of self rather than a continuous butting against the already floundering client. The puzzled life of a person with the label "chronic" can often be given a more even tenor with fewer limitations through the persistent practice of nursing within a durable, solid relationship. Growth is possible for all human beings. Reliance on the potential of human growth can be the mainstay of the nurse.

The long-term nursing situation leaves no room for self-doubt. Commitment to growth through care, concern, nurturance, and applied theoretical knowledge is the core component in helping others in difficulty disentangle their lives.

Mental health is an individual asset; it fluctuates with new situations and new insights in each person's life.

Stress can alter an individual's functioning, adjustment, and adaptation, calling forth new methods of coping with situations that rely on old strengths.

Perception and integration of messages when high stress is present can alter functioning. A client can feel pushed under, unable to function properly, unable to rely on old methods, and needing new strength.

Mental health is a dynamic process. It is built with care and love and is sustained by love and care from within and without. It is tested in life by the process of living. One may fumble in reaching or grasping for a way to protect the self, and in so doing can usually find new strengths and a firmer base of mental health.

It is the application of one's personal and nursing philosophy that engenders the tremendous power to assist another human being cope on a level of increased health that makes the difference among nurses. All nurses have learned how to help clients cope; all nurses can choose to practice this client-centered skill. The nurse who assists clients to cope with life's realities is truly a practitioner of nursing.

If one wishes to make a change or support a transition, if one wishes to do something new, one must have commitment to an idea. One must be willing, whether it is comfortable or uncomfortable to demonstrate one's skills, to be responsible for one's actions, to try not to feel threatened or be threatening, and to have objective theory and data to support one's method of operation.

Several years before I was granted privileges (individual practice privileges in a health care organization), I learned that in order to be of any value to my patient/client, I had to be able to forget totally about myself when I exercised my professional skills. This was difficult for me to learn, but I have learned it so well that when I am in a professional relationship with a patient/client, I first of all turn all my thoughts to the patient/client and off myself. When I turn to my client and give nursing care, I make every effort to remain open to questions or peer evaluation. If I've done well, or done poorly, I can evaluate with ease because my concern has not been for me but for my patient/client. My concentration level and listening ability have increased with this "other centeredness."*

The often missed beauty of nursing process is its built-in reinforcement for one's self both personally and professionally while offering an objective umbrella of "other centeredness." Nursing process is a thinking, action-oriented, professional activity leading to observable behavioral outcomes. For purposes of this book I subscribe to the four-step method of nursing process. Nursing process is implemented as *assessment* of the client, *diagnosis* of the problem areas, *intervention*, or actual nursing care planned and administered, and *evaluation* of concrete outcomes.

The essence of the material presented here assumes the reader's extensive knowledge base and theoretical foundation. The substance of the case format is intervention strategy and implementation requiring basic philosophy and principle supplementary to nursing formulation and action.

I wish to express my sincere appreciation to numerous colleagues, students, and clients, both past and present, and to devoted family and friends whose encouragement, insights, and collaboration have inspired and fortified me to

---

*From Rowan, F. P.: The privileged nurse. In American Nurses' Association: Power nursing's challenge for change, Kansas City, Mo., 1979, The Association. Reprinted with permission of the American Nurses' Association.

complete my task. I am especially indebted to Bernard A. Schultz, my mentor for this project, who not only inspired growth but insisted on development and maturation of my written communication skills. The conscientious support of Frances M. Ludwig, R.N., M.S.N., urged persistence and validated my commitment to the value of this book. Cynthia Braem, secretary-typist, adjusted her time to my needs and to the completion of the task not only without complaint, but with a smile and words of encouragement. Christine M. Wolohan, R.N., B.S., provided reliable, organized reference research in a limited time period.

Frances Power Rowan

CONTENTS

NURSING PHILOSOPHY, CONCEPTUAL HYPOTHESIS OF PRACTICE, AND A PERSONAL CONTEMPLATION

Nursing process is a systematized thinking and action-oriented method that lends credence and refinement to nursing practice. For the methodology of nursing process to be learned effectively, it must be broken down into segments of the whole. All the pieces can be then viewed by the nurse as separate entities. Data collection, for example, is done to obtain pertinent information. Later, these data become part of the assessment, and much later, the assessment becomes part of the whole or total of nursing process. Many of the segments of nursing process are learned as paper-and-pencil exercises and must be transferred to a flowing-thinking exercise executed in one's mind and delivered through one's nursing skills. The quality of one's nursing practice should be measured through the individual application of nursing process to one's practice.

Nursing process is an intellectual method that nurses are educated and disciplined to apply to the practice of client care. In-service education, continuing education programs, and current professional literature regularly provide refinements and perspectives on nursing process.

Hypothetically, the currently accepted information and application of nursing process will always be necessary to nursing practice. Presumably access to and knowledge of all current nursing process information *can affect* one's nursing practice, *but it does not necessarily or automatically* do so. It is the implementation and skillful application of nursing process that refine and give credibility to one's nursing practice.

Nursing process *is not* choosing to follow a memorized one-, two-, three-, four-step procedure or a five-step procedure, or is it the implementation of an eight-step procedure. Nursing process is a circular, ongoing thinking and doing process activated by extensive, applied specific and general knowledge of one person toward another person or persons within the confines of an interpersonal relationship. It produces growth if the elements of caring, discriminating communication techniques, and scientific skills are employed by the caregiver-nurse.

The total objective application of nursing process allows the nurse to review actual practice with immediate answers or explanations for the outcomes of the given care. Evaluation and continual assessment remove ambiguity about the whys and wherefores of the nursing outcomes. The answers are evident to the open, questioning, and evaluating mind. Mistakes, wrong conclusions, and misinformation are readily corrected when nursing process is continually and systematically applied. Renewed nursing efforts are methodically practiced until the end goals or outcomes of nursing action are assured, objectively aborted, or redirected.

Evaluation lends objectivity to limited progress in the long-term client relationship and the slow-paced therapy movement that the clinician confronts daily in routine encounters with long-term psychiatric clients. This phase of nursing process monitors nursing action to aid in preventing stagnation and feelings of helplessness. The use of the methodology itself provides a control over one's practice. A mode of regulation gives power to the clinician in preventing or dispersing the apathy and helplessness that can cripple both clinician and client.

Proficient, ongoing assessment as part of nursing process is a highly functional key to progress in long-term psychosocial nursing situations. The umbrella-like nature of continual assessment ensures an active process that is always alert to new behavior, change, and growth whether it be toward or away from health. Assessment does not stop once all apparent data have been collected by the clinician or when nursing diagnosis is concluded. It brings continuity accompanied by growth, productivity, and a more holistic quality to the client care. With long-term psychosocial nursing situations it can prevent stagnation and entrenchment in unhealthy behavior and reliance on ineffective coping patterns. The constant assessment factor unearths new, relevant data. Validation of coping styles, interacting manners, and behavior patterns is derived through steady, repeated, and persistent appraisal of the observable data, client and nurse perception, and the execution of the client's life stance.

Psychosocial nursing diagnosis is a statement of essential groupings or a compilation of significant assessed data, both objective and subjective, obtained from a relevant investigation of the client. Nurses obtain these data within the scope of the established interpersonal relationship from both verbal and nonverbal communications. Other pertinent facts are gathered from available records, collaboration with other reliable professionals involved with the client, family members, and other significant relationships. Relevant, significant data are then converted to short, descriptive, identifying themes on which nursing intervention is based. Nursing diagnosis may be viewed as the core of nursing interventions. Colloquially, nursing diagnosis is a "springboard" to nursing intervention.

Three nursing diagnoses consistently applied in each case are essential components of the fundamental dilemma of the chronically distressed client. They are anxiety, dependence/independence struggle, and low self-concept. Intrinsic and extrinsic conflicts produce an unremittingly high anxiety level that is intensified by lack of conflict resolution, uncertainty, and discomfort. In the client a relentless life quandary between dependence and independence with a usual nonautonomous stance is reinforced by an essentially reliant nature, supported by negative and uncertain feedback and a diminished level of functioning. Low self-concept is a perceptual disturbance that is strengthened and replenished by the process of chronicity, the nonautonomy, perplexing and irresolute life stance, and lack of significant person associations. The nurse's relationship with the client must facilitate differentiation of the self while fostering healing and growth, adaptation, and change.

The term "nursing diagnosis" in long-term psychosocial nursing situations is extremely relevant to practice. Psychosocial nursing is a broad area that reaches from the heights to the depths of human behavior. Nursing diagnosis in the case material encompasses symptoms of emotional distress such as anxiety; descriptions of the clients' prominent behaviors, such as lack of insight; and simplistic descriptions of core pathology, such as inability to grieve. (See Appendix A.) Simple, descriptive, recognizable terms that apply to a client's particular dilemma based in observable reality are a nursing diagnosis of choice. Nursing diagnosis must be relevant to the client's current situation, mandating nursing intervention. The application of nursing process is based on knowledge, theory, proficient and skillful communication, and practice experience. In addition, the knowledgeable application of nursing process methodology, professional and self-motivation, a care-concern quality for other individuals, a refined innate sensitivity (or "gut-level" instinct), and the courage to apply one's proficiency with dis-cretion to another human being are all germane components to the nursing process. This task often looms as formidable. The risk lies in daring to begin, to evaluate, and to stay with the process until the outcome is satisfactory to both practitioner and client. The level and objectivity of commitment help to differentiate and identify nursing practice as a professional alliance.

In the case examples of intervention in psychiatric nursing, the process is a continuously applied, four-step method of assessment, diagnosis, intervention, and evaluation to assist an individual to cope with life as evidenced in behavioral outcomes. Additionally, the nursing process is further implemented *at selected points* in a step-by-step procedure, *beginning with* evaluation, renewed assessment, diagnosis, and intervention. The format of the application of the process is elaborated in Table 1.

Table 1. Psychosocial nursing process methodology (adapted from four-step nursing process format and problem-oriented medical record format)

Nursing process step	Methodology
IV Evaluation	**1**—Evaluation yields the following data: 　Nursing diagnosis (N.D.) 　　Subjective component (S) 　　Objective component (O) 　　Actual outcome evaluation
I Assessment	**2A**—Continual assessment yields additional data: 　Nursing diagnosis (N.D.) 　　Subjective component (S) 　　Objective component (O) **2B**—Continual assessment yields data validated by repetition of behavior: 　Nursing diagnosis (N.D.) 　　Subjective component (S) 　　Objective component (O)
II Diagnosis	**3**—Additional nursing diagnosis conclusions
III Intervention	**4A**—Intervention is predicated on nursing judgment of the following: 　1. Evaluation data 　2. Assessment data 　3. Selected nursing diagnosis

Continued.

Table 1. Psychosocial nursing process methodology (adapted from four-step nursing process format and problem-oriented medical record format)—cont'd

Nursing process step	Methodology
III Intervention— cont'd	4. The presence (positive) or absence (negative) of the influence of the following client variables: Reality timing $+5+4+3+2+1$ $0-1-2-3-4-5$ Relationships $+5+4+3+2+1$ $0-1-2-3-4-5$ Stressors and/or crisis $+5+4+3+2+1$ $0-1-2-3-4-5$ Coping resources $+5+4+3+2+1$ $0-1-2-3-4-5$ Significant emotional strength $+5+4+3+2+1$ $0-1-2-3-4-5$ Significant emotional limitations $+5+4+3+2+1$ $0-1-2-3-4-5$ Therapy relationship $+5+4+3+2+1$ $0-1-2-3-4-5$ Physical health status $+5+4+3+2+1$ $0-1-2-3-4-5$ Physical and emotional readiness dimension $+5+4+3+2+1$ $0-1-2-3-4-5$ Available support systems $+5+4+3+2+1$ $0-1-2-3-4-5$ Meaning significance $+5+4+3+2+1$ $0-1-2-3-4-5$ Values and beliefs impact $+5+4+3+2+1$ $0-1-2-3-4-5$ Other, if applicable 5. Additional knowledge Nursing diagnosis (N.D.) 6. Analysis and synthesis Nursing diagnosis (N.D.) **4B**—Intervention activity is supported by nursing judgment conclusions resulting in a design of action: Nursing diagnosis (N.D.) 1. Plan 2. Strategy 3. Expected outcomes 4. Criteria

Measurement scale

| Positive, or presence of health potential | | | | | | | | | | Negative, or absence of health potential |

← +5   +4   +3   +2   +1   0   −1   −2   −3   −4   −5 →

| strongest | | stronger | | strong | | weak | | weaker | | weakest |

Fluid line

In the left-hand column the Roman numerals indicate the more usual order of the four-step methodology. It is underscored that the initial *implied* case application of nursing process was the more usual order of assessment, diagnosis, intervention, and evaluation. The case material focuses on intervention, and it is after initial assessment, diagnosis, and intervention that the methodology is first elaborated at selected points. Assessment is basic to intervention, but it is not the focal point of the client's case study when life stance modification is germane to health and growth. Initial assessment content includes all data described prior to the point of stated nursing diagnosis. Furthermore, assessment is a continuous core element of all psychosocial nursing. In the actual application of nursing process over extended periods, the resumed intellectual implementation of the nursing process occurs during the evaluation step, then proceeds to a renewed assessment, diagnosis, and intervention effort by the nurse. Skilled nursing activity is rooted in this refined intellectual methodology called nursing process. The case studies have been constructed to portray this circular, *ongoing thinking/action* methodology *focusing* on restorative, replenishing, *intervention* endeavors.

The intellectual component of nursing process is implemented at selected points in the case material with emphasis on assessment and planning, but in no way do these points represent the only appropriate or significant periods of intervention. Both the depth and breadth of the implementation could be increased. Methodology applications were selected to demonstrate initial, intermediate, and extended progression in the therapy. Selection criteria were also the intensity of an interaction, the duration of the relationship, and the repetition of the intervention needed to achieve an end goal. The final implementation of the selected methodology does not include evaluation. It is suggested that enough data have been provided to complete this element. A paper-and-pencil

approach would be most useful. An additional suggested exercise would be the selection of a new or alternate area in the case to apply the espoused methodology. Performance of this intellectual task in a simulated situation extends proficiency and skill into the actual nursing situation requiring practitioner action.

The client variables identified in Table 1 are instruments of nursing judgment. They are elements of change that alter the essence of a situation and apply to the predictability of a psychosocial nursing intervention. There is a subjective element in judging or qualifying these variables. Objectivity can be acquired and refined through practice. The proficiency of observation skills and the intensity, duration, and quality of the helping relationship refine the clinician's impersonal, unbiased judgmental abilities.

The selected variables are chosen as factors that influence and complicate one's nursing intervention in long-term psychosocial nursing but do not have scientific validity or reliability. The need for refinement of the variables as a tool for psychosocial assessment is acknowledged. Distinct, discriminating definitions of the terms in ascending and descending order need to evolve. The elementary identification of relevant areas is hypothesized as a baseline in need of standardization.

A rating scale of both positive and negative scores was chosen to show the actual deficits as well as positive force factors in operation within the client's life. The *individual score* of each variable *is significant* in itself. Each area represents one influencing life factor. The standardization of terms, definitions, and measurement would clarify more clearly the interdependence of the variables themselves.

An overall balance score of positive, negative, or balance indicates the presence or absence of potential for change or adaptation. A composite numerical score is not applicable in the present form of the instrument. The tool has not been tested for reliability or validity. Other rating scales might lend themselves better to standardization; however, it is important to acknowledge that clients have both positive and negative forces affecting their functioning. Therefore an alternate choice of the sole criterion of a plus scale or minus scale may not portray the actual life position of the client.

In addition, the variables have value only at the point in time of judgment. A quantitative composite of several numerical scores over time would not necessarily indicate growth or lack of growth. For example, a lower quantitative composite score after 2 years of therapy when crisis factors are prominent does not preordain a decrease in coping ability or interacting manner or an increase in reliance on negative behavior patterns. It may only represent the presence of increased stress factors activating pathology. The client may be ready to experience the learning of new, more effective coping, open interacting methods, and new positive behaviors to alleviate the stress. A lower composite score may also suggest a new or increased willingness to engage in life struggles and not retreat to a state of negative polarization. This client willingness may not be accompanied by functioning ability. The nursing intervention plan and activity become the map to experience positive outcomes. The identified variables are road signs to help chart the chosen course of action for a unique client, with a particular set of circumstances, at a specific point in time.

The necessary nursing judgments can be defined as follows:

1. Reality timing—selecting the proper moment for doing a task or beginning an intervention to achieve the desired objective. An example of reality timing at a -3 level is choosing a point to begin a therapy goal when some objective data exist that will interfere with goal initiation or achievement.

2. Relationship—an association or connection between people. Such an alignment, if positive, usually has a quality of supportiveness and emotional involvement. An example of a relationship at a $+5$ level is a select number of people in one's personal territory, both familial and nonfamilial. Such a relationship is of an emotionally intimate nature. Several associate or comrade relationships exist that are of a social nature.

3. Stressors and/or crisis—equilibrium factors that are both intrinsic and extrinsic to the balancing of life forces. Crisis is a condition of instability in the life factors. Crisis can be considered a turning point in life, leading to a new direction that can be either positive or negative in nature. An example of stressors and/or crisis at a 0 level is a balance in the presence of life pressuring forces, not causing undue anxiety. The lack of current or impending crisis in one's life is also an example of a judgment at 0 level.

4. Coping resources—available capabilities to contend with the life problem at hand. An example of coping resources at a -3 level is when few adequate supports are available to meet the continual demands or pressures of life over an extended time.

5. Significant emotional strength—prominent feelings of affective force or energy or the deficiency or a fragility of such energy or force. An example of significant emotional strength at a $+5$ level is an observable identified positive force in more than one area of living. The reverse, or a -5 level, is an observable identified deficiency of a positive force or emotional fragility in more than one area of living.

6. Significant emotional limitations—prominent lack of emotional capacity or an inability to feel; a restrictive affective weakness. An example of a significant emotional limitation at a 0 level is the absence of an observable identified obstacle or boundary to self-disclosure within the therapy relationship.

7. Therapy relationship—the essence of the bond between client and nurse. The association denotes an emotionally intimate level of connections. Overriding qualities of rehabilitation, a healing or curative nature, client self-disclosure, and clinician skill are apparent to the

observer. An example of the therapy relationship at a 0 level is one in which the identified qualities exist but the relationship lacks the quality of endurance over time and observable, measurable, objective progress in the client. No deterrents to the relationship are identified.

8. Physical health status—the soundness of the body; an indication of the lack or presence of a physical disease condition or process. An example of physical health status at a −2 level is the presence of a transient viral infection.

9. Physical and emotional readiness dimension—a synchronization of body and emotions. Somatic and psychic forces become involved in the task at hand and in the achievement of the desired objectives and identified goals. An example of the physical and emotional readiness dimension at a −4 level is the presence of identifiable physical health problems and of identifiable intrinsic and extrinsic anxiety.

10. Available support systems—the existence of or accessibility to methods or structures of sustenance, maintenance, assistance, or strength. An example of an available support system at a −5 level is the absence of an identifiable structure offering strength at a high point of stress.

11. Meaning significance—indicative interpretation or important implication of a life factor. Meaning is often subjective to the client and may be a covert element. An example of meaning significance at a −5 level is a client's pervading and unshakable perception or interpretation that originates in his psychopathology.

12. Values and belief impact—an intrinsic and extrinsic thrust of personal ideals and convictions and societal norms. The person holding these values and beliefs accepts them as authentic, factual, and basic to life. An example of values and belief at a +3 level is convictions founded in reason and realism that have a positive force toward the client's health. The degree of impact will change the level.

All nursing judgments are relative to the specific situation of each client. The degree of balance depends on the time, place, interdependence of the identified variables, and presence or absence of psychopathology.

One's use of nursing process comes from within oneself. One's talent, knowledge, and skills applied to each situation will provide a unique contribution for a nurse practitioner. The other-centered approach to nursing care is a communication tool applied to enhance the relationship through the nursing process by providing comfort and objectivity both to the nurse and to the client.

The implementation of nursing process as a decision-making tool allows for a broadness of one's nursing practice. The science of nursing has a comprehensive and diversified knowledge base requiring extensive practice skills for each individual nurse. Astute assessment of one's client allows for individualized treatment supported by data about a person or group at a specific point in the process that considers all of the applicable variables of a situation. The clinician's acute observation aptitude further validates the client's behavior by ongoing assessment of the dynamic client profile.

Frequently, in the treatment of clients for emotional problems or mental illness, the therapist employs only a narrow philosophy or one treatment modality in the expectation that it will improve the problem. Treatment goals and health outcomes for a client or group often depend on the therapist's astuteness, combined person and knowledge complexities, and skill rather than on the discipline, philosophy, or specific treatment modality. No amount of knowledge, no single philosophy, and no single treatment modality provide a panacea for a successful client outcome. Growth, change, and healing occur within the scope of a relationship. The relationship combined with proficient assessment and skilled intervention supercede the choice of professional discipline, treatment philosophy, and/or curative modality.

Nurse-psychotherapy is a broadly based,

helping-healing process, accomplished within the confines of an interpersonal relationship, that encourages the client, guided by the nurse, to unfold and experience life, emotions, and feelings. The process provides for the client a reality validation for his unstable life position and stance. Initiation of the therapy relationship lends credence to the client's potential for growth and hope for a renewed existence. The relationship between client and nurse creates the force to direct energy into a growth orientation. Nursing process methodology regulates the intellectual and activity course of the interpersonal relationship.

The essence of helpful nurse psychotherapy is in astute assessment, on which is based individualized treatment, accompanied by sound theoretical knowledge applied through the framework of nursing process to fit the assessed needs of the client. The therapist should not attempt to fit the client into a predetermined philosophy, belief, or treatment modality. Nursing process allows for a broad philosophy and flexible treatment plan chosen to fit the client's total present situation.

Psychosocial nursing is applied by means of nursing process to promote or maintain the mental health of clients under a nurse's care, whatever the setting. No matter what the problem may be—a transient, limited disease process, an educational need, a disabling illness, an adjustment transition, a terminal disease process, a complex growth phenomenon, or the implementation of a preventive measure—it is how one assists the client to cope with the demands of the situation that will make the difference both in the client's ability to live here and now and in the quality or level of one's nursing practice.

It must be recognized that all human beings have potential and strengths, but no acceptable substitute for the term "mental illness" and "psychopathology" can be given credence when one is working with long-standing individual limitations and incapacities for which no

healing or change or growth is possible *without* knowledge and understanding of the dynamics of identified psychopathology. Chronically emotionally disabled individuals have coped ineffectively for years, this negative coping style being self-reinforcing. Society has reinforced their impaired interacting manner with negative self-concept ideations. Negative behavior patterns have provided insulation or protective shielding from confrontation with the real world. Until someone can provide a better framework for the understanding of the long-term emotionally disabled individual and a functional basis for the implementation of therapeutic interventions for this rooted group of people, maintenance of a firm stance in the use of the term "mental illness" is indispensable.

For purposes of clarification, the term "mental illness" is defined as noticeable behavioral deviations (beyond the normal range) that indicate a degree of self-disintegration accompanied by a degree of functioning impairment within the culturally accepted norm of a community. The intensity and aberration of the erratic behavior may vary according to person and lifestyle. Mental illness is more than the lack of mental health; it encompasses behaviors that impede or deter self-growth, positive coping skills, and productive life choices. Mental health is a relative balance of intrinsic and extrinsic psychic life factors. Mental illness is the relative imbalance of these same life factors. It is more than a fluctuation of psychic balance.

Phenomenologically, a picture of mental health is viewed as a precariously balanced seesaw, changing from moment to moment. The fluid line between health and illness is invisible. On any given day one's emotions fluctuate on this balance scale. It is when the balancing factors weigh in a negative direction over a long duration, without positive self-affirmation, corrective feedback, and supportive relationships that chronic imbalance results in self-disintegration and decompensation episodes with its accompanying deviant behaviors. This self-disintegration guise precipitates and reinforces a manner of thinking referred to as psychopathological.

Professional relationships with long-term psychosocial clients are characterized by the qualities of duration, constancy, and intensity. The depth of the relationship is indicative of the emotional involvement, privations, and abilities of the client and the relevancy, homogeneity, and alliance bonding of the professional affiliation. The reciprocal interchange and dynamic movement between two people with a common goal form a professional kinship with a poignant power to achieve emotional health and healing. This strong relationship is the pivot for the modification of divergent behaviors, the revealing of untapped personal resources, and the alteration of divergent life-styles.

The clinician confronted with the client's long-term pathology and limited prognosis may retreat from the overwhelming feelings of the situation rather than rise to its challenge. The therapist needs a certain, unshakable sense of self and self-assurance, patience, maturation, stability, and wisdom of foresight.

Frequently, the nurse must empathize with rather unappealing people. A sense of sadness can pervade the nurse's care and concern if the reality is viewed as hopeless rather than with a sense of potential for change. The frequent, competent, intricate judgments involved in choices related to the nurturing aptitude and the "doing of" tasks are not usual to nursing, but they are basic to teaching life-style adaptations and the learning of daily living skills and social modification for the client. The weighty client dependence/independence struggle within the relationship is taxing on the nurse. One can easily overreact and place unrealistic expectations and demands on the client when feedback from peers and from objective data is limited. The task of caregiving to long-term emotionally unstable individuals requires one to confront core pathology on a most dynamic yet simplistic level. The nurse's proficiency, excellence of skills, and competency are judged by the artistry and craftsmanship demonstrated to meet the client at a mutually acceptable beginning point with an extended goal encompassing an increased quality of life, emotional healing, and a renewed level of health.

For the therapist, long-term client care requires a philosophy of realism, but *tempered* realism sensitized by idealism. The nurse cannot work effectively with the client without accepting the reality of the client's present lifestyle, choices, and prevalent psychopathology. Reality does lock one into time and space, often decreasing the growth potential of the client and suffocating the initiative of the nurse. If the clinician is to dwell within the boundaries of reality, she must allow for hope for a better future to provide a satisfactory medium for healing, and for an ultimate improved level of health. To dream is to grow and to achieve. An honest balance between a clear perception of the graphic real world and the broad hope for a better tomorrow encourages a positive attitude for the clinician. Realism is often grim. The clinician's imagination can foster creativity. Vision for the future and fantasy often are divided by a fine fluid line. Absolute truth can poison hope. The clinician must always be imbued with hope to kindle confidence and optimism in the client concerning his present living situation and future life.

SUGGESTED READINGS

Aguilera, D.: Review of psychiatric nursing, St. Louis, 1977, The C. V. Mosby Co.

Altschul, A. T.: Use of the nursing process in psychiatric care, Nursing Times **73:**1412-1413, Sept. 8, 1977.

Aspinall, M. J.: Nursing diagnosis—the weak link, Nursing Outlook **76:**434-437, July, 1976.

Aspinall, M. J., Jambruno, N., and Phoenix, B.: The why and how of nursing diagnosis, The American Journal of Maternal Child Nursing **2:**354-358, Nov./Dec., 1977.

Collins, M.: Communication in health care, St. Louis, 1977, The C. V. Mosby Co.

Craig, A., and Hyatt, A.: Chronicity in mental illness: a theory on the role change, Perspectives in Psychiatric Care **16:**139-154, May-June, 1978.

Davis, J.: The rights of chronic patients, Hospital and Community Psychiatry **29**:38, Jan., 1978.

Doona, M., et al.: Professional affirmation in nursing care, Journal of Psychiatric Nursing **15**:16-23, Aug., 1977.

Durand, M., and Prince, R.: Nursing diagnosis: process and decision, Nursing Forum **5**:50-64, April, 1966.

Finkelman, A. W.: The nurse therapist: outpatient crisis intervention with the chronic psychiatric patient, Journal of Psychiatric Nursing **15**:27-32, Aug., 1977.

Gebbie, K., and Lavin, M. A.: Classifying nursing diagnoses, American Journal of Nursing **74**:250-253, Feb., 1974.

Gebbie, K., and Lavin, M. A., editors: Classification of nursing diagnosis, St. Louis, 1975, The C. V. Mosby Co.

Gordon, M.: Nursing diagnosis and the diagnostic procedures, American Journal of Nursing **76**:1209-1300, Aug., 1976.

Grahan, K.: Problem solving as a therapeutic process, Journal of Psychiatric Nursing **14**:37-39, Nov., 1976.

Gurevitz, H.: Caring for chronic patients: some cautions and concerns, Hospital and Community Psychiatry **29**:42, Jan., 1978.

Hall, E.: The hidden dimension, Garden City, N.Y., 1963, Doubleday & Co., Inc.

Harris, T.: I'm OK—you're OK, New York, 1967, Harper & Row, Publishers.

Henderson, V.: The nature of nursing, American Journal of Nursing **64**:62-68, Jan., 1964.

Jahoda, M.: Current concepts of positive mental health, New York, 1958, Basic Books, Inc., Publishers.

Jourard, S.: Transparent self, Princeton, N.J., 1964, Van Nostrand Co.

Keener, M. L.: The public health nurse in mental health follow-up care, Nursing Research **24**:198-201, May/June, 1975.

Kerr, N.: Anxiety: theoretical considerations, Perspectives in Psychiatric Care **16**:36-46, Jan.-Feb., 1978.

Levine, J., et al.: The nurse practitioner: role, physician, utilization, patient acceptance, Nursing Research **27**:245-254, July/Aug., 1978.

Lipp, M.: What's in it for the therapist? Hospital and Community Psychiatry, **29**:40, Jan., 1978.

Little, D., and Carnevali, D.: Nursing care planning, Philadelphia, 1976, J. B. Lippincott Co.

Marriner, A.: The nursing process, St. Louis, 1975, The C. V. Mosby Co.

McCaie, R.: Nursing by assessment—not intuition, American Journal of Nursing **65**:82-84, April, 1965.

Mereness, D., and Taylor, C.: Essentials of psychiatric nursing, St. Louis, 1978, The C. V. Mosby Co.

Minckley, B.: Space and place in patient care, American Journal of Nursing **68**:510-516, March, 1968.

Mitchell, P.: Concepts basic to nursing, New York, 1973, McGraw-Hill Book Co.

Mundingir, M. E., et al.: Developing a nursing diagnosis, Nursing Outlook **75**:94-98, Feb., 1975.

North, G.: The concepts of mental illness and disability, Occupational Health Nursing **25**:12-14, July, 1977.

O'Brien, M.: Communications and relationships in nursing, ed. 2, St. Louis, 1978, The C. V. Mosby Co.

Orlando, I.: The dynamic nurse-patient relationship, New York, 1961, G. P. Putnam's Sons.

Peplau, H.: The work of the psychiatric nurse, Psychiatric Opinion **4**:5-11, Feb., 1967.

Peplau, H.: Professional closeness, Nursing Forum **8**(4):342-360, 1969.

Peplau, H.: Psychotherapeutic strategies, Perspectives in Psychiatric Care **6**:264-270, Nov.-Dec., 1969.

Peplau, H.: Psychiatric nursing: role of nurses and psychiatric nurses, International Nursing Review **25**:41-47, March/April, 1978.

Report to the President from the President's Commission On Mental Health, Vol. I, Washington, D.C., 1978, Government Printing Office.

Report to the President from the President's Commission On Mental Health, Vol. II, Washington, D.C., 1978, Government Printing Office.

Rogers, C.: On becoming a person, Boston, 1961, Houghton-Mifflin Co.

Rowan, F. P., Theurer, L. S., and Welch, M. R.: Psychosocial nursing skills, Winona, Minn., 1976, Nursing Consultation, Inc.

Roy, C.: A diagnostic classification system for nursing, Nursing Outlook **75**:9-94, Feb., 1975.

Satir, V.: Conjoint family therapy, Palo Alto, Calif., 1967, Science & Behavior Books, Inc.

Satir, V.: People making, Palo Alto, Calif., 1972, Science & Behavior Books, Inc.

Selye, H.: The stress of life, New York, 1976, McGraw-Hill Book Co.

Snyder, J., and Wilson, M.: Elements of a psychological assessment, American Journal of Nursing **77**:235-239, Feb., 1977.

Sundeen, S., et al.: Nurse-client interaction, St. Louis, 1976, The C. V. Mosby Co.

Szasz, T.: The myth of mental illness, New York, 1961, Harper & Row, Publishers.

Topalis, M., and Aguilera, D.: Psychiatric nursing, ed. 7, St. Louis, 1978, The C. V. Mosby Co.

Travelbee, J.: Intervention in psychiatric nursing, Philadelphia, 1969, F. A. Davis Co.

Weinberg, J.: The chronic patient: the stranger in our midst, Hospital and Community Psychiatry **29**:25-28, Jan., 1978.

CHAPTER 2

RATIONALE FOR INTERVENTION AND AN APPROACH TO CLIENT CARE

To give concise meaning to the case history format applied, certain terms and concepts must be detailed. The initial case description— a person with ineffective coping style, impaired interacting manner, and negative behavior patterns that *foster* specific life force turmoil and difficulties of living—is delineated with terms characterizing negative life-style actions.

These terms separate problematic life conduct. One such area of behaviors multiplies others. Negative development of one category of action reacts negatively with the other indexed actions so that, for example, an impairment in interacting or communication reinforces and compounds already existing negative behavior patterns. In the reverse, hypothetically, if one identified life-style action can be altered or substituted in other than the defined destructive deviation, the negative patterns become weakened and healthy new actions or behaviors can evolve. This indicates that an effective coping measure will foster positive interpersonal interactions.

Coping is a dynamic skill for encountering or contending with life that changes to meet life's demands and goals. An ineffective coping style can be defined as an unproductive manner of relating to life experiences. Each individual possesses a repertoire of coping skills that he or she uses to relate to life experiences or to attain desired life conclusions.

All human beings communicate and interact with their environment. An impaired interacting manner is a weakened, reduced, or damaged style or method of interchange or person association. It is a communication breakdown in message clarification, translation, and integration between the sender and the receiver-perceiver of the message.

Negative behavior patterns are dissenting or inaccurate forms or modes of conduct that are not in accord with accepted societal norms. The action does not usually achieve the desired end or goal, resulting in increased anxiety, frustration, and negative reinforcement.

An introductory and summary profile is set forth in the outline on p. 12 to present a systematized and comparative sketch of the targeted client.

Personal profile*

Social adjustment
   Subjective component
   Objective component
Emotional health status
   Subjective component
   Objective component
Physical health status
   Subjective component
   Objective component
Spiritual dimension
   Subjective component
   Objective component
Daily living skill performance
   Subjective component

   Objective component
Coping skill repertoire
   Subjective component
   Objective component
Maturational struggle according to
   Erikson's developmental stages
   Subjective component
   Objective component
Self-integration
   Subjective component
   Objective component
Quality of life
   Subjective component
   Objective component

---

*Profile employed as a comparison tool applied to assist in judging holistic growth from the formation (introductory profile) of the nurse-client relationship to the termination (summary profile) of this relationship. Significant variables are the congruence or incongruence of the subjective and objective components of assessment at the introductory level and at the summary level, and the comparison of congruence or incongruence between the two profiles.

The profile operationalizes accepted qualitative categories of person and action description congruent with the stated philosophy. Quality of life and maturational struggle, according to Erikson's developmental tasks, will be further developed. A subjective and objective delineation is utilized to classify the introductory and summary assessment into areas of clearly defined interpretations.

Assessment is a compilation of data collected by the clinician to begin or complete a client profile. Client appraisal is both objective and subjective in nature. Accurate data gathering depends on the disciplined and sensitive practice skills of the clinician.

The objective element of initial assessment is a collection of all observable data concerning the client. One does a cephalocaudal (systematic head-to-toe) evaluative observation, noting the norm, incompatibility, and incongruence with the norm as a baseline of physical, psychological, spiritual, and social assessment. A collection of environmental data and a historical, physical, and psychosocial inventory, with emphasis on the present life status, complete a baseline personal profile.

The subjective element of assessment at any stage of the process is gathered through observation or the application of the therapist's sensory aptitude—sight, sound, smell, touch, and taste. Active listening, a qualified "sixth sense," an educated intuitive intelligence for the problem, and an expertness are qualities that the astute clinician working with long-term emotionally disabled clients must develop. Dexterity of applying these qualities lends mastery to the therapist's assessment skills. Clinical assessment qualities remain credible through practice and established feedback mechanisms from both client and peer.

Recognition of both verbal and nonverbal client messages are of immediate consequence.

It is mandatory for the clinician to give importance to the nonverbal client messages if assessment is to be concluded with a profile of solidarity and sufficient data for nursing diagnosis and corrective intervention measures.

Assessment of one's client is an open-ended, ongoing procedure. Space must always be available for new data and/or validated information relevant to life, growth, adaptation, or crisis through new or renewed appraisal efforts. This is an example of the refined intellectual methodology of nursing process producing applicable practice knowledge for nursing action.

Quality of life is often viewed as only subjective and is related to the human values of the observer. The index chosen is used to describe a broad scope of change or improvement in the client's life-style and human comfort. If one makes esthetic environmental alterations such as painting walls or adding curtains to windows, it can enhance one's pleasure. If one changes from a thin, worn mattress and wire mesh springs to a thick, firm mattress and box spring, it can provide a positive change in physical comfort. Diet modification can produce a health adaptation that improves a person's self-image, physical mobility, and energy level. Renewed gratification, contentment, and personal solace may signify quality-of-life alteration. The quality-of-life measure cannot be what the therapist would subjectively or objectively choose for a personal style of living, but what the client chooses to enhance personal comfort, effective coping style, and need satisfaction.

Developmental maturation of the eight stages of man and resultant "favor ratio" or "basic virtues" signifying maturational development or strength gained through experiencing the conflict or struggles of basic task achievement, as defined by E. H. Erikson, are as follows:

1. Basic Trust vs. Basic Mistrust: Drive and Hope
2. Autonomy vs. Shame and Doubt: Self Control and Will Power
3. Initiative vs. Guilt: Direction and Purpose

4. Industry vs. Inferiority: Method and Competence
5. Identity vs. Role Confusion: Devotion and Fidelity
6. Intimacy vs. Isolation: Affiliation and Love
7. Generativity vs. Stagnation: Production and Care
8. Ego Integrity vs. Despair: Renunciation and Wisdom*

Many developmental theories are available from which to choose a framework. Erikson's theory provides both breadth and depth and is readily applicable to nursing. He asserts that there exists a continuous thread of life events in each individual's life history. Furthermore, affective or emotional process is believed to be the basic motivational factor for all human behavior. Each individual is to be understood in his own unique but complex life situation.

Erikson believes that life unfolds in an orderly process. Maturation is on a growth continuum, and life is represented as a synthesis of maturational tasks in a hierarchy of stages. It is an orderly process. Each new developmental phase gives an opportunity to correct past incomplete tasks of maturing. This process is lifelong, not necessarily completed in a defined period. Setbacks and reversals are recognized as essential. Regression is a constant variable and an accepted deviation from the norm. Trust in adaptive powers is the key to maturational achievement.

Erikson explores adult development and considers adolescence below the adult developmental level. He asserts that one's self-awareness and understanding continues throughout a person's life. Polarity or a relative mix of all identified task achievement is present at all times in a person's life. The stages are interdependent, and each stage is in relationship to the other stages. No one achieves complete

---

*From Erikson, E. H.: Childhood and society, ed. 2, 1963, New York, W. W. Norton & Co., Inc., Publishers, and London, The Hogarth Press, Ltd., p. 274.

mastery of any polarity before progressing to the next plateau.

There can be a struggle in the maturational process between two opposing internal pulls until polarization may occur. Each new conquest in polarity becomes the foundation for a new phase of development. Independence, trust, and interpersonal relationships result from successful outcomes of conflicting pulls. Stress is put on each ''favorable ratio'' development.

The acceptance of these beliefs concerning personal growth and maturation lends an ease to involvement with long-term clients whose life maturation process often lacks polarity and positive orderliness and demonstrates poor adaptation to life demands. The nurse-clinician rarely discerns polarity of developmental tasks when involved in therapy with long-term clients, rather the nurse engages the client in the struggle of opposing forces and guides the client's action to positive outcomes.

A strong degree of commitment within the interpersonal relationship by both client and nurse is necessary to fulfill established goals. This commitment encompasses both intellectual and emotional involvement by the clinician. An intellectual commitment of effort to knowledge and quality can facilitate modification in lifestyle. An emotional commitment or appreciation is an intricate quality of person power, not an entanglement to an end goal or even to health itself. The complex meaning of this personal involvement is hope for a better measure of life and an overall personal growth in life skills for the client entrusted to one's care.

The rooted and disorganized state of the long-term client lends a perplexing nature to therapy encounters. Lack of insight, vagueness, apathy, other-person reliance, pervading anxiety and vulnerability, and an inadequate sense of self perpetuate the client's mazelike, complicated existence. These characteristics can spill over to the therapy encounter, often yielding unclear data that will uncloud only with the duration of the interpersonal relationship and the client's healing and growth. The sensitivity of the therapist allows the actuality of this condition. Acceptance of the client in his current state grants needed permission for the client-initiated, internal self-approval and emergence of new behaviors, and it provides a baseline for therapy growth and evolution of the needed distinct, understandable data. A structured therapy format helps to disentangle the intricate detail of the individual client who is in a vulnerable state of chronic distress.

A nursing approach to long-term psychosocial care almost always involves an extended task focus to promote daily living skill performances. A former task avoidance stance by the client impeded personal growth and fostered withdrawal from life responsibilities, and it also allowed undue and extensive self-absorption and the maintenance of psychopathology. These ''doing'' interventions or nursing activities are usually slow, tedious achievements, requiring the clinician to adjust to the client's often apathetic and lethargic pace while maintaining a posture of sensitivity, supportiveness, reassurance, and confident belief in the realization of the identified positive expectations. Tasks are chosen to facilitate fulfilling life priorities and responsibilities, and/or to impede pathological behaviors, and/or to achieve a satisfying life experience or experiences, and/or to accommodate or realize a client's life choice. Often, the client's life posture determines the choice of the task and may even complicate the assignment. Respect for the selection and preference of the client is mandatory. The client's acknowledgment of the nurse's judgment is also mandatory in regard to health decisions and healing directions. Task achievement creates a climate of safety for clients to express their emotions within the professional relationship, often culminating in a new and more intense level of interaction.

Communication may be defined most simply as a system of sending and receiving messages. It is an interchange of knowledge, opinions, and thoughts. Communication may be verbal (talk) or nonverbal (gestures or writing). Human communication is more explicitly described by Shapiro as occurring any time that one (sender) does or does not do something (message) and this is interpreted by someone else (receiver-perceiver), whose interpretation has an effect on an interpersonal relationship or the accomplishment of a task. The context evaluation of the communication is vital to comprehension of the intended message. Communication is considered successful only when understanding occurs. In the therapy situation the client often discloses information of an intensely personal nature. The revealed statements usually have previously had a covert nature, and the revelations usually present some perceived risk of exposure to the personhood of the client.

Communication feedback is essential to therapeutic interaction. Feedback provides sustenance and understanding through returning of the observed *or perceived* behavior (output) sent by the receiver to the (input) sender. Feedback gives a frame of reference for recognizing messages and assigning meaning.. Professional helpers must understand both the connotative, or internal, emotional, personal attributes and the denotative, or cultural, objective, observable attributes of the client's messages.

Feedback is objective, action-oriented communication or positive person-oriented communication (affirmation). Employment of feedback techniques by a proficient clinician provides strength for the client's personhood and helps the client know if his response is correct. It reinforces and encourages behavior and ego strength and promotes understanding. This system of interacting influences or modifies behavior through knowledge by allowing a medium for the understanding of cause and effect.

Meaning is a cognitive interpretation. It is the significance of the implication to the individual. Meaning is located in both external or observable responses and in internal or obscure mes-

sages. An explanation of meaning is understood through feedback and context evaluation for latent communication themes. Frankl calls meaning the psychic energy for a situation. Meaning is achieved through experience and can provide motivation to an individual. One gives meaning by ascribing traits or qualities to an index. Often the experienced clinician develops a ''praecox feeling'' or inner sense for the meaning at a relevant point in the therapy relationship. This refined subjective meaning quality comes with proficiency in nurse-client interrelating at an advanced level or intense degree of shared emotional intimacy. This is an integration of true other-centeredness.

Nursing process employs restrictive communication by its use of strategy or plan, its evaluative component, and its attempt to structure or direct the interaction. Restrictive communication can limit feedback. Such restrictions can be countered with a true care-concern quality, active listening, an other-centeredness, personal flexibility and warmth, and role adaptability. A climate of trust and emotional security will foster open communication. One must be sensitive to the fact that an individual intentionally communicates only that which he feels safe in revealing. Rewards for client feedback must be. established to cultivate maturation of the professional relationship and progress toward positive outcomes in therapy. The client must develop his own ''bank account'' of positive feedback (ego strength), which will give him emotional energy to take relationship risks required by the therapy situation. Self-disclosure is threatening to an already emotionally compromised and vulnerable individual. The nurse's sensitivity to actualities of the client's life and emotional capability is essential to therapeutically touching the previously hidden, hurting self.

Self-disclosure is a communication skill learned within a relationship that is often missing from the repertoire of living skills of the long-term, emotionally disabled client. The introduction of a self-disclosure element within the bonds of a secure professional relationship may often be perceived as difficult, frightening, and/or impossible by the client who has spent 30 or more years withholding self-revelation. Avoidance of this emotive sharing is common, and the task of learning is tedious. The slow, uneven tenor of each client's life and adherence to the protective shield from life events demand a deliberate, controlled intervention stance from the clinician. Self-disclosure information applied to healing intervention within the relationship increases trust and decreases the uncertainty and perceived hurt associated with personal revelations and emotional intimacy.

Nurse psychotherapy provides for emotional experiences that furnish a medium for feeling growth. Emotional experiences are an openness to live the pain, discomfort, trauma, anxiety, or healing associated with the encounter. These experiences have a replenishing effect for the client and establish a base for realization of new feelings and self-knowledge. They also provide for the professional maturation of the nurse. When the client braves the emotional encounter, a new sense of self can be sustained or enjoyed. The experiences provide a process of realization of human feelings in a condoned, protected climate.

In the majority of case studies, a regularity of progression in the relationship occurs. Initial focus (1) is physical health maintenance and medication assessment. The intermediate therapy focus (2) is a task-centered supportive approach, concentrating on work responsibility and recreational activities. The extended focus (3) is relevant to the emotional self, personhood, and growth struggles of the client. This progression seems to provide a safe climate to the chronically distressed, vulnerable client.

The initial and intermediate steps are an action-oriented intervention that validates genuine interest in the client's welfare. Physical health concerns are usually expected to be a nursing focus. These tasks can be performed efficiently and create a climate of security and low self-risk. Fulfilling health work and task concerns free emotional energy that enables the client to become intellectually and emotionally involved in therapy. These initial and intermediate concerns are usually objective pursuits that develop a true aura of safeness within the interpersonal relationship, fostering a climate of self-disclosure and emotional expression. In some relationships the client reverses this order of progression and requires that the therapist begin early intervention measures at the emotional self level. This circumstance is a testing of the nurse's proficiency, trustworthiness, and skill. It also provides a prematurely expanded assessment arena for the clarification of the strengths, limitations, verbal skills, accessibility, and needs of the client.

The major theoretical nursing concept for intervention in the case material is similar to what Peplau calls an investigative approach in which current interpersonal problems are resolved. Through assessment and decision making the nurse examines the problem from the onset. Problematic behaviors, environmental observations, meanings for the client, supportive resources, and alternative behaviors are explored in the therapist's prior preparation and by the client and therapist planning together. This results in decisions about therapy focus, therapy goals, and expected outcomes. Therapy agreements may be verbal or written contracts, depending on the nature of the situation, persons involved, and specific end goals. A limited supportive emotive approach is implemented to free energy, foster emotional development and self-esteem, and expand a restricted client self-concept. The level of the client's insight and emotional accessibility qualifies or circumscribes the amount of convergence in this emotive approach. Real changes must be an outcome of this concentration with the client in examining the ineffective coping styles, the impaired interacting manner, and the negative behavior patterns that interfere with healthful living. The result of an investigative emotive approach to nurse-client therapy is for the client to adapt alternate coping styles, untried communication methods, and new behaviors with guidance and support from the nurse. The "trying on," or experiencing, of these coping styles, communication methods, and behaviors by the client is a measurement of progress in therapy. Often the essence of the chronic emotional disability of the client presents a perceived high risk for the client's becoming involved in such proceedings. The doing of tasks fosters pride and self-respect from the achievement, producing a positive feeling and enhancing the client's sense of self. Completed, task-centered interventions often assist the client to become more accessible to an emotive level of interaction with the therapist. Concrete, objective, measurable task achievement within an investigated nursing process format is more readily accepted, operationalized, and integrated by the long-term emotionally disabled client. A limited emotive approach is defined by the essence of the person and by the client's pathological structure, problems, and availability to the mode of nursing intervention. The client's accessibility to a sensitive nurse-therapist, demonstrating a true care-concern quality and other-centered focus within the professional relationship, further defines the therapy direction.

An essential component in the nurse's fundamental knowledge and belief is an intellectual and emotional acceptance of the fact that therapy progress with long-term emotionally disabled clients is extremely slow paced and is measured in quarter inches or even millimeters. The trudging movements, interactions, and activities must be accepted as a beginning of therapy and as an actuality of the client's lifestyle. The nursing relationship endeavors to add a deliberate approach to this slow, languid life stance. The clinician who is eager to change the disruptive inactivity will quickly fail in these efforts. Assessment will validate a required adaptation by the clinician to the realities of the

client psychopathology, actual limitations, and life stance to create a common ground and mutual bond for a cohesive beginning of health work, healing tasks, and future chosen life goals and adaptations for the client, whose efforts will be guided to fruition by the clinician.

SUGGESTED READINGS

Aguilera, D.: Review of psychiatric nursing, St. Louis, 1977, The C. V. Mosby Co.

Blair, K.: It's the patient's problem—and decision, Nursing Outlook **19**:587-589, Sept., 1971.

Collins, M.: Communication in health care, St. Louis, 1977, The C. V. Mosby Co.

Craig, A., and Hyatt, B.: Chronicity in mental illness: a theory on the role change, Perspectives in Psychiatric Care **16**:139-154, June, 1978.

Davis, J.: The rights of chronic patients, Hospital and Community Psychiatry **29**(1):39, Jan., 1978.

Erikson, E.: Childhood and society, New York, 1963, W. W. Norton & Co., Inc., Publishers.

Frankl, V.: Man's search for meaning, New York, 1959, Washington Square Press.

Fromm, E.: Man for himself, Greenwhich, Conn., 1947, Fawcett Publications, Inc.

Fromm, E.: The sane society, Greenwich, Conn., 1955, Fawcett Publications, Inc.

Fromm, E.: The art of loving, New York, 1956, Harper & Brothers, Publishers.

Gaylin, W.: Caring makes the difference, Psychology Today **10**:34-39, Aug., 1976.

Gregg, D.: The therapeutic roles of the nurse, Perspectives in Psychiatric Care **1**:18-24, Jan./Feb., 1963.

Gurevitz, H.: Caring for chronic patients: some cautions and concerns, Hospital and Community Psychiatry **29**:42, Jan., 1978.

Harris, T.: I'm OK—You're OK, New York, 1967, Harper & Row, Publishers.

Jahoda, M.: Current concepts of positive mental health, New York, 1958, Basic Books, Inc., Publishers.

Jourard, S.: Transparent self, Princeton, N.J., 1964, Van Nostrand Co.

Kennedy, E.: The pain of being human, New York, 1974, Doubleday & Co., Inc.

Kratz, C.: Planning nursing care for the chronic sick, Nursing Times **74**:9-12, Jan. 26, 1978.

Lipp, M.: What's in it for the therapist? Hospital and Community Psychiatry **29**:40, Jan., 1978.

Maslow, A.: Toward a psychology of being, Princeton, N.J., 1962, Van Nostrand Co.

May, R.: The meaning of anxiety, New York, 1977, W. W. Norton & Co., Inc., Publishers.

Mayeroff, M.: On caring, New York, 1971, Harper & Row, Publishers.

O'Brien, M.: Communications and relationships in nursing ed. 2, St. Louis, 1977, The C. V. Mosby Co.

Orlando, I.: The dynamic nurse-patient relationship, New York, 1961, G. P. Putnam's Sons.

Osgood, C.: The nature and measurement of meaning, Psychological Bulletin **49:**197-237, 1952.

Osgood, C., Succi, G., and Tannenbaum, P.: The measurement of meaning, Urbana, Ill., 1967, University of Illinois Press.

Peplau, H.: Interpersonal relations in nursing, New York, 1952, G. P. Putnam's Sons.

Peplau, H.: Basic principles of patient counseling, Philadelphia, 1964, Smith, Kline & French Laboratories.

Peplau, H.: The work of the psychiatric nurse, Psychiatric Opinion **4:**541, Feb., 1967.

Peplau, H.: Psychotherapeutic strategies, Perspectives in Psychiatric Care **6:**264-270, Nov./Dec., 1969.

Report to the President from the President's Commission on Mental Health, Vol. I, Washington, D.C., 1978, Government Printing Office.

Report to the President from the President's Commission on Mental Health, Vol. II, Washington, D.C., 1978, Government Printing Office.

Rogers, C.: On becoming a person, Boston, 1961, Houghton Mifflin Co.

Satir, V.: Conjoint family therapy, Palo Alto, Calif., 1967, Science & Behavior Books, Inc.

Satir, V.: People making, Palo Alto, Calif., 1972, Science & Behavior Books, Inc.

Seeger, P.: Self-awareness and nursing, Journal of Psychiatric Nursing **15:**24-26, Aug., 1977.

Sencicle, L.: Taking the labels off, Nursing Times **74:**52, Jan. 12, 1978.

Shapiro, G.: Interpersonal communication in the modern organization, Englewood Cliffs, N.J., 1968, Prentice-Hall, Inc.

Simon, S.: Caring, feeling, touching, Niles, Ill., 1976, Argus Communications.

Skinner, B. F.: Beyond freedom and dignity, New York, 1971, Alfred A. Knopf, Inc.

Sundeen, S., et al.: Nurse-client interaction, St. Louis, 1976, The C. V. Mosby Co.

Toews, J.: Community psychiatry: a re-examination of some concepts, Canadian Mental Health **25:**3-4, Dec., 1977.

Topalis, M., and Aguilera, D.: Psychiatric nursing, ed. 7, St. Louis, 1978, The C. V. Mosby Co.

Travelbee, J.: Interpersonal aspects of nursing, Philadelphia, 1966, F. A. Davis Co.

Veninga, R.: Communications: a patient's eye view, American Journal of Nursing **68:**758-762, April, 1978.

Watzlawick, P., Beavin, J., and Jackson, D.: Pragmatics of communication, New York, 1967, W. W. Norton & Co., Inc., Publishers.

The case material in the following chapters focuses on persons with *ineffective coping style, impaired interacting manner,* and *negative behavior patterns* that *foster* specific life force turmoil and/or difficulties of living. These manifestations of problematic life conduct are identified as vital limitations created by the client's self-reinforced mazelike network of existence.

Significant data have been altered to protect the anonymity of the clients. Case material is written from recall rather than from the records of any agency. Incidents are composites of and/or facsimile material from experience. None of the persons cited exists per se.

CHAPTER 3

MAZIE W *manifests*

PROBLEMATIC LIFE CONDUCT

evidenced by

UNRESOLVED GRIEF AND DEPRESSION

INTRODUCTORY PERSONAL PROFILE

Social adjustment

S "I've always had a hard time making friends." "No, I don't talk to the neighbors anymore." "People look at me. It bothers me." "I can't call my son."

O Extreme motor activity influencing interpersonal relationships. Withdrawal from social encounters and avoidance of interpersonal contacts.

Emotional health status

S "Sometimes I don't sleep well." "I eat enough." "My stomach hurts." "I can't always remember." "I'm so nervous." "I don't know why I'm nervous, do you?"

O Extreme motor activity. Sleeping and eating pattern indicative of depression. Memory loss. Sad, drawn expression. Approximately 6 weeks after electroshock therapy. Unresolved grief work and role transition. Husband's death $2^1/_2$ years previously.

Physical health status

S "Sometimes I don't sleep well." "I eat enough." "I don't care to cook anymore." "My stomach hurts." "I get so tired."

O Extreme motor activity. Early morning rising with few sleep hours. Sluggish bowel. Blood pressure and pulse within norms. Height 5 feet, 7 inches. Weight 155 pounds. Approximately 6 weeks' postelectroshock therapy. Memory loss. Fatigue level high in relation to activity.

Spiritual dimension

S "I don't go to church as much as we used to." "I get nervous with people." "I can't stay and talk."

O Regular church attendance. Several church-related activities.

Daily living skill performance

S "I washed early today. Don't have many clothes when you live alone." "This house isn't very neat. I need to work at cleaning more often.''

O Clean environment. Good personal grooming. Responsible management of home and finances but not of personal needs and requirements.

Coping skill repertoire

S ''I just can't go out.'' ''Oh, now I couldn't do that.'' ''I don't know how.'' ''Do you really think so?'' ''I just can't help myself.''

O Ineffective in sustaining personal integration. Negative patterns of behavior reinforced with negative feedback and withdrawal from the mainstream of living.

Maturational struggle according to Erikson's developmental stages

S ''Oh, I can't do that.'' ''We were happy.'' ''I don't understand why he left me.'' ''Nothing seems to help.'' ''This is Mrs. Abraham W'' (In telephone conversation.)

O Basic trust vs. basic mistrust.
   Autonomy vs. shame and doubt.
   Identity vs. role confusion.

Self-integration

S ''Sometimes I wish I had died, too.'' ''We did everything together.'' ''We were happy.'' ''I don't understand why he left me.'' ''I forgot.'' ''I don't know.'' (Related to feelings.)

O Fluctuating level of psychic balance. Identity crisis related to role transition and unresolved grief remain prominent despite $2^{1}/_{2}$-year time span.

Quality of life

S ''It's OK.'' ''I don't need anything.'' ''I just sit here lots of time.''

O Withdrawal, loneliness, chronic psychic distress. Somatic discomfort. Limited financial resources.

Time span: 6 years

Mrs. W is a 60-year-old, widowed, white female. She is 5 feet, 7 inches in height and large boned. She weighs 155 pounds and is bulky in appearance. She is grey haired and pale, and her small brown eyes rarely meet one's glance. She appears to exhibit extreme symptoms of extrapyramidal syndrome, although she receives a minimal dosage of thioridazine, 50 mg t.i.d., along with biperiden, 2 mg t.i.d., to counteract this syndrome.

Mrs. W's husband had died of a sudden massive cerebral hemmorrhage $2^{1}/_{2}$ years before her first meeting with the therapist. She talked very little about her husband but always identified herself as Mrs. Abraham W despite her given name of Mazie. The little information she gave about her marriage led one to conclude that there was an exclusive interdependence for Mr. and Mrs. W, so much so that they had few separate interests, hobbies, activities, or friends. Mr. W's death was a blow that Mrs. W was unprepared to cope with. She did not perceive herself as existing without her husband. The reality of a separate existence was a traumatic life experience that Mazie had been unable to integrate successfully into her being. When Mr. W died, Mazie, a lifetime teetotaler, used brandy and sleeping pills to ease her psychic pain and feelings of loss and to help her sleep.

Mrs. W has two adult sons, Abraham, Jr., and Arthur, both of whom are married. Abraham, Jr., a professional man and the father of eight children, lives a thousand miles from his mother. He calls her once a month and visits her home with his wife for a few hours once a year. This son sends his mother lovely gifts and money on all the right occasions—Christmas, Mother's Day, and Easter. Mrs. W had many pictures of her eight grandchildren. There is a hint of sparkle and pride in her eyes when she shows these pictures. The second son, Arthur, lives within 20 miles of his mother, but he seems to make as few contacts as possible with her. Her state of health seems to embarrass Arthur and his wife.

Despite approximately 10 contacts with these young men and their wives over the 6 years that Mrs. W was in therapy, all attempts to bridge the gap in the mother-son relationships were futile. Physical distance and telephone conversations are not conducive to bridging carefully created family emotional distance. There was no viable opportunity to pursue family therapy per se.

Mrs. W owns her own home, an old, clean, simply furnished structure, small but comfortable and adequate for her. Financially, she has a small savings account, receives Social Security benefits, and is comfortable according to her frugal standard of living, although she is not secure financially by accepted economic standards.

Each time she was visited by the therapist, Mrs. W was clean in appearance and dressed neatly, usually wearing a faded cotton housedress, a beige cardigan sweater, brown oxford shoes, and dark nylon stockings. She exhibited severe neurological extrapyramidal symptoms as evidenced in *akathisia,* that is, jitteriness, motor restlessness, and anxiety-associated behaviors; *tardive dyskinesia,* swallowing difficulties and protrusion of the tongue; and *pseudoparkinsonism,* masklike facies, tremors, and shuffling gait. The excessive prominence of these symptoms interfered with her already faulty interpersonal relationships. These relationship difficulties were viewed simply by Mrs. W, who would say ''I've always had a hard time making friends.'' Her uncontrolled body movements aggravated her existing relationship problems in all of her associations and increased her prevailing low self-concept.

At 60 years of age Mazie W was first seen by a mental health professional and hospitalized for situational depression in a state mental hospital for a 6-week duration. At 62 years she was again hospitalized and received a course of twelve electroshock treatments. She was discharged from the hospital with no relative

change after 5 months of confinement. The discharge date was not clearly specified in available data but was judged to be within a relative time span of 3 weeks after electroshock therapy. It was at this point in her life that she began weekly nurse psychotherapy in her home.

Nursing diagnosis of Mrs. W includes the following:

Anxiety
Dependence/independence struggle
Low self-concept
Inability to complete the grieving process
Unhealthy learned behavior
Loneliness
Trust/mistrust struggle
Faulty support system
Interpersonal relationship disturbance
Lack of insight
Short concentration span
Transient memory loss
Passive resistance

Mrs. W, at her first meeting with the therapist, on questioning, decided she would like to be called Mazie, although she rejected use of the therapist's first name. Somehow, using the surname seemed to provide needed security, furnish an authority figure, and allow a healthy dependency for her.

The first months of therapy were difficult for Mazie. The acceptance of this client in her current state of functioning, ability to evaluate nursing intervention, and insight were valuable devices for the bonding of this professional relationship. Mazie was uncomfortable with the therapist, with herself, and with the therapy situation. Furthermore, she was uncomfortable with life and living.

The usual meeting place was Mazie's living room. She chose the seating arrangement to keep herself at a 20-foot distance across and at opposite ends of the room from the therapist. Her territorial space was not to be readily invaded. The living room was drab and uncomfortably warm, and it had a loudly ticking antique grandfather clock. Mazie's body movements were distracting, her voice lacked inflection, and her movements increased if the therapist paced the process faster than Mazie could extend herself.

Granting silence was essential to a climate of acceptance and rapport. Slow, quiet talking, repetition, and a calm voice were all part of forming the relationship. The therapist's own body language reflected control to give a message of calmness and security. The frequently long, 10-minute silences were communication maneuvers by the client to test the safety of this new and threatening relationship.

At the end of each interview, Mazie wanted to know if and when the nurse would return. It was the only clue to her acceptance of the therapy situation. At the end of 6 months of therapy, Mazie took the initiative to call to state she forgot the appointment, or she would ask, "When will you come?" at the termination of a therapy session.

Mazie's progress was extremely slow. A noninsightful, apparently very ill woman of 62 years does have intrinsic value. The therapist let her know in a nonthreatening manner that she liked Mazie, and certainly Mazie needed to know that someone liked her. With concentration one could block out her body movements but at the same time remain aware that increased motor activity did signal increased inner tension.

After six 1-hour weekly therapy visits, Mazie did not increase her motor activity during the visits. At this point the therapist chose to move from her accustomed end of a long couch to the reverse end. This decreased the distance by 5 feet, while continuing to keep the client and nurse at opposite sides but not at opposite ends of the room. Mazie now allowed the therapist into her personal territorial space (Figure 1). The polarity of positions had created a barrier to communication, a restraint to the interpersonal

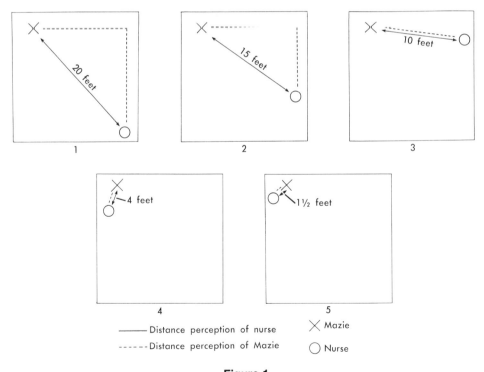

Distance perception of nurse
Distance perception of Mazie

✕ Mazie
◯ Nurse

Figure 1

relationship, and a hindrance to the therapy movement.

During the seventh visit, the therapist asked for a tour of Mazie's home. Mazie evidenced increased comfort as she smiled hesitantly and increased the speed and tone of her speech; her gait was more controlled as she proceeded to "show and tell." This interview was marked by increased verbal exchange. Mazie spoke of her husband and his death in an unemotional, flat tone of voice, but she could say it was "awful that he was gone." Ever so slowly, progress was being made and some feelings were surfacing in a climate of openness, warmth, guidance, and caring.

The therapist investigated Mazie's medication regimen. Thioridazine, 50 mg t.i.d., and biperiden, 2 mg t.i.d., had been prescribed by her physician. She often forgot to take her "pills" as prescribed. During each day she frequently wondered *if* she took them and/or *when* she really did take them. Together, Mazie and the therapist wrote big notes to post on her refrigerator to remind her to take one of each tablet (specifying by color) at 9:00 A.M., 2:00 P.M., and 7:00 P.M. It was agreed that the therapist would count her medication at each weekly visit. Unfortunately, the "big note" was not a successful nursing measure. In the next weeks it became a systematized chart, which needed a check after each pill was taken. This chart method was relatively successful as measured by counting medication regularly in maintaining proper medication management for Mrs. W.

PROCESS IMPLEMENTATION

1 — Evaluation
N.D.   *Anxiety*
    S   It's "awful that he is gone."
    O   No increased anxiety on entering personal territorial space observed. Extreme motor activity. Smiled hesitantly. Increased speed and tone of voice. Gait more controlled.
N.D.   *Trust/mistrust struggle*
    S   "When will you come?"
    O   Increased appropriate conversation. Increased amounts of verbal dialogue. Responses increased from one word to phrases to sentences

of three to six words. No increased anxiety observed on entering personal territorial space.
N.D.   *Interpersonal relationship disturbance*
    S   "When will you come?" "Call me Mazie." "I've always had a hard time making friends." "People stare at me."
    O   No increased anxiety observed on entering personal territorial space. Extreme motor activity.
N.D.   *Dependence/independence struggle*
    S   "When will you come?" "Call me Mazie."
    O   Initiative to validate appointment time. Decided to be called by first name. Decision took 20 minutes. Decided to address therapist by surname. Decision took 25 minutes.
N.D.   *Unhealthy learned behavior*
    S   "I can't sit still." "People stare at me."
    O   Thioridazine 50 mg, biperiden 2 mg. Akathisia. Tardive dyskinesia. Pseudoparkinsonism. Extreme motor activity. No increased anxiety observed on entering personal territorial space.
Actual outcome
Basic relationship bonding between the client and nurse.

2A — Assessment
N.D.   *Anxiety*
    S   "I'm just so nervous." "I can't sit still."
    O   Extreme motor restlessness. Unable to follow oral or written directions.
N.D.   *Unhealthy learned behavior*
    S   "I'm just so nervous." "I can't sit still."
    O   Continued akathisia, tardive dyskinesia, and pseudoparkinsonism after decrease in drug ingestion and also after lengthy drug withdrawal.
N.D.   *Short concentration span*
    S   "I can't remember if I took my pills." "What did we talk about when you were here last time?"
    O   Relative time after electroshock therapy 5 weeks. Unable to follow oral or written directions.
N.D.   *Transient memory loss*
    S   "I can't remember if I took my pills." "Maybe I took them this morning when I got up." "What color pill do I take at 9:00 A.M.?" "Oh, the time is written out for me."
    O   Relative time after electroshock therapy 5 weeks. Not taking medication as prescribed. Not remembering therapy appointments.
N.D.   *Low self-concept*
    S   "I want this to stop but I can't." "I just can't help myself."

O In public situations people stare, point, and comment, "Look at that strange lady," or "That lady isn't very ladylike when she chews gum." Difficulty interacting with therapist.

N.D. *Passive resistance*

S "I just don't know when I took my pills." "I want this to stop but I can't." "I just can't help myself." "You do it with me."

O Not taking medicine as prescribed. Not remembering therapy appointments. Lack of follow-through or completion of expected tasks between therapy appointments. Verbal agreement but no action on agreed tasks.

2B — Validation by assessment

N.D. *Short concentration span*

S "I can't remember if I took my pills." "What did we talk about when you were here last time." (Repeated several times each visit.)

O Comments reduced with increased length of time since EST and reduced internal and external stimuli.

N.D. *Transient memory loss*

S "I can't remember if I took my pills." "Maybe I took them this morning when I got up." (Repeated several times each visit.)

O Comments reduced with increased length of time since EST and reduced internal and external stimuli.

3 — Additional nursing diagnosis

None.

4A — Variables

Reality timing	+5
Relationships	−5
Stressors and/or crisis	0
Coping resources	−4
Significant emotional strength	−2
Significant emotional limitations	+2
Therapy relationship	0
Physical health status	0
Physical and emotional readiness dimension	0
Available support system	+1
Meaning significance	+3
Values and belief impact	0
Other	
BALANCE	0

Additional specific knowledge

See case material.

Analysis and synthesis

N.D. *Anxiety.* Perpetuation of this chronic state depends on reinforcement of negative behaviors. Decrease of this state is necessary for beginning movement in therapy.

N.D. *Unhealthy learned behavior.* No attention is received for positive behavior. Negative verbal and nonverbal reinforcement is given to client for motor restlessness. Negative behavior must be controlled or limited. Medium for positive affirmation must be created and maintained.

N.D. *Short concentration span.* Problem is partially self-limiting and related to time span post-EST. Mental and physical exercises or tasks must be created to lengthen concentration span.

N.D. *Transient memory difficulties.* Problem is partially self-limiting and related to time span post-EST. Mental and physical exercises or tasks must be created to assist with memory retention.

N.D. *Low self-concept.* No support is received for positive behavior. Negative verbal and nonverbal reinforcement is given to client for motor restlessness. Negative behavior must be controlled or limited. Medium for positive affirmation must be created. Verbal feedback for positive behavior must be given readily, and reinforcement of all behavior must be a priority of care.

N.D. *Passive resistance.* Assistance to begin and complete simple tasks must be given, followed by reward for behavior. This is a difficult area to grapple with because confrontation medium is absent and client's excuses are many and frequent, some of which are reality based. Reality reasons must be sorted carefully.

4B — Design of action

N.D. Anxiety, unhealthy learned behavior, short concentration span, transient memory loss, low self-concept, passive resistance.

1. Plan
   a. Body control exercises.
2. Strategy
   a. Begin defined exercise with client and therapist practicing together.
   b. Supportive corrective and affirming verbal and nonverbal feedback.
   c. Direct that exercises be done routinely at first by client and therapist. Later, by client autonomously.
   d. Transfer exercise to new environment to control.
3. Expected outcome
   a. Increased control over motor activity, allowing extension of life to new and broader environment.
   b. Improved positive self-concept.

c. Increased concentration span.
d. Increased memory retention.
e. Increased self-discipline.
4. Criteria
a. Visible body control.
b. Fewer negative comments by other persons.
c. Verbal positive self-comments.
d. Increased measurable concentration span.
e. Increased measurable memory retention.
f. Less passive resistance to new ideas and expectations.

As Mazie's sensorium cleared after electroshock therapy, the medication chart became less necessary. During times of increased stress, Mazie's retention of information and ability to follow direction would become a problem. The structure of returning to the medication chart would help facilitate functioning until the current anxiety or stressor leveled for her.

The procedure of counting medications and the implementation of medication charts were the first objective indications that Mazie's extrapyramidal symptoms were at least partially a misnomer. There was no alteration in her drug-associated behavior when she did not take the thioridazine. Later, it was discovered that her behavioral symptoms of motor restlessness— akathisia, tardive dyskinesia, and pseudoparkinsonism—remained prominent after lengthy withdrawal from all major tranquilizing drugs. Anxiety, stress, and tension seemed to affect her body language more than did the ingestion of drugs. The therapist came to regard Mazie's body language as unhealthy learned behavior of psychogenic origin rather than an extrapyramidal syndrome. Therapy within a relationship could help to modify her body language. Withdrawal from all major tranquilizers and changing her symptomatic drug treatment from biperiden to benztropine mesylate and finally to diphenhydramine hydrochloride caused little or no behavior change. Relationships were a stressor for Mazie, now negatively controlled, since she had learned how to keep people at a distance and to receive needed feedback despite its negative nature with her odd body movements. This was one more example of how insecure and frightened she really must have been. Negative feedback was better than no feedback, creating an obscure relationship to her environment, and this element increased Mazie's need to maintain her controlling behavior. Retention of this regulating stance would intensify her other maladaptive behaviors.

One trouble area that the therapist had to focus on with a very direct approach was Mazie's tardive dyskinesia. This syndrome, characterized by rhythmical involuntary movements of her tongue, face, and jaw, was distracting in any interpersonal encounter and negatively strengthened Mazie's already faulty self-concept. A clinical consideration of importance is the fact that her symptoms would probably remain persistent and could even be considered irreversible.

Eighteen months into the nurse-client relationship and at a time when she was withdrawn from major tranquilizers, the topic of her constant chewing movements, puckering mouth, and occasionally protruding tongue was introduced. Mazie discussed the issue readily. She was aware of the problem, embarrassed by her behavior, and willing to try suggestions to help modify this unpleasant state. The feelings of embarrassment and awareness of the condition were self-motivating factors for her to begin new behaviors. She could gain relative control. Neither her physician nor her nurse-clinician believed that this identified behavior was totally drug related, but self-discipline would be a tedious task for client and nurse.

Despite her high degree of motivation, Mazie felt that she could not help herself. "I want this to stop but I can't," or "I just can't help myself," were typical rejoinders. One solution to the problem was to have Mazie chew gum or suck on hard candy when she was in a public or social situation. This did reduce the unkind remarks from others to a less destructive level.

Unkind comments improved from "Look at

that strange lady" to "That woman isn't very ladylike when she chews gum." Unfortunately, Mazie's teeth showed a large increase in the number of dental caries, and she was told by her dentist, "Only sugarless gum" and "No candy."

The passing of time and the bonding of the relationship between nurse and client allowed a freer movement within Mazie's territorial space. Now one could often move a chair within 2 feet of her during a conversation. Direct eye-to-eye contact became more frequent in this close personal proximity (Figure 1). Unless other stressors influenced her behavior, Mazie's posture during therapy was relatively tranquil except for slow, continuous foot swinging, and limited chewing movements with her mouth. In this relative calm, client and nurse began to practice body control exercises.

At first the nurse chose to sit in front of Mazie and to do the exercises with her. She was cooperative, thought it was "a bit funny," but showed trust enough to begin. The key to a degree of cooperation and success was to work in short time spans and to give generous quantities of accurate, sincere supportive verbal and nonverbal feedback at appropriate times.

Exercises began with deep breathing. Rarely did Mazie expand her lungs to capacity or breathe from her diaphragm. Five deep breaths made her feel good and helped her to sit straight and more erect. Next, both feet were placed flat on the floor and a straight and quiet posture was held for 2 minutes. This maneuver was practiced by both parties during each visit for the next 3 months. On most days Mazie could gain control of her body during these exercises, and she became proud of this accomplishment. This achievement intensified the bonds of the nurse-client relationship. She could laugh and smile again.

In due course, Mazie was able to lengthen the time span to 10 minutes of sitting quietly with both feet flat on the floor. Once each day between visits she did the relaxation and control exercise. She reported that it was more difficult to do it alone, but she seemed proud to relate her accomplishment. She smiled as she told how she had sat in restrained activity every day and that she had decided to use a timer to help her remain within an identified time span.

Periodically, Mazie, motivated by loneliness, ventured into new environments. As this activity became more frequent, she would relate her self-consciousness and the hurt she felt from unkind remarks. She perceived herself in a tight double bind. Her desire to do more and to reach out as opposed to the discomfort of her negative acceptance by others caused painful conflict. It was time for Mazie to begin a transfer of her private quiet sitting exercise to public situations. Mazie found it difficult at first, but as she continued to employ this unostentatious exercise and found she could sit still at church or at a neighbor's home, the positive effects of appearing more tranquil increased her self-concept. The therapist no longer needed to reinforce the fact that Mazie could control her body. Mazie would boast that she had accomplished self-restraint. She was also developing autonomy.

Mazie would still be described by others as "having difficulty sitting still." Some might describe her as "fidgety" or "nervous." Her therapist would describe her as unruffled, one who had enough self-confidence and self-determination to win a difficult victory. Mazie's self-concept was becoming broad and increasingly realistic. She did not perceive as much hurt in occasional negative comments from others.

PROCESS IMPLEMENTATION

1—Evaluation

N.D. *Anxiety*

    S "I want this to stop." "I just can't help myself." "I can do it." "Look! I did it." "I exercise away from here—in church."

    O Slow, continuous foot swinging. Limited chewing movements. Laugh. Smile. Sitting straight and erect. Transference of control to public setting.

N.D. *Unhealthy learned behavior*
S "I want this to stop." "I can't help myself."
O Akathisia, tardive dyskinesia, and pseudo-parkinsonism remain prominent after lengthy drug withdrawal. Relationships negatively controlled; other persons remain distant. Limited control of behaviors through relaxation and concentration. Transference of control to public setting.

N.D. *Short concentration span*
S "It's difficult but I do it."
O Practiced exercises for 10 minutes. Time lapse post-EST now more than 6 months. Employment of timing device. Actual involvement in exercise. Transference of control to public setting.

N.D. *Transient memory loss*
S "Yes, I did the exercise every day, sometimes twice a day."
O Time lapse post-EST now more than 6 months. Transference of control to public setting.

N.D. *Low self-concept*
S "It's a bit funny." "I can do it." "Look! I did it." "It's not too hard."
O Cooperative with exercises. Laugh. Smile. Sitting straight and erect. Smiling; voice inflection when reporting on exercise practice. Transference of control to public setting.

N.D. *Passive resistance*
S "I want this to stop." "I just can't help myself." "Yes, I did the exercise every day, sometimes twice a day." "It helps this exercise you make me do."
O Cooperative with exercises. Employment of timing device. Less verbal resistance. Follow-through of activity in therapist's absence.

Actual outcome
Ability to limit or control motor activity, allowing extension of life to new and broader environment. Increased concentration abilities and memory retention. Limited positive self-concept expansion. A new sense of self-discipline and self-control.

2A—Assessment

N.D. *Dependence/independence struggle*
S "It makes me feel good."
O Defensive, angry when confronted with alcohol content of cough medicine. Withheld negative emotions.

N.D. *Lack of insight*
S "Drinking brandy to sleep." "I can't do that anymore." "It makes me feel good." "Yes, I have a cough."

O Over-the-counter cough medicine emptied in kitchen and bathroom waste basket. No observable respiratory symptoms.

N.D. *Low self-concept*
S "It makes me feel good."
O Lack of emotional support and affirmation in environment. Withheld negative emotions. Positive self-expression absent from life.

N.D. *Inability to complete the grieving process*
S "It makes me feel good."
O Lack of medium to facilitate and support grief. Increased stress from lack of resolution. Withheld negative emotions.

N.D. *Loneliness*
S "It makes me feel good."
O Lack of emotional support and affirmation in environment. Positive self-expression absent from life.

2B—Validation by assessment

N.D. *Lack of insight*
S "Drinking brandy to sleep." "I can't do that anymore." "It makes me feel good." "Yes, I have a cough."
O Over-the-counter cough medicine emptied in kitchen and bathroom waste basket. No observable upper respiratory symptoms. Inability to correlate or integrate brandy episode and cough medicine episode.

3—Additional nursing diagnosis
None.

4A—Variables

Reality timing	0
Relationships	−3
Stressors and/or crisis	−2
Coping resources	+2
Significant emotional strength	+2
Significant emotional limitations	−2
Therapy relationship	+3
Physical health status	0
Physical and emotional readiness dimension	0
Available support system	−5
Meaning significance	+4
Values and belief impact	+5
BALANCE	+

Additional specific knowledge
See case material.

Analysis and synthesis
N.D. *Dependence/independence struggle*. There is continual emergence of unmet dependency needs. Ambivalence in struggles increases anxiety and lack of resolution. It is impor-

tant to continue struggle for eventual autonomy to emerge.

N.D.   *Lack of insight.* Client has lifelong values and beliefs in negative aspect of alcohol consumption. Ambivalent pull between value, beliefs, and need to feel good. Stressors have slowed intellectual capacity.

N.D.   *Low self-concept.* The chemical effects of alcohol temporarily enhance the positive self, but perception is unrealistic. Often depression follows elation. Benefits are only temporary. Introduction of new avenues to enhance positive self is a must.

N.D.   *Inability to complete the grieving process.* The chemical effects of alcohol depress initiative to cope with the emotion involved in the process and promote avoidance.

N.D.   *Loneliness.* The chemical effects of alcohol decrease the void feelings and decrease the need to reach outside the self. Introduction of other modes to promote "good feelings" is a must.

4B—Design of action

N.D.   Dependence/independence struggle, lack of insight, low self-concept, inability to complete the grieving process, loneliness

1. Plan
   a. Confront the alcohol ingestion.
2. Strategy
   a. Acknowledge observations to client.
   b. Correlate observations with brandy episode as related by client.
   c. Begin examining new modes of positive interaction available to client.
3. Expected outcomes
   a. Acknowledgement of facts.
   b. Intellectual and emotional acceptance of the detrimental use of cough medicine.
   c. Increased self-disclosure.
4. Criteria
   a. Dialogue of facts.
   b. Removal of cough medicine containers.
   c. Free expression of both positive and negative emotions related to episode and therapist confrontation.
   d. Verbal acceptance of *idea* to *explore* new tasks in therapy.

One early symptom of Mazie's difficulty was her chemical dependency. Her mismanagement of psychotropic drugs did not seem to be related to dependency or abuse but rather to memory loss. During the years of nurse psychotherapy in her home, Mazie had no prescribed drugs other than what was supervised. As far as could be determined through observation, she also kept no alcoholic beverages in her home.

Mazie mentioned several times during her grief work of "drinking brandy to sleep," that "it makes me feel good," and of admitting, "I cannot do that any more." On two occasions, during her high stress periods, several large, empty bottles of over-the-counter cough medication were noticed in Mazie's kitchen waste basket, and her bathroom waste basket contained several additional empty cough medicine bottles.

On the day of the second observation, a trip to shop for clothing was made. Mazie stopped at the drug store to buy cough syrup during the outing and was asked if she had a cold or a cough. She said yes, she did. The therapist responded that there were no apparent or visible symptoms of such distress. Mazie countered that the medicine "helped" her dry mouth.

Later, sitting in her home, Mazie was asked to produce the cough medicine for the therapist, which, as was suspected, had a high alcohol content. Mazie was informed that the nurse was aware of her large consumption of this medicine. At first, she was defensive, even angry, as she stated that the medicine made her feel good.

The nurse explained about the alcohol content of the cough medicine and correlated it to the brandy episode. Mazie had really had a cough; the medicine made her feel good, and she continued to use it. Client and therapist had to examine the current stressors, evaluate the present living situation and proceed from there. Mazie needed increased emotional support, additional explicit verbal feedback and affirmation, and increased encouragement to express herself in therapy to help ameliorate her negative feelings. The safe confines of the therapy relationship provided her with space to receive healing strokes and the fortitude to continue her progress toward an increased healthy existence.

This was the only occurrence of overt chemical dependency during the years of the relationship. The clinician was continually aware of the possible problem and of Mazie's high need to "feel good" or avoid "feeling bad." Mazie's life-style, age, sex, and even her person helped conceal her possible alcoholic problems. Clients who cope with altering a self-destructive coping pattern such as chemical dependency can be effectively supported in the strength of a positive relationship. Home-based therapy does broaden the nurse's awareness of current problems. Previous observations in Mazie's home provided sufficient data for the clinician to confront the "cough medicine episode" when it was occurring. The behavior was episodic, and early confrontation of her ineffective coping did not allow the pattern to become entrenched in her life-style.

PROCESS IMPLEMENTATION

1—Evaluation

N.D.   *Dependence/independence struggle*
   S   "It makes me feel good." "I can keep myself busy when I try." "When he was alive, life was better."
   O   Less defensive. Anger resolved. Evident beginning of self-disclosure in therapy.

N.D.   *Lack of insight*
   S   "It makes me feel good." "I couldn't sleep last night so I read." "No one feels good all the time." "When he was alive, life was better."
   O   No observed cough medicine containers.

N.D.   *Low self-concept*
   S   "It makes me feel good." "I don't like being alone." "When he was alive, life was better."
   O   Evident beginning of self-disclosure in therapy. More alert and involved during therapy.

N.D.   *Inability to complete the grieving process*
   S   "I don't like being alone." "When he was alive, life was better."
   O   Evident beginning of self-disclosure in therapy.

N.D.   *Loneliness*
   S   "It makes me feel good." "I don't like being alone." "When he was alive, life was better."

Actual outcome
   Although protective of self, Mazie did begin intellectually and emotionally to accept that she

could not drink cough medicine to make her feel good. (Cough medicine containers were emptied and removed.) The confrontation itself produced a new level of self-disclosure. The idea of exploring new tasks in therapy was introduced. No further evidence of chemical abuse was noted.

2A—Assessment

N.D.   *Low self-concept*
   S   "Do you really think so?" "You did?" "You do?" "You will?"
   O   Slow, tedious, toilsome task of choosing an activity. Resistance to group eating and socialization.

N.D.   *Interpersonal relationship disturbance*
   S   "No" in regard to dinner guests.
   O   Foot swinging. Chewing movements. Subject changing. Prominent unrestrained body behavior. Fragmented thinking in a large, loud group. Observed protecting her isolation with verbal maneuvers when suggestions were made to open her life to others. Absence of viable friendship.

N.D.   *Anxiety*
   S   "I'm sick to my stomach." "I'm too sick to eat." "I have a headache."
   O   Cancellation of appointments. Prominent unrestrained body behavior. Increased fatigue. Fragmented thinking in a large, loud group.

N.D.   *Unhealthy learned behavior*
   S   "I'm sick to my stomach." "I'm too sick to eat." "I have a headache."
   O   Foot swinging. Chewing movements. Subject changing. Prominent unrestrained body behavior.

N.D.   *Passive resistance*
   S   "I'm sick to my stomach." "I'm too sick to eat." Relating being cold in evening and needing a new robe. "I have a headache."
   O   Foot swinging. Chewing movements. Subject changing. Cancellation of appointments.

N.D.   *Faulty support system*
   S   "Do you really think so?" "You did?" "You do?" "You will?"
   O   No observable or acknowledged significant other persons in environment. Observed protecting her isolation with verbal maneuvers when suggestions were made to open her life to others.

N.D.   *Trust/mistrust struggle*
   S   "Do you really think so?" "You did?" "You do?" "You will?" Relating being cold in

evening, needing a robe, and disclosing returned gift.

O Cancellations of appointments. Hesitant acceptance of affirmation.

N.D. *Dependence/independence struggle*

S "Yes, I sew." "I like to knit and quilt." "I used to crochet." Relating being cold in evening and needing a new robe.

O Involvement in brochure, pamphlets, and reading material to choose an activity. Slow, tedious, toilsome task of choosing an activity.

N.D. *Loneliness*

S "I used to cook for Abraham." "Food doesn't taste good any more." "No" in regard to dinner guests.

O Observed protecting her isolation with verbal maneuvers when suggestions were made to open her life to others. Fragmented thinking in a large, loud group.

3—Additional nursing diagnosis
None

4A—Variables

Reality timing	0
Relationships	−5
Stressors and/or crisis	−3
Coping resources	−3
Significant emotional strength	+2
1 Significant emotional limitations	3
Therapy relationship	+5
Physical health status	0
Physical and emotional readiness dimension	0
Available support system	−5
Meaning significance	+3
Values and belief impact	+3
Other	
BALANCE	−

Additional specific knowledge
See case material.
Analysis and synthesis

N.D. *Low self-concept.* Increased social contact, positive task completion of daily living, and a more adequate diet are necessary. Promotion of self-esteem, an expanded self-image, and feelings of importance are needed. Client is less fragile than at therapy initiation. There is increased potential for self-discipline.

N.D. *Interpersonal relationship disturbance.* An absence of necessary social interaction skills must be countered in therapy. A lack of practice in conversation skills only promotes increased withdrawal and negative feedback in social situations.

N.D. *Anxiety.* Stressors from therapy expectations and new situations increase feelings of insecurity and promote self-protection through flight. Actual task achievement will decrease stress.

N.D. *Unhealthy learned behavior.* Anxiety of new and threatening situations would always cause a regression to this pattern of coping. Initial regression should be allowed. Control through learned exercise must be encouraged.

N.D. *Passive resistance.* Habitual indirectness as a life coping pattern is prominent when change is an issue. Confrontation of reality, expectations of directness, and learning a new coping pattern of confronting issues and feeling must be encouraged.

N.D. *Faulty support system.* No support system will develop unless client is forced to confront reality and social relationships. This must be done slowly and with guidance.

N.D. *Trust/mistrust struggle.* Trust will develop if client is forced to struggle through the dilemma. Support and a medium for experience must be provided.

N.D. *Dependence/independence struggle.* Autonomy will develop if enough can be given to allow the struggle between the forces. Trust resolution should precede this struggle. Social situations will provide learning medium.

N.D. *Loneliness.* Discomfort in the isolation can motivate the client to seek socialization or stop avoiding social settings. Is loneliness the result of many other life choices?

4B—Design of action

N.D. Low self-concept, interpersonal relationship disturbance, anxiety, unhealthy learned behavior, passive resistance, faulty support system, trust/mistrust struggle, dependence/independence struggle, loneliness.

1. Plan
   a. Facilitate social interaction.
2. Strategy
   a. Expect compliance in regular attendance at senior citizens' luncheon group.
   b. Confront situations calling for resolution through task performance and social interaction.
   c. Allot time in therapy to learn social interaction skills.

    d. Involve client in task research and task choice and expect action based on the decisions.
    e. Provide accurate, sincere, and explicit corrective feedback and person affirmation.
  3. Expected outcomes
    a. Regular attendance at senior citizens' luncheon group.
    b. Increased daily living task completion and socialization.
    c. *Beginning* comfort and proficiency in social interaction in therapy situation.
    d. Beginning decision making demonstration.
    e. Increased autonomy.
  4. Criteria
    a. Regular attendance at senior citizens' luncheon group.
    b. Responsible daily living task completion.
    c. Increased dialogue in therapy. Initiation of conversation and topics.
    d. Beginning decision making and autonomous action.

The next focal point in therapy was nutrition. Mazie was a good cook, but she had no motivation to prepare food or to eat nourishing meals while she was living alone. Nutritionally, she ate inadequately, although her body weight remained stable. Mazie consumed sufficient daily calories, but her nutrient intake was poor. Discussion centered around food for many weeks. In guided meal planning, Mazie learned to make her own T.V. type of frozen dinners out of the larger meals she prepared for herself. She reported that she followed the menus as planned and that she ate more balanced meals. She even began to bake cookies for the therapist's visits. The suggestion of inviting her son, Arthur, and his wife, or her sister, or a neighbor in for a meal met with quiet, but strong, verbal answers of "no," increased foot swinging, and other bodily gestures indicating agitation and resistance to the social maneuver.

After approximately 3 years of therapy and one more hospitalization, Mazie was expected to join the senior citizens' lunch group Monday through Friday. This was a project for several months, during which time she struggled with the idea because it would require a modification in her pattern of living and force previously avoided social encounters. After she finally agreed to try eating with the group only if the therapist would take her and remain with her, there was a series of her canceling appointments or of her being "sick to her stomach" or of being "too sick to eat" when it was time for the scheduled meal. The first day she attended the group lunch, it was such a stressor that her body activity was again extremely unrestrained. Many people stared at her, talked about her, even pointed at her, and avoided contact with her. The therapist supported Mazie's positive behavior of doing something new, although it was difficult and frightening to her. What a tremendous step this was for her in therapy and in life. When the therapist chanced to encounter Mazie for the last time, Mazie was leaving the senior citizens' group, busily talking with two companions, and her body language was positively controlled. She stopped to say hello for a brief period, but she had to hurry off to another group activity with her two friends. Slowness and the early prodding in a relationship can have ultimate benefits for the client. Proper timing, guidance, and support in a new therapy situation can be prime factors to extensive growth and goal achievement.

An established pattern of regular meals helped Mazie with her memory loss difficulties. Mazie appeared to be healthier when she ate a well-balanced diet, as evidenced by her decreased fluctuating fatigue level. She had fewer "stomach aches" and fewer problems with bowel elimination. Interaction aids digestion and absorption. It is sound nutritionally as well as psychologically to include socialization and pleasant atmosphere in a mealtime climate. The discipline of meals at scheduled intervals adds structure and purpose to daily living routines. Basic physiological need satisfaction allows the client to concentrate energy on psychological resolution of problems. The dietary benefits supported the therapy goals of a continual thrust to elevate and expand Mazie's self-concept. It produced positive objective behaviors that would be reinforced verbally with comments such as, ''You look attractive today, Mazie,'' ''Your eyes sparkle so brightly,'' and ''That color dress compliments your eyes.''

Self-imposed isolation was a difficult early block to continuous progress in therapy. Mazie saw the therapist weekly, and she seemed to enjoy most of the time together. She conversed more readily as weeks became months. Yet Mazie would have been very satisfied to remain at home. The therapist's weekly visits seemed to reinforce Mazie's negative behavior of isolation. As the relationship evolved, it became clear that dialogue and self-disclosure would never culminate in a reaching out for other relationships. A pattern of withdrawal, dependence, and aloneness reinforced by emotional deprivation existed as a lifetime coping style for this client. A here-and-now attempt for Mazie to become involved in the peripheral world was the necessary goal to establish and pursue if a level of autonomy was to occur.

Therapy interaction regarding goals always found the therapist setting the objectives, Mazie agreeing to them but verbally unable to set a goal with the therapist. Goal activation sets up continuous power and control struggles like that in the senior citizens' lunch project. Each struggle provided Mazie with the basis for grappling with stressors and learning to cope with anxiety on a new and more healthy level. She also gained some needed independence and a degree of control over her unhealthy learned body language.

The first successful attempt to get Mazie out of the house involved Mazie's son, Abraham, who had sent her a lovely bath robe for Christmas. Mazie did need a new robe. However, this gift was a size too small for her. Abraham told his mother where he had purchased the gift, to return it for one that did fit her, and not to be concerned about any increased cost. The bath robe remained in the gift box for many months. During one of the therapist's regular home visits, Mazie told of being cold in the evening, her need for a new robe, and the unreturned gift. It was easy to suggest that they exchange the gift together, but it was difficult to bring about this project.

Again the ''sick stomach'' ploy, the added ''headache,'' and even the canceled visit came into play. It was easier for Mazie to telephone the therapist than to go shopping with her. Yet, the telephone call itself was a positive step. Finally, all excuses were invalidated and Mazie knew there would not be any alteration of the plan to help her exchange the robe. With a great deal of encouragement and supportive presence, Mazie completed the task of exchanging her small yellow robe for a comfortable, warm, blue robe that she liked.

Mazie's inappropriate body movements while completing this exchange were distracting and subject to comment. Positively, she had accomplished a simple task of daily living, but one not perceived as a simple task by her. The robe exchange was another observable action for which positive feedback could be given. The therapist was proud of Mazie and told her so. Even Mazie's son in his own way expressed pleasure. Mazie did not appear as anxious as she had during the first visits, as measured by motor activity and body movements. She seemed to be in a state of restoration, and she was told that she appeared ''better.'' For the first time she smiled as she responded, ''Do you really think so?'' That question was to be repeated many times for the duration of therapy. The answer was always honest, considering her present state of rehabilitation.

Affirmation was hesitantly accepted by Mazie. The therapist always told her simply and noneffusively when it was an enjoyable session. ''I enjoyed visiting with you today, Mazie,'' or ''Our time seemed to go very fast today. I do like being with you,'' or ''I'll look forward to seeing you again.'' Such comments were frequently greeted with ''You did!'' ''You do?'' or ''You will?'' A simple ''yes'' usually got a smile. When Mazie smiled, one could really feel her radiated warmth. As the relationship intensified, the therapist would take Mazie's hand upon leaving to reinforce the "I like you" message. Her smile showed that she had heard the intended message, and sometimes a broad smile indicated that she was learning to believe in herself.

Social interaction was part of the relationship and a medium for Mazie's learning conversation skills. Comfortable chatting about the day's happenings or the week's events strengthened Mazie's value as a person and gave her experience and example in "how to talk with others." Mazie was delighted to relate a piece of community news or some recent gossip. At times she seemed eager to recount a piece of news before the clinician had heard it from any other source.

One never believes the number of activities a community provides until one has the opportunity to investigate. After the first year of therapy, goals were focused on increasing Mazie's independence and decision-making skill. For months the therapist came to interviews armed with pamphlets and newspaper articles dealing with current events and activities. Together, the two sorted this information and talked of their interests and interesting activities. It was learned that Mazie possessed talent in sewing, quilting, knitting, and crocheting. She played cards well and enjoyed light reading, but it took months of careful, slow, deliberate plodding and encouragement for Mazie to choose an activity that she would like to do outside of her home.

Bingo was Mazie's choice, but bingo was not what Mazie expected it to be. The room was crowded; the activity was loud and, verbally and intellectually, moved too swiftly for her. It fragmented her thinking, increased her anxiety, and increased her body movements and personal agitation despite the therapist's presence and support. It was determined that bingo was not a favorable activity, and both parties returned to the reading material for other ideas.

Mazie's second choice was not made for another 2 months. She chose to join a small needlework class composed of women within her age range. The therapist, too, joined this class. Stress was apparent in Mazie's body language, but she remained with this group for an hour, joined in a needlework project, made limited attempts at conversing, and chose to return alone to the group the following week. Mazie became one of the stable, core members of this continuous, open-ended, task-centered group for several years. Belonging helps one to view one's self more positively. Mazie's self-concept was enhanced by this group association and task productivity.

PROCESS IMPLEMENTATION

1—Evaluation

N.D. *Low self-concept*

    S   "*I* decided to join a new church group." "*I* didn't like the food they served today."

    O   Revealing need to exchange robe. Well-balanced diet and socialization promoted self-esteem. Hesitant acceptance of affirmation. Broad smile when person affirmation expressed. Increased frequency of word "I" and introducing herself by first name rather than Mrs. A. W.

N.D. *Interpersonal relationship disturbance*

    S   "*I* met a new lady today. We talked about . . ."

    O   Revealing need to exchange robe.

N.D. *Anxiety*

    S   "I'm sick to my stomach."

    O   Increased exploration of new milieu despite the high stressors perceived and experienced in social situations. Extreme motor activity when client experienced stress.

N.D. *Unhealthy learned behavior*

    S   "People don't talk about me so much now."

    O   Increased but limited control of motor activity.

N.D. *Passive resistance*

    S   "I have a headache." "I'm sick to my stomach."

    O   Therapy encounter forced more direct effective coping measures. Behavior remains prominent under stress or pressure to change.

N.D. *Faulty support system*

S ⎫
O ⎭ No change noted.

N.D. *Trust/mistrust struggle*

S "I decided to join a new church group." "I met a lady today . . ." "That lady I met at lunch came here for coffee."

O Revealing need to exchange robe. Broad smile when person affirmation expressed.

N.D. *Dependence/independence struggle*

S "I decided to join a new church group." "I didn't like the food they served today."

O Completed task of exchanging small yellow robe for a comfortable blue robe.

N.D. *Loneliness*

S "I was so busy yesterday." "Time passes more quickly now." "That lady I met at lunch came here for coffee."

O Time spaces relatively filled with activity, task completion, and socialization.

N.D. *Transient memory loss*

S Decreased number of "I forgot" statements.

O Decreased fluctuating fatigue level. Regular eating pattern. Increased balance in diet.

N.D. *Short concentration span*

S "We talk for 10 minutes." "I read the newspaper for half an hour last night."

O Lengthened concentration span when involved in structured activity. Regular eating pattern. Increased balance in diet.

Actual outcome

Regular attendance at senior citizens' luncheon group with increased socialization. Completion of gift exchange. Decision and beginning execution of bingo activity and subsequent decision and execution of needlework class activity. Less dependency on therapist when entering new or threatening social milieu.

2A — Assessment

N.D. *Inability to complete the grieving process*

S "It's awful that he's gone."

O Longer, more stable sleep patterns. More verbal awareness of everyday activity such as the arrival of spring weather. New neighbors. Interest in returning to church activity. Wearing a small amount of makeup. Reading the daily newspaper. Increased attention span. Memory recall of recent events. Interest in T.V. Referring to herself when making an appointment as Mazie W instead of Mrs. Abraham W. Less silence during therapy sessions. More controlled body behavior.

N.D. *Lack of insight*

S "Do I really look like that?"

O Lack of comprehension or understanding of the facts regarding her recent past.

N.D. *Trust/mistrust struggle*

S "Will you attend church services with me?" "Do I really look like that?"

O Risk taking in relationships defining boundaries. Increased but limited self-disclosure in therapy.

N.D. *Dependence/independence struggle*

S "It would be nice to see you, but I have other plans."

O Did not alter plans. Defined boundaries for visiting. Defined limits for another person regarding her person.

N.D. *Low self-concept*

S "Do I really look like that?" "It would be nice to see you, but I have other plans."

O Did not alter plans. Defined boundaries for visiting. Defined limits for another person regarding her person.

N.D. *Passive resistance*

S "Do I really look like that?" "It would be nice to see you, but I have other plans."

O Direct questioning of concern issue. Did not alter plans. Defined boundaries for visiting. Defined limits for another person regarding her person.

3 — Additional nursing diagnosis

None

4A — Variables

Reality timing	+2
Relationships	+2
Stressors and/or crisis	0
Coping resources	+3
Significant emotional strength	+3
Significant emotional limitations	−2
Therapy relationship	+5
Physical health status	+2
Physical and emotional readiness dimension	+4
Available support system	−1
Meaning significance	+3
Values and belief impact	+3
Other	
BALANCE	+

Additional specific knowledge

See case material.

Analysis and synthesis

N.D. *Inability to complete the grieving process.* An opening of the self to feelings of loss and resolution of grief is promoted through deliberative, supportive therapy relationship. Adaptation in behavior, coping, and interacting resulted in new person strength.

N.D. *Lack of insight.* Increased trust, autonomy, and positive self emotions create a decrease of self-protection measures, allowing new understandings, acceptance of truth, and resolution of stressors and conflict.

N.D. *Trust/mistrust struggle.* Developing renewed sense of trust promotes willingness to become involved in grief process, experience feelings of loss, and attempt resolution.

N.D. *Dependence/independence struggle.* Developing sense of autonomy allows for new level of interaction, relationships, and insight. A renewed independence fosters self-concept expansion and growth.

N.D. *Low self-concept.* Developing sense of autonomy allows new unfolding of more secure self. A new openness to interaction, relationships, and life involvements. Acceptance of the reality of her loss and its resultant emotional turmoil.

N.D. *Passive resistance.* Emergence of new positive behavior. Direct coping and confrontation with life and living increasingly possible. Decrease in avoidance of emotions and issues promotes comfort.

4B — Design of action

N.D. Inability to complete the grieving process, lack of insight, trust/mistrust struggle, dependence/independence struggle, low self-concept, passive resistance.

1. Plan
   a. Assist client to feel loss, resolve grief, and proceed with experiencing life in the present.
2. Strategy
   a. Continue response to question, "Do I really look like that?" with accurate, knowledgeable statements. Cite objective data then move to subjective facts.
   b. Assume a caring and supportive stance. Speak clearly, distinctly. Carefully assess client response to therapist's message through astute observation and client feedback.
3. Expected outcomes
   a. "I do look better now than in that picture." "I wish I could have it retaken." Willing examination of feelings of loss and related life resolutions.
   b. Implementation of exercises when stress re-

sults in increased motor activity. Limited control of body language.
   c. "I miss him." "I wish we had more time." "Sometimes I expect him to be here when I come home. I catch myself saying hello."
   d. Increased self-initiated involvement and enjoyment in activities with people.
4. Criteria
   a. Therapy interaction denoting and connoting grief resolution, especially significant and relevant verbal feedback.
   b. Nonverbal feedback indicates emotional comfort or anxiety, especially motor activity.
   c. Emotive expression of feelings of loss, such as tears.
   d. Increased quantity, quality, and involvement in task, life actions, and person interaction will indicate grief resolution.

Grief work for Mazie was slow, tedious, and directed inward. Self-expression was difficult for her, and feeling expression was not familiar to her during the first half of her life. She rarely talked about her husband, and when she did, she exhibited increased distracting nonverbal behavior. She experienced sleep disturbances during her long static state of bereavement. Her grief resolution was measured by longer, more stable sleep patterns, more verbal awareness of everyday activity such as the arrival of spring weather, new neighbors, interest in returning to church activity, wearing a small amount of makeup, reading the daily newspaper, increased attention span, memory recall of recent events, interest in T.V., referring to herself as Mazie W instead of Mrs. Abraham W, when making an appointment, less silence during therapy sessions, and more controlled body behavior. This healing and resolution unfolded over $4^1/_2$ years. More verbal resolution of her grief was desirable but was hampered by a limited self-disclosure aptitude. Her husband's death with its resultant demands was the trauma that intensified ineffective coping patterns, resulting in depression. Reexamination of the nursing diagnosis determined an overall goal in which Mazie had to learn and relearn adequate coping behavior within a structured relationship to achieve a level of physical and psychic comfort and functional abilities in her present reality. She had to be helped in therapy to feel her loss, to resolve her grief, and to continue with the tasks of living.

Toward the end of the therapy relationship, Mazie's life was relatively complete with activities that kept her busy and provided a sense of fulfillment for her. Occasionally, Mazie's level of insight was cause for concern. As her growth in therapy was evaluated, analysis revealed that time had been filled with activity. As her readiness developed, time would be spent discussing feelings and relationships and assisting with the development of her self-disclosure aptitude.

As nurse and client were about to launch into an examination of the scope of Mazie's activities and begin to explore emotive readiness, she stopped the interaction by revealing an incident that had occurred during the previous week. Abraham, Jr., had called one evening to say he would be arriving the following day for a few hours' visit. Mazie very matter-of-factly told him that it would be "nice" to see him but that she had other plans for the next day. She did not change her plans, and her son did not visit. However, a month later, she received yet another call from him a week in advance of an anticipated visit, and both she and her son enjoyed this visit.

Mazie could now fend for herself in significant relationships, indeed, in all relationships. She *had* increased the level of her insightfulness, and there was no demand to explore her relationships in other than the sphere already defined. Life adaptation had occurred through her involvement in personal action and activities, through clinician role modeling, and from within the secure confines of the nurse-client relationship. Task-oriented interventions in psychosocial nursing situations are highly effective actions to promote maturation.

One nursing activity was to allow the clinician to share an emotional growth experience with Mazie that the usual office-centered, talking situation would not have provided. Mazie and the clinician subscribed to different religious beliefs and practice. As Lent approached that year, Mazie wished to go to church but felt that she could not attend a service alone. She asked the therapist to accompany her to her church on Ash Wednesday, and the invitation was accepted.

After the religious service the congregation was invited to the church auditorium to view pictures of the congregation. The pictures had been taken 10 months previously to be used as a new congregation directory. Mazie did not mingle with the group but stood for several minutes in front of her picture. She turned to the therapist and, with a puzzled expression, asked, "Do I really look like that?"

Mazie's picture portrayed her pervading feelings of depression, sadness, and grief. It depicted her as she had appeared in the depth of her illness, but it was a faulty, inferior likeness of the face of Mazie here and now.

Mazie and the therapist chose to walk home slowly and to continue the conversation over tea at her home. Slowly, distinctly, and caringly, Mazie's question: "Do I really look like that?" was answered. The therapist's remarks that evening were more active than they had been in any other encounter between the two. The therapist explained the differences in Mazie's behavior during the previous years and spoke simply, accurately, and knowledgeably about mental health and mental illness. Mazie's growth and her present health were stressed. The two looked into the mirror, and the therapist pointed with certainty to the difference in Mazie's appearance compared with the picture published in the church directory.

Mazie seemed to absorb the discourse but with little comment. In the weeks that followed, she questioned the events of that evening and the therapist's comments. Mazie greeted harsh reality that particular evening, eased by the guidance and support of the therapist, and she gained insight from the experience of confronting truth. The impact and seeming shock value of this encounter could not have been recognized had the nurse not been a participant-observer in the situation.

Mazie did learn to cope effectively through trusting herself and others. She learned to reach out by giving and receiving. She gained a concept of "I am" and "I have worth." Even so, Mazie's relationships with others could not be described as emotionally intimate. She would not have been termed an insightful person. Today, Mazie is active, her days are full, she laughs and initiates conversations with neighbors and friends. In a word, she has a sense of fulfillment and relative happiness. She describes herself as happy. She takes no medication, although sometimes she is anxious. On occasion, Mazie has loud, distracting body language, but this phenomenon is less frequent and of shorter duration. Mazie herself decided she was too busy for nurse psychotherapy. This new sense of independence and self-initiated decision making was a mark validating the soundness of her decision to terminate the relationship.

Psychosocial nursing intervention can be less complicated than many nurses choose to believe. Mazie's growth to relative balance or relative emotional health was fostered by a continual intense interpersonal relationship and a deliberate, thoughtful implementation and evaluation of communication within the framework of conscious and knowledgeable application of nursing process. In addition, there was the willing risk to care for and become involved with Mazie. Finally, there was the living commitment to the human value of another person. Psychosocial nursing performance is guided by a continuous, conscious system of thought. When the intellectual and action components of nursing process are cohesively combined in practice with a true "other-centered" interpersonal approach, they foster growth, healing, and health through new person interac-

tions, through abdicating destructive behaviors, and through learning or relearning methods of coping with one's present life situation.

SUMMARY PERSONAL PROFILE
Social adjustment

S   "Sometimes I have trouble sitting still." "Did you know that . . . ?" "I heard Mr. S . . ."

O   Laughing. Smiling. Controlled body posture. Regular involvement in group lunch project. Involvement in social conversation. Involvement in several group activities. Less noticeable memory loss.

Emotional health status

S   "Sometimes I have trouble sitting still." "I will be busy that day." "Do I really look like that?" "I'll try." "I never used to sleep that well."

O   Laughing. Smiling. Controlled body posture. Regular involvement in group lunch project. Less noticeable memory loss. Grief resolution. Decision-making skills. Autonomous actions.

Physical health status

S   "Sometimes I have trouble sitting still." "The food was good at lunch today." "I never used to sleep that well. I didn't wake up until 8:30 A.M."

O   Controlled body posture. Regular involvement in group lunch project. Less fatigue. Improved skin color and turgor. Fewer complaints of 'stomach ache.' Bowel tone improved. Less noticeable memory loss.

Spiritual dimension

S   "I like the 10:00 A.M. service—that's the one I always attend. "I do my exercise when I feel nervous." "We had coffee and donuts after church last Sunday."

O   Regular church attendance and involvement. Several new church-related activities.

Daily living skill performance

S "I only wash once a week." "I baked for the church bazaar. I can't afford to give money." "I used to keep a neater house, but it's comfortable and OK for me."

O Clean environment. Good personal grooming. Responsible management of person, home, finances.

Coping skill repertoire

S "I'll try." "I like that group. They're nice women there." "The food was good at lunch today." "I have other plans for the day." "I feel uncomfortable when . . ."

O Sufficient and effective coping methods to sustain personal integration and growth. Positive patterns of behavior reinforced with positive feedback, personal growth, and involvement in the mainstream of living. Decision-making skills. Autonomous actions. Beginning self-disclosure development.

Maturation struggle according to Erikson's developmental stages

S "I am going to Ladies' Aid tomorrow." "I'd like you to come at a later time next week." "Yes, this is Mazie." (In a telephone conversation.)

O Basic trust vs. basic mistrust—developing hope.
Autonomy vs. shame and doubt—limited self-control and developing willpower.
Identity vs. role confusion—developing fidelity.

Self-integration

S "I'll try." "I had a good time at . . ." "Sometimes I have trouble sitting." "I do my exercises when I feel nervous." "I feel good when . . ."

O Fluctuating level of psychic balance. Identity and grief-crisis resolution. Increased efficiency in coping with distress, anxiety, and daily living demands. Decision-making

skills. Autonomous actions. Beginning self-disclosure development. Self-direction.

Quality of life

S "I had a good time yesterday." "I like the 10:00 A.M. service . . ." "I'll try." "Sometimes I'm lonesome." "Did you know that . . ." "I like being busy."

O Involvement in present reality, self-acceptance, transient psychic distress.

SUGGESTED READINGS

American Nurses' Association: Standards of psychiatric mental-health nursing practice, Kansas City, 1973, The Association.

Bowlby, J.: Attachment and loss, New York, Vols. I and II, 1969, 1973, Basic Books, Inc., Publishers.

Costello, C. G.: The adaptive function of depression, Canadian Mental Health **25**:20-21, Dec., 1977.

Crill, M. E.: In bereavement, Journal of Practical Nursing **27**:22-25, Oct., 1977.

Fell, J.: Grief reactions in the elderly following death of a spouse: the role of crisis intervention and nursing, Journal of Gerontological Nursing **3**:16-20, Nov./Dec., 1977.

Flynn, G.: The development of the psychoanalytic concept of depression, Journal of Psychiatric Nursing **6**:138-149, May/June, 1968.

Govoni, L., and Hayes, J.: Drugs and nursing implications, New York, 1971, Appleton-Century-Crofts.

Hall, E.: The hidden dimension, New York, 1966, Doubleday & Co., Inc.

Hitchens, E. A.: Helping psychiatric outpatients accept drug therapy, American Journal of Nursing **77**:1144-1148, July, 1977.

Horoshake, I.: Suicide: how to spot and handle high risk patients, RN **40**:58-63, Sept., 1977.

Jones, C.: The nursing process—individualized care, Nursing Mirror **145**:13-14, Oct. 13, 1977.

Kalisch, B.: What is empathy? American Journal of Nursing **73**:1548-1552, Sept., 1973.

Kline, N. and Davis, J.: Psychotropic drugs, American Journal of Nursing **73**:54-63, January, 1973.

Kolb, L.: Modern clinical psychiatry, Philadelphia, 1977, W. B. Saunders Co.

Kubler-Ross, E.: On death and dying, New York, 1974, John Wiley & Sons, Inc.

Lovett, R. M.: Assessment: a many headed process, Nursing Mirror **146**:41-42, June 15, 1978.

McAfee, H.: Tardive dyskinesia, American Journal of Nursing **78**:395-397, March, 1978.

McCawley, A.: Helping patients cope with grief, Consultant **17**:64-66, Nov., 1977.

McShea, M.: Clinical judgement: an ethical issue, Journal of Psychiatric Nursing **16:**52-55, March, 1978.

Mitchell, C.: Assessment of alcohol abuse, Nursing Outlook **24:**511-515, 1976.

Mitchell, H., et al.: Nutrition in health and disease, Philadelphia, 1976, J. B. Lippincott Co.

Ray, O.: Drugs, society, and human behavior, ed. 2, St. Louis, 1978, The C. V. Mosby Co.

Roberts, S. L.: Territoriality: space and the schizophrenic patient, Perspectives in Psychiatric Care **7**(1):28-33, 1969.

Rubin, T.: The angry book, New York, 1969, Collier Books.

Stillman, M. J.: Territoriality and personal space, American Journal of Nursing **78:**1670-1672, Oct., 1978.

Synder, L.: Environmental changes for socialization, Journal of Nursing Administration **8:**44-50, Jan., 1978.

White, C. L.: Nurse counseling with a depressed patient, American Journal of Nursing **78:**436-439, March, 1978.

Wilken, D.: Community care of the mentally handicapped . . . family support, Nursing Mirror **146:**39-40, April 27, 1978.

CHAPTER 4

HILARY N *manifests*

PROBLEMATIC LIFE CONDUCT

evidenced by

ISOLATION AND A DISRUPTED LIFE-STYLE

INTRODUCTORY PERSONAL PROFILE
Social adjustment

S   "I'm really a late bloomer." "I choose to be a loner." "I'm not a very social person." "I can't" messages.

O   Demonstrated exceptional scholastic ability in high school, college, and law school. No extracurricular activities during educational experiences. No male or female relationship ties in adolescent or early adult years. Choice of solitary activities and social relationship avoidance.

Emotional health status

S   "I'm really a late bloomer." "I choose to be a loner." "I don't have a high level of energy. I tire easily."

O   Coping pattern of living a narrow, carefully ordered existence, using intellectual abilities to achieve and receive approval, to initiate and maintain interpersonal relationships, and to contain emotional experiences. Choice of solitary activities and social relationship avoidance.

Physical health status

S   "I don't have a high level of energy. I tire easily."

O   Height 5 feet, 5 inches. Weight 110 pounds. Dull, lusterless eyes. Rigid gait. Limited extrapyramidal syndrome from continuous large dosage of phenothiazine preparations. Drug-induced photosensitivity.

Spiritual dimension

S   "Sometimes I pray, but I'm not very religious." "Our family went to church on Christmas and Easter."

O   Does not subscribe to a defined religious denomination or belief.

Daily living skill performance

S   "I choose to be a loner." "Yes, I like my work." "I seem to stay busy."

O   Personal appearance neat, well kept, and stylish. Slow, deliberate, structured work pace, yielding quality output. Ordered financial management.

Coping skill repertoire

S "I'm really a late bloomer." "I choose to be a loner." "I seem to stay busy." "Well, we'll have to set a specific day and time for our appointment each week." "I don't know what you can do for me that my doctor can't do." "I'm not a very social person."

O Coping pattern of living a narrow, carefully ordered existence, using intellectual abilities to achieve and receive approval, to initiate and maintain interpersonal relationships, and to contain emotional experiences. Choice of solitary activities and social relationship avoidance. Intellectualization.

Maturational struggle according to Erikson's developmental stages

S "I'm not a very social person." "Sometimes I don't know what to do with myself." "I choose to be a loner."

O Basic trust vs. basic mistrust.
Dependence vs. independence.
Intimacy vs. isolation.

Self-integration

S "I choose to be a loner." "Well, we'll have to set a specific day and time for our appointment each week."

O Intellectualization. Coping pattern of living a narrow, carefully ordered existence, using intellectual abilities to achieve and receive approval, to initiate and maintain interpersonal relationships, and to contain emotional experiences.

Quality of life

S "I am comfortable." "Sometimes I don't know what to do with myself." "I stay busy." "Yes, I like my work."

O Ordered financial management, a pattern of saving, allowance for comforts and pleasures. Restricted interpersonal relationship.

Work focus of life. Intellectual achievements focus of reward.

Time span: 2 years

A close inspection of Hilary N reveals an average young woman, whose appearance is enhanced by full, blonde, wavy hair and a flair for color and coordination in clothes, makeup, and accessories. Often she could be described as striking.

Hilary N is a single, professionally educated woman, 31 years of age. She stands 5 feet, 5 inches tall, she weighs 110 pounds, and she is small framed and rather fragile looking. Her carefully applied makeup veils her sallow, pale complexion and augments the oval shape of her face and her clean, well-styled hair. Her blue contact lenses assist her appearance and mask the dull, lusterless, sad eyes that reveal her highly medicated state. Hilary's gait has a rigid quality, adding a degree of dignity to her well-dressed appearance. This covert measure superimposes any extrapyramidal syndrome experienced from a continuous large dosage of phenothiazine preparations. This young woman is a frightened person, who is experiencing persistent thought disorder. Hilary's coping mechanism is one of structure, order, and control in her life-style to maintain a semblance of self-integration.

Her inner emotional state is difficult for her to experience. The essential painfulness of feeling experiences and a coping pattern of living a narrow and carefully ordered existence, using intellectual abilities to achieve and receive approval, to initiate and maintain interpersonal relationships, and to contain emotional experiences further block emotional growth. Realistically, Hilary has dealt well with her many problems of living and has actual achievements beyond those of other women of a comparable age group.

Hilary is the oldest of four children. Two brothers and a sister were born to her parents in the 4 years immediately following Hilary's birth. Her young sister and her maternal grandparents died in a car accident when her sister was just 4 years of age. One brother died in a swimming accident at 9 years. Her only living sibling, Thomas, is 28 years old. He has maintained an estranged relationship with both his parents and Hilary for the past 10 years. Hilary's parents are retired, and they live in a southern retirement community. They travel frequently and maintain a geographic-social-emotional distance from their daughter. They call her at various times each month, and they have established a substantial trust fund for her. Several years ago they made a down payment on a patio home for their daughter, and they continue to provide an adequate insurance program for her.

Hilary demonstrated exceptional scholastic ability as a student, graduating in the top 5% of her high school class. She then attended a small private women's college, again graduating at the top of her senior class with an overall G.P.A. of 3.98 and receiving several scholastic honors for her intellectual achivements. Hilary reports few happy memories from high school or college experiences. She did not participate in extracurricular activities and maintains no ties, male or female, from these years. She describes herself as a late bloomer and a loner.

After college graduation, Hilary entered law school and excelled academically for the first year. During her second year she was confined for 3 months in a private psychiatric hospital in what was described as a grossly psychotic self-disintegration episode, accompanied by fragmented thinking and severe reality distortion. On discharge Hilary continued outpatient psychotherapy, returned to law school, and with a tremendous energy expenditure, graduated in 2 years, maintaining a grade-point average of 3.01. Hilary was admitted to the bar 6 months later, and she was employed by a small law firm in a metropolitan suburban area.

Hilary functioned relatively well in her first 2 years as a practicing attorney. She seemed to enjoy the research and preparation of client data material. In fact, she excelled in her work. The stressors of being forced into more public situations, client contact, any person-focused situations, and her perceived stress from legal practice precipitated another episode that required 3 months of confined psychiatric care. This episode involved treatment with a course of electroshock therapy. Hilary continued outpatient psychotherapy on discharge, but her sensorium impairment did not allow her return to work for another 3 months. Hilary's memory loss was severe, her sensorium slow to clear, and her impaired functioning abilities noticeable at the time of her discharge from the hospital.

A significant variable at that time was Hilary's employer, who provided the most kind, caring, and honest support she had ever experienced. She was given freedom to choose projects, a relative lack of pressure, and flexibility in schedules and deadlines when she returned to work. This atmosphere without criticism or judgment was provided for 1 year, when changes had to be made as decided by both parties. Hilary could produce neither at an expected professional level nor in a necessary competitive business manner. Her peers could no longer maintain the slack load, and conflicts concerning Hilary arose among both the professional and clerical office staff, necessitating resolution.

Hilary had enough insight, reality orientation, and limited autonomy to cope with the employment problem. This was a growth experience for her in which feelings and intellectual activity were combined to produce a solution. Hilary terminated her association with the firm and secured a half-time research position in a larger law firm. This employment arrangement decreased Hilary's stress level. She functioned by producing in-depth, thorough, high-quality researched materials, often choosing to increase her daily work schedule from 4 to 6 hours because of her slow, deliberate, structured pace. Between her parentally endowed trust fund and this half-time position, Hilary was able to manage a comfortable existence. An ordered financial management controlled stress in this area of her life and allowed for a pattern of saving and even some comfort and pleasures in her life-style.

It was at this point that Hilary was referred for supportive outpatient nurse psychotherapy. The initial interview was distant, intellectual, and uncomfortable for her. Early communication was marked by a strong tug-of-war between Hilary's communication distance maneuvers and the therapist's attempt to establish an interpersonal-relationship base. Hilary quickly established a fast-moving intellectual game of reasoning for and against a nurse-client relationship. Objective defining of general goals and purposes of such an encounter helped persuade Hilary to begin a nurse-client relationship. Hesitantly, she allowed nursing visits, contracted on the basis of one home visit a week for a 3-month period.

After the intake interview, a review of her available records, and collaboration with her psychiatrist, the following nursing diagnosis was concluded:

Anxiety
Dependence/independence struggle
Low self-concept
Suicide potential
Thought disorder
Interpersonal relationship disturbance
Psychotropic medication side effects
Loneliness
Unrealistic self-expectations
Rigid life stance
Faulty support system
Short concentration span
Lack of insight
Intellectualization
Trust/mistrust struggle
Intimacy/isolation struggle

The establishment of trust was found to be less difficult than the intake interview predicted.

Hilary discovered a bond in age similarity. She respected the therapist's educational level and professional credentials, although her need to question the therapist's qualifications proved trying. This exchange validated the therapist's competence and credibility, establishing Hilary's trust in the nurse's professional abilities and bonding the interpersonal relationship.

Conversations remained on an intellectual level for several visits. This level of interaction was allowed until the timing, readiness, and trust level of the relationship would allow exploration into new territory, more threatening to Hilary. Emotional closeness and expression and even superficial self-disclosure were approached by Hilary with extreme caution. This remained true during the entire duration of her treatment.

Intellectualization is a difficult defense mechanism for a clinician to confront effectively in the therapy situation. Theorists often advise therapists against allowing or encouraging clients to engage in this usually skillful mechanism of avoiding disclosure of feelings. Knowledgeable practitioners often advise quick eradication of this self-protective mechanism if a client is to make any degree of healthy progress. All behavior employed by clients should be evaluated as to their protective or destructive factors, purposes, strength, usefulness, and available positive substitutions. Hilary's intellectualization methods were rarely destructive to her person and on occasion even promoted personal growth. It served a purpose for her productivity in society and could be directed toward her emotional maturation. Most importantly, no positive substitute for this mental mechanism was readily available. Client assessment data can overrule the normative therapy procedure.

At first fears, mistrust, and concerns about the actual confidentiality of the professional relationship created ambivalence for Hilary. Ethical practices and beliefs in keeping a confidence were discussed factually during a half dozen interviews. Honesty with her about record keeping and the therapist's collaborative efforts with Hilary's psychiatrist were constant elements in the encounters. She signed confidential information releases, allowing the therapist to collaborate with her psychiatrist and to examine her medical and psychiatric records. Hilary was informed by the therapist prior to each collaborative visit with her physician, and after such collaboration frank discussion of these efforts and resultant goals were included in nurse-psychotherapy sessions. This allowed Hilary's active involvement in the direction and implementation of her overall psychiatric care. On two occasions, client, nurse, and physician met to plan and evaluate Hilary's progress, satisfactions, and dissatisfactions with therapy. This type of inclusion increased Hilary's trust, self-confidence, self-esteem commitment, and self-concept. It was a medium for positive feedback, active client involvement, and cohesion of the therapy approach. It also utilized Hilary's strength of intellectual coping abilities and newly forming emotional coping abilities.

Hilary received massive dosages of major tranquilizing drugs or antipsychotic agents, minor tranquilizing drugs or antianxiety agents, and antidepressant medications. These were prescribed in maximum daily dosages. Hilary frequently asked to have her medications reduced. Perceptually, she equated taking medications with *being* ill rather than with the reality of their being supportive measures to promote her present and future health.

Data from Hilary's records documented that each time a medication was reduced, she soon developed episodic behavior that indicated decompensation and self-disintegration. Her psychiatrist believed that a medication reduction was not indicated. Her current regimen might need to remain as a maintenance dosage for many years.

To assist Hilary in understanding and accepting this vital fact, data were gathered from her records regarding the four periods of time that medication reduction had been attempted, and the resulting behavior, distress, and life disruptions. These negative data were balanced with the positive behavior, growth, and achievement during the previous 10 months and during other treatment periods of a noninterrupted medication regimen combined with psychotherapy. (See Table 2.) It became clear to Hilary that her choice for the present was to continue with the current therapeutic dosage rather than take the high risks involved in medication reduction.

The idea of "drug holidays" of some duration is being espoused for clients who have received treatment both over a long duration and in maximum quantities with the antipsychotic drug preparations. With severe thought disorders such as Hilary's, maintenance dosages of phenothiazine preparations should be given in dosages as low as possible while the clinician continues to assist the client with the maintenance of self-integration and reality functioning. Unfortunately, Hilary's complex psyche did not allow reality functioning without continued high level dosages of phenothiazine preparations. Growth and healing were being slowly achieved through intensive psychotherapy. Insight gains, emotional unburdening, and interpersonal expansion were progressively increasing Hilary's psychic equilibrium, enlarging her coping skills, providing new successful communication patterns, and expanding her reality-oriented behavior base. Medication reduction accompanied by self-integration and a satisfactory and functional life-style would always be a primary consideration in the therapy goal decision-making process.

Hilary had few medication side effects other than some rigidity, well controlled by benztropine mesylate, and some telltale signs in her eyes. Her major adverse side effect was the problem of photosensitivity. She sunburned rapidly and intensely. This curtailed outside summer activities. A sunscreen lotion and makeup protected her sensitive skin and allowed limited outdoor activities. Hilary used

Table 2. Data comparison sample*

Point in time	Overt behavior problems exhibited during medication reduction process	Overall growth and terminal goals achieved during medication maintenance regimen as measured by the following behaviors
Reduction 1 Reduction time: 2 weeks Time interval: 18 months	Concentration problems Decreased G.P.A. Weight loss Intellectual retention problems Temper outburst problems Fragmented thinking Relationship difficulties Withdrawal	
Reduction 2 Reduction time: 6 weeks Time interval: 36 months	Same behaviors as in Reduction 1 Increased withdrawal Active psychotic process necessitating hospitalization and treatment with electroshock therapy with resultant memory impairment interrupting her chosen life-style	Return to law school Graduation from law school Successful completion of bar examination Practicing attorney Job reevaluation and relocation Competent financial mangement Satisfying social activities Growth through psychotherapy Increased decision-making ability Absence of rehospitalizations Employment stability, satisfaction, and success Absence of blatant psychotic process
Reduction 3 Reduction time: 3 weeks Time interval: 12 months	Withdrawal Employment-related problems Intellectual retention problems Concentration problems Fragmented thinking Relationship difficulties	
Reduction 4 Reduction time: 3 weeks Time interval: 12 months	Withdrawal Employment-related problems Intellectual retention problems Concentration problems Fragmented thinking Relationship difficulties	
Current time interval on maintenance drug	*No overt behavior interfering with her chosen life-style*	

*Significant variable is the short duration period before overt behavior problems emerge. Note correlation between longest reduction period and resultant rehospitalization.

her fashion flair to camouflage her skin with attractive coverup, light-weight clothing, hats, and large stylish sunglasses. She stated that she missed the summer tan of her teen years but planned her time to swim, bicycle, and play tennis on warm summer evenings.

Hilary did enjoy the challenge of circumventing her limitations. She was sufficiently informed to understand that if she had been emotionally distressed to this extent before the chemical advance of tranquilizing medication, she would have been hospitalized on a long-term basis.

PROCESS IMPLEMENTATION

1—Evaluation

N.D.   *Low self-concept*
   S   "Do I look all right in this new makeup? It seems so heavy." "The chart shows I'm better, doesn't it?" "I should be able to do it without drugs."
   O   Client equated taking medications with being ill rather than with the reality of their being supportive measures to promote health.

N.D.   *Psychotropic medication side effects*
   S   "I bought this pale blue, long-sleeved blouse for summer." "Do you like my sunglasses?" "A lot of women are wearing big hats again." "I don't mind putting my exercise off until evening."
   O   Rigidity. Dull eyes. Photosensitivity. Application of sunscreen lotion and makeup. Attractive coverup clothing. Swimming, bicycling, and playing tennis during evening hours. Drug prescription for benztropine mesylate.

N.D.   *Lack of insight*
   S   "Yes, I've read several books about my drugs." "I don't mind putting my exercise off until evening." "Your chart helped." "I should be able to do it without drugs."
   O   Client equated taking medications with being ill rather than with the reality of their being supportive measures to promote health. Intellectual and emotional understanding and acceptance of the need for psychotropic medication and the consequences of not maintaining the drug regimen.

N.D.   *Intellectualization*
   S   "Yes, I've read several books about my drugs and I know I must take them." "Your chart helped."
   O   Client equated taking medications with being ill rather than with the reality of their being supportive measures to promote health.

N.D.   *Unrealistic self-expectations*
   S   "I should be able to do it without drugs."
   O   Client equated taking medications with being ill rather than with the reality of their being supportive measures to promote health.

Actual outcome
   Emotional and intellectual understanding and acceptance of data comparison sample (Table 2). Continues to take medication as prescribed. Less questioning of medication rationale.

2A—Assessment

N.D.   *Anxiety*
   S   "You mean I really don't have to give a reason?" "I don't always know what to say."
   O   Controlled territorial distance of 3 to 4 feet. Trembling voice, finger tapping, foot swinging when in company of unfamiliar persons.

N.D.   *Interpersonal relationship disturbance*
   S   "I don't know how to make friends." "I guess I've never had a friend." "You mean I don't have to give a reason?" "I don't always know what to say."
   O   Controlled territorial distance of 3 to 4 feet. Trembling voice, finger tapping, foot swinging when in company of unfamiliar persons. Declined invitations from social acquaintances.

N.D.   *Loneliness*
   S   "I don't know how to make friends." "I guess I've never had a friend."
   O   Declined invitations from social acquaintances. Extended time periods spent alone.

N.D.   *Unrealistic self-expectations*
   S   "You mean I really don't have to give a reason?" "I don't always know what to say." "I wish I could adjust more quickly."
   O   No allowance given for her sheltered growth and development years. Unfavorable comparisons between her-self and others frequently emphasized by client.

N.D.   *Trust/mistrust struggle*
   S   "I don't know how to make friends." "I don't always know what to say."
   O   Controlled territorial distance of 3 to 4 feet. Declined invitations from social acquaintances.

N.D.   *Dependence/independence struggle*
   S   "Could you help me make friends?"
   O   Continual ambivalent pull between reaching out for social contact and withdrawal from social contact.

N.D. *Intimacy/isolation struggle*
- S "I've never dated." "Yes, I think I'd like to date." "I don't always know what to say."
- O Controlled territorial distance of 3 to 4 feet. Declined invitations from social acquaintances.

N.D. *Lack of insight*
- S "I don't always know what to say." "You mean I really don't have to give a reason?" "I wish I could adjust more easily."
- O Intellectual understanding of life situations but inability to integrate the knowledge emotionally.

3 — Additional nursing diagnosis
None

4A — Variables

Reality timing	+4
Relationships	−4
Stressors and/or crisis	+2
Coping resources	0
Significant emotional strength	+2
Significant emotional limitations	−4
Therapy relationship	+3
Physical health status	+2
Physical and emotional readiness dimension	+4
Available support system	−2
Meaning significance	+3
Values and belief impact	+1
Other	
BALANCE	+

Additional specific knowledge
See case material.

Analysis and synthesis

N.D. *Anxiety*. Related to conflict regarding socialization and isolation. New social skills and experiential medium to "try on" skills will reduce overall stress and insecurity.

N.D. *Interpersonal relationship disturbance*. Had limited life relationship. Past stroking had been gained from intellectual achievements and academic success rather than from within a relationship. Methods of relating must be learned and experienced, and rewards from this method achieved.

N.D. *Loneliness*. Discomfort from her aloneness is a motivator to reach out and experience new modes of living.

N.D. *Unrealistic self-expectations*. Client's usual self-comparison to peers is not valid. Perception of others and self will moderate as social growth is initiated and relationships are experienced.

N.D. *Trust/mistrust struggle*. Lack of social and in-

teraction skills, high anxiety level, and lack of belief in self increase the trust/mistrust conflict.

N.D. *Dependence/independence struggle*. Lack of belief in herself coupled with perceived life failures, especially mental illness, decrease an ability to assume an autonomous stance.

N.D. *Intimacy/isolation struggle*. Discomfort associated with closeness and a life pattern of withdrawal and false security from this stance block attempts to initiate relationships and also increase the inner struggle.

N.D. *Lack of insight*. Client self-knowledge is related to emotions experienced while encountering a situation. Increased person association will broaden self-realization.

4B — Design of action

N.D. Anxiety, interpersonal relationship disturbance, loneliness, unrealistic self-expectations, trust/mistrust struggle, dependence/independence struggle, intimacy/isolation struggle, lack of insight.

1. Plan
   a. Develop client's social skills and interaction skills.
2. Strategy
   a. Create a medium for learning social and interaction skills within the therapy situation, that is, discussion of methods, norms, and functions of a social relationship.
   b. Encourage self-disclosure within the therapy relationship. Reinforce emotional expression with feedback.
   c. Expect client to choose and partake in social activities.
   d. Support involvement in social activities no matter how limited the experience may be.
3. Expected outcomes
   a. Regular discussion of social experiences.
   b. Increasing comfort and involvement in emotional self-revelation.
   c. Participation in several social activities.
4. Criteria
   a. Initiative in choosing therapy discussion topics.
   b. Decreased observable anxiety during self-disclosure in therapy.
   c. Relating experiences from social activity.
   d. Acknowledged learnings and insights from activity and related therapy discussions.

Many of the factual elements dealt with in Hilary's beginning therapy encounters cemented the professional interpersonal relationship.

The therapist remained matter-of-fact but warmly responsive during nursing visits. The usual territorial space distance of 3 to 4 feet controlled by Hilary offered her security. Touching, supportive measures with hands as well as with words can threaten some clients. The therapist touched Hilary only once with the hand as a social gesture, and that was at the termination of the relationship.

With a climate of trust and security established within the confidential relationship, Hilary began occasionally to disclose her emotions. She revealed she had never dated. She thought she might like to date but did not know how to behave with men. She had declined invitations from acquaintances "to have a drink after work" because she knew she could not combine alcohol with her drugs. The therapist introduced the idea of her having a nonalcoholic beverage and commented on Hilary's strengths in making social conversation. She was rather astounded by the fact that one can, for example, simply say "no" and refuse an alcoholic beverage without the need to offer reasons. Some matters need not become the business of other individuals. Hilary offered the insight that when a relationship threatened her, she most often blocked the other person with an acceptable, intellectual "I can't" message as a coping measure.

Some weeks later, Hilary joined a singles social group, and many of her therapy sessions were used to discuss the happenings of these social activities. She remained on the periphery of this group and chose to join only activity-centered gatherings. Her circle of acquaintances was broadened, and her time alone and living experiences were expanded.

Hilary reestablished her contract for therapy five times during a 2-year period. Except for the first contractual reestablishment, she initiated the procedure. She also took the leadership in determining the termination of the nurse-client relationship. The termination issue was reasoned according to her belief of having outgrown the need for the defined relationship, which was, in reality, true. Jointly decided nursing therapy goals had been achieved. Termination was also spurred by a recognized valid need for emotional closeness that Hilary knew she must begin to secure in the nonprofessional realm. For Hilary the mental illness experience was being directed for positive, creative, and freeing realization.

Friends were missing from Hilary's life. The developmental experiences of making friends, having friends, losing friends, and making new friends seemed to have been absent in her early years, especially during her adolescence, the expected period for this task achievement. Hilary perceived that her parents, hurt by the losses of their other children, succeeded in putting her under a "bushel basket," so to speak. It was a kind of protective canopy devoid of emotion. The nurse-client relationship offered Hilary a medium in which to discuss her experiential learnings about life and an encounter in which to solve the problem of how to acquire and judge friendships.

Hilary sought friendship from within a helping relationship. One professional mark of a relationship is its quality of other-centeredness. Friendships have a joint character of trusting, sharing, self-disclosure, giving and taking, and disagreeing. This alliance proceeds with free-floating emotional entanglements, invaded freedom, varying degrees of commitment for each individual, and expectations that are not always clearly defined. Friendship usually lacks an authority atmosphere, often a quality of the professional interaction. Professional relationships are marked by clearly defined boundaries with stated expectations, stated roles, stated goals, and a stated degree of involvement and of commitment. These qualities should be explicitly interpreted in the beginning stages of a relationship. The rules of the professional encounter are established and agreed on, whereas other life relationships often have covert game rules or no established contractual relationship agreements.

The therapist offered to teach Hilary how to be a friend, thus providing defined therapy relationship boundaries, an experimental field for learning about interpersonal relationships, new social interaction skills, and guidance in reaching out to the social world. The variables in this therapy task were its other-centeredness, the explicit goals and defined game rules of the therapist's own degree of self-disclosure, and the acknowledged dimensions of Hilary's own expectations. This established the professional relationship boundaries and provided guidance and space for Hilary to discuss and test behaviors within secure relationship limits. Hilary was expected to learn, question, and experiment. When she felt ready to become a friend to someone, she would have the therapist's support and guidance.

In some of the encounters, there were discussions of the methods, norms, and functions of social relationships. These intellectual exercises led to Hilary's experimenting in other encounters and then questioning the results for corrective feedback or personal affirmation. She often wondered what the therapist would do in a similar situation or if another person had such experiences. A limited sharing of like circumstances helped her to understand that other human beings felt as she did. The therapist would say, "That would embarrass me also," or "Yes, I have felt uncomfortable in a similar group." When called on to relate a similar incident from life experience, the therapist must always use judgment and caution not to expound on an incident or issue simply for the need to share or for one's own self-gratification.

Hilary bought a sewing machine and enrolled in a sewing class. For her this was a thought-out but personally perilous venture. Her classmates were friendly and outgoing, the class was small, and Hilary expressed pleasure in participating. She needed reinforcement to begin, to continue, and to complete this 12-week course. Hilary probably would never be an accomplished seamstress, but she could follow a pattern, hem, sew on buttons, replace a zipper, and make simple repairs and alterations. In her course she made an attractive skirt. Hilary usually took pride in her appearance and began using two afternoons a month to repair and maintain her wardrobe by using her new skill.

Hilary reported more frequent interactions with fellow employees. She became less anxious about coffee breaks and lunch times, and she even reported transient superficial encounters with clients. She revealed that although she did not enjoy these experiences, she did not feel impelled to avoid them as she had in the past. The process of reaffirming the value and dignity of an individual is a slow and often tedious task for the clinician but of infinite worth for movement toward therapy goals.

Hilary joined an indoor tennis club with a woman she met while doing research at a library. Her new friend was a library assistant, and they played tennis weekly. Hilary's involvement in this activity took great energy, since her agility was impaired by her medication; her determination to play tennis was not in the least impaired, however. The two women played several sets of tennis every Wednesday night. Their relationship seldom involved any other activity or encounter except for an occasional cup of coffee or soft drink after their game. Hilary felt less alone by participating in this regularly scheduled tennis game. Some of her daily accumulated anxiety had a positive outlet as well.

Hilary also enjoyed bicycling, which she could acceptably do alone and in the latter part of the day, preventing direct exposure to the sun. It also provided an adequate energy outlet for her built-up anxiety. Both tennis and bicycling assisted in remedying transient constipation problems produced by her sedentary lifestyle and side effects of her prescribed medications.

Hilary diligently sought and found healthy ways to fill her increased time spaces as she pursued her career on a part-time basis. Gradually, she achieved a positive balance for her time spent alone and time spent with other people. Comparison of time ratios spent alone as opposed to time spent with others was approximately 4:1. Before Hilary participated in nurse psychotherapy, she had maintained a hermitlike existence and had expended much energy to continue this lonely existence.

PROCESS IMPLEMENTATION

1—Evaluation

N.D. *Anxiety*
- S "Have you ever felt that way?" "I had a good time last night."
- O Less observable anxiety (body gestures and speech) when relating to the therapist. Client encounters. Interactions with other employees at coffee break.

N.D. *Interpersonal relationship disturbance*
- S "Have you ever felt that way?" "I had a good time last night." "Can you tell me what it means when someone says . . ."
- O Remained on periphery of singles group and chose to join activity not social gatherings. Client encounters. Interactions with other employees at coffee break. Joined tennis club with a female companion.

N.D. *Loneliness*
- S "I had a good time last night." "I don't feel so alone anymore."
- O Spent less time alone. Interactions with other employees at coffee break. Joined tennis club with a female companion.

N.D. *Unrealistic self-expectations*
- S "Have you ever felt that way?" "It's OK to go at my own pace."
- O Remained on periphery of singles group and chose to join activity not social gathering.

N.D. *Trust/mistrust struggle.*
- S "Have you ever felt that way?" "It helps to talk to you." "I feel . . ."
- O Increasing amounts of self-disclosure in therapy regarding new learnings, insights, and emotions. Client encounters. Interactions with other employees at coffee break.

N.D. *Dependence/independence struggle*
- S "I had a good time last night." "I decided to . . ." "I don't feel so alone any more."
- O Joined a singles group. Bought a sewing machine and enrolled in sewing class. Joined a tennis club. Resumed bicycling.

N.D. *Intimacy/isolation struggle*
- S "I had a good time last night." "I feel . . ."
- O Remained on periphery of singles group and chose to join activity not social gatherings. Interactions with other employees at coffee break. Joined tennis club with a female companion.

N.D. *Lack of insight*
- S "I just say I can't when I don't know what to do." "Maybe I don't have to say I can't." "I feel . . ." "It's OK to go at my own pace."
- O Insights carried over to actions, that is, decreased "I can't" excuses. Initiative to renegotiate therapy four times.

Actual outcome

Joined a singles group, enrolled in a sewing class, joined a tennis club, and resumed bicycling. Initiated reestablishment of therapy contract four times. Discussion of new activities, person association, and resultant feelings in therapy. Increasing amount of self-disclosure in therapy regarding new learnings, insights, and emotions. Less observable anxiety when relating to therapist.

2A—Assessment

N.D. *Dependence/independence struggle*
- S "I didn't have much to say about this house." "I guess it needs something but I don't know what."
- O Had not been involved in the purchase or furnishing of her home. Reserved second bedroom for parents' occasional visits. Chose not to invest emotional energy, time, or money in living accommodation. Increased amounts of conversation about home environment.

N.D. *Loneliness*
- S "I don't have much need to do anything with the house. You're the only one who comes here."
- O Chose not to invest emotional energy, time, or money in living accommodation. Low-stimulus home environment that maintains and supports isolation.

N.D. *Low self-concept*
- S "I didn't have much to say about this house." "Sometimes I'd like to decorate, but I really don't know how."
- O Chose not to invest emotional energy, time, or money in living accommodation. Expressed a desire to redecorate home but uncertain about doing as she wished. Increased amounts of conversation about home environment.

N.D. *Lack of insight*
- S "Sometimes I'd like to decorate, but I really don't know how."

O Expressed a desire to redecorate home but uncertain about doing as she wished.

3 — Additional nursing diagnosis
None

4A — Variables

Reality timing	+3
Relationships	+3
Stressors and/or crisis	0
Coping resources	+1
Significant emotional strength	+1
Significant emotional limitations	0
Therapy relationship	+4
Physical health status	0
Physical and emotional readiness dimension	+4
Available support system	0
Meaning significance	+4
Values and belief impact	+2
Other	
BALANCE	+

Additional specific knowledge
See case material.

Analysis and synthesis

N.D. *Dependence/independence struggle.* Budding initiative in new life areas. Desire to make some decisions about self and response to self-gratification needs.

N.D. *Loneliness.* New activities and association aided realization of how others live. Less need for isolation and low-stimulus environment.

N.D. *Low self-concept.* Increased sense of security and new ability to allow self-gratification and comfort.

N.D. *Lack of insight.* Unable to view any potential she has in new, untested life areas. Realization will occur from ''doing'' and experiencing new modes of coping and emotions.

4B — Design of action

N.D. Dependence/independence struggle, loneliness, low self-concept, lack of insight.

1. Plan
   a. Support client decision and actions in redecorating home environment.
2. Strategy
   a. Assist with planning.
   b. Affirm positive decisions and actions.
   c. Encourage self-comfort and self-gratification measures.
3. Expected outcomes
   a. Redecoration of home environment in various stages to final completion.
4. Criteria
   a. Involvement in planning changes and purchases.

b. Execution of actual changes.
c. Discussion and display of redecoration at various stages and at completion.

Hilary's patio home could be described as adequate. It contained two medium-sized bedrooms, an eating area, a kitchen combined with laundry facilities, a medium-sized living room, and a small bath. There were many windows, allowing the brightness of sunshine to warm the place on most days. Her furniture was of good quality and construction. Accent furnishings such as pictures, decorator items, or pieces with sentimental value did not appear in any room. There was no esthetic display in her home, in direct contrast to her flair for clothes and stylish personal appearance.

It was revealed that Hilary had never lived in a place that she had considered her own. Her parents chose and bought the house, and her mother carpeted the floors, draped the windows, and purchased necessary furniture. Hilary was not asked to become involved in this activity and chose not to invest emotional energy, time, or money in this dwelling other than to use it as a living accommodation.

As Hilary's life began to have some semblance of stability, she expressed in her therapy sessions a desire to change her living environment. She also expressed a feeling of not knowing how to do this or even where to begin. Attention was focused on her expressions of what she wanted to do. Responding to her own wants and needs was a new and uncertain experience for Hilary, as was redoing anything previously done by her parents.

Hilary began by adding some accent pieces to her living room and bedroom. The therapist reinforced Hilary's activity as a positive action of self-gratification and initiative. Hilary could understand that her thrifty nature and monetary security would allow her to make purchases of choice without causing financial difficulty. The therapist correlated Hilary's flair for personal style in her appearance with her dormant ability to decorate her home, using her innate artistic talents. In due course she purchased an oil painting, a decorator lamp, an elegant crystal vase that she filled with soft-colored silk flowers, ornamental fragrant candles, and other pieces that made her feel more comfortable. As Hilary's own person expanded, so did the personality of her private environment.

This decorating effort provided actual visible achievement and self-affirmation, offering feedback for her initiative, talents, choices, and increased self-expansion. Months later, Hilary was to risk inviting her tennis partner into her now warm, inviting, and comfortable home.

Hilary wished to redecorate her rarely used second bedroom, which she perceived as an uncertain undertaking. The room was closed off and saved for her parents' semi-annual visits. With tremendous trepidation, ambivalence, and need for support, Hilary acted on her desire to transform this room. She sold the old furniture by means of a newspaper advertisement, bought new drapes, a queen-size hide-a-bed, a desk and chair, a lamp, a rocker, a large bookcase, a small T.V., and stereo equipment. She placed her sewing machine in this room and arranged the space into a combined study-recreational area for her personal enjoyment.

This room, Hilary said, provided considerable comfort and space to pursue some of her chosen activities. When Hilary's parents announced their intention of visiting, she felt guilt, anxiety, and fear at their approaching arrival. Supportive nurse-psychotherapy visits were increased to help avoid the perceived crisis. There was no crisis. In fact, little parental comment, either negative or positive, was made concerning Hilary's change in her own home.

The week before her parents' visit provided some strained moments for Hilary. During the actual visit, however, her job performance did not vary, and she weathered the visit with increased strength, self-assurance, insight, and autonomy.

The concept of providing experimental space for a client to experience new modes of coping was highly applicable to Hilary and gave her both an emotional and a social growth medium. The experience of "going through the motions," a "trial-and-error" situation, or a "test flight" and the random sampling of perceived life ordeals helped Hilary attempt new life situations with less apprehension. As time passed, she groped less while investigating new experiences. Security in other-person encounters came with the verification that she could do as she perceived others doing. Feedback from within the nursing relationship validated for her the realization that she was indeed "OK" as a person. Experience in feeling good about herself as a person was not only new, but it was also a seemingly hazardous concept for her. Allowing the feeling experience to happen in a positive atmosphere is a necessary component of achieving healing and emotional growth. These experiences are a fertile field for development of insight and self-realization, often waiting to be cultivated in community, home-based psychosocial nursing interventions.

PROCESS IMPLEMENTATION

1—Evaluation

N.D.   *Dependence/independence struggle*

S   "My new study is comfortable. I spend a lot of time there." "I asked . . . to visit after tennis last night." "I decided to buy a . . ." "I've made quite a few decisions lately."

O   Inviting tennis partner into home. Sold old furniture bought new drapes, hide-a-bed, desk, chair, lamp, rocker, bookcase, T.V., and stereo. Placed sewing machine in study-recreation room. Purchased and placed decorator items.

N.D.   *Loneliness*

S   "I asked . . . to visit after tennis last night." "Time seems to go so fast when I'm in my study." "I enjoyed . . ."

O   Invited tennis partner into home. Created an environment of comfortable stimuli.

N.D.   *Low self-concept*

S   "My new study is comfortable. I spend a lot of time there." "I asked . . . to visit after tennis last night." "I decided to buy a . . ." "I feel good about . . ." "I enjoyed . . ."

O   Inviting tennis partner into home. Developed artistic talents. Effectively coped with parents' visit.

N.D.   *Lack of insight*
  S   "Once I started this decorating, I liked it." "I've made quite a few decisions lately." "I'm not so afraid of new things now."
  O   Completion of a new task potential. Realization of new skills and acknowledgement of person potential.

Actual outcome
  Redecoration of home environment to produce comfort and adapt to changing life-style. Many therapy hours spent in planning, observing, and affirming transition over several months.

2A—Assessment

N.D.   *Suicide potential*
  S   "It's hard to continue living like this."
  O   No history of suicidal gestures. Contracted to call therapist if feeling self-destructive.

N.D.   *Thought disorder*
  S   "It's hard to continue living like this." "I guess I didn't hear you." "I don't know where my thoughts were." "Did you tell me to . . . no, it wasn't you."
  O   Forgotten appointment, usually neat appearance disheveled, eyes swollen and reddened. Dwelling dark. Unsuccessful at regaining composure. Fear and apprehension noticed in voice and eyes.

N.D.   *Short concentration span*
  S   "What did you say?" "I don't know how I forgot the appointment."
  O   Forgot the appointment. Infrequent but recurring lost train of thought.

N.D.   *Faulty support system*
  S   "You're the only one I really talk to." "I'm not close to anyone."
  O   Unable to unburden her stress to another. No viable sharing relationship present in her life.

N.D.   *Rigid life stance*
  S   "You're the only one I really talk to." "I'm really very busy. I don't have time for friends."
  O   Time spaces filled with tasks. Ordered, routine daily life pattern.

N.D.   *Thought disorder*
  S   "What did you say?" (Repeated four times per visit.) "I guess I didn't hear you." "I don't know where my thoughts were." "Did you tell me to . . . no, it wasn't you." (Repeated four times per visit.)
  O   Infrequent but recurring lost train of thought. Appeared distant during intense encounters. Increased interaction problems. Fear and apprehension noticed in voice and eyes six times per visit.

3—Additional nursing diagnosis
None

4A—Variables

Reality timing	+5
Relationships	−5
Stressors and/or crisis	−4
Coping resources	+2
Significant emotional strength	0
Significant emotional limitations	−3
Therapy relationship	+4
Physical health status	0
Physical and emotional readiness dimension	+4
Available support system	−5
Meaning significance	+3
Value and belief impact	0
Other	
BALANCE	+

Additional specific knowledge
See case material.

Analysis and synthesis

N.D.   *Suicide potential.* Always a potential problem when hallucinatory material is prominent. Assess and plan verbally with client.

N.D.   *Thought disorder.* Symptomatic of increased stress perceived by client and an inability to cope effectively with the stressors. Emotions controlled or withheld rather than expressed. Fragmented thinking.

N.D.   *Short concentration span.* Symptomatic of increased stress perceived by client. Transient symptom will be relieved by decrease of perceived stress and renewed coping measures.

N.D.   *Faulty support system.* Therapy relationship offers needed support to confront crisis. Other person support could help abort future similar incidents. No medium for emotional sharing viable in client's life other than therapy relationship.

N.D.   *Rigid life stance.* Inability to maintain the needed order increases stress. Assist to regain control. This coping mechanism helps client remain intact. Begin to evaluate for initiation of beginning flexibility in life-style to produce some balance and offset future similar crisis states.

4B—Design of action
N.D.   Suicide potential, thought disorder, short concentration span, faulty support system, rigid life stance.
  1. Plan
     a. Offer supportive measures to strengthen self.
     b. Assess for coping strength and reality orientation.

2. Strategy
   a. Supportive review of accomplishments, positive coping with daily living, self growth while focusing on health.
   b. Offer no judgment concerning present behavior.
   c. Assess reality orientation, limitations, strengths, and suicide potential.
   d. Confront suicide issue. Confront distress and ineffective coping as control returns and feelings emerge.
3. Expected outcomes
   a. Restore needed control, order, and structure to client's person.
   b. Contract to contact therapist if suicidal feelings persist.
   c. Discussion of perceived life stressors.
   d. Feeling disclosure.
4. Criteria
   a. Observable return of usual control in speech, manner, and posture.
   b. Execution of verbal contract to contact therapist when suicidal feelings persist.
   c. Revealing current life stressors.
   d. Self-disclosure of troubling emotions.

On six evening occasions after the initial 6 months of therapy, the therapist arrived at Hilary's home to find her highly distressed. On each of the occasions she had forgotten the appointment, her usually neat appearance was disheveled, her eyes were swollen and reddened as if she had been crying, and her house was dark.

On the first such meeting, Hilary struggled desperately but unsuccessfully to "pull herself together," but fragmented thinking prevented composure. The security of her relationship with the therapist allowed her to begin to unburden herself, and she proceeded slowly and cautiously. As a rule, Hilary expected unrealistic performance from herself. She was bright, and she had excelled academically during most of her life, but she did not give herself any leeway for error. Indeed, she did not even give herself space to be human.

Hilary also spent a large portion of her psychic and physical energy maintaining a posture of control. Her life was rigidly structured to maintain order. She filled her time with tasks not only to prevent others from entering her personal space but also to prevent unstructured time alone with herself.

Hilary experienced auditory hallucinations when stress in her life increased. She was time structured, carefully controlled in speech, manner, and posture, and infrequently but recurrently she lost her train of thought. She appeared distant at intermittent intervals, noticeably during intense encounters. It was not clinically sound for the therapist to confront her with suspicions of thought disorder. In a collaborative effort, Hilary's psychiatrist expressed the same "praecox feeling" as the nurse had experienced. Based on these stated data, nursing interventions were supportive of time structuring and maintenance of a client-controlled environment balanced by a focus on realistic self-expectation and social-emotional strength development, healing, and self-disclosure.

Suicide potential is a constant variable when thought disorder and blatant psychopathology such as hallucinations persist. During one evening visit when she was unusually distressed, suicide was discussed in a matter-of-fact manner. Hilary denied any actual suicidal thoughts or plans, but she offered, "It is hard to continue living like this." The therapist was alert to the continuous potential of self-destructive behavior. At points of high stress, it was decided to increase therapy hours and contact times. A verbal contract was made with Hilary, asking her to call the nurse when she felt it "hard to continue like this." She agreed to the contact, but she never executed it. She had no history of suicidal gestures. She did allow the therapist to spend time with her when she regressed into aloneness and self-disintegration, thus not totally closing out reality as she had done in the past.

The encounters on the six evenings when she was experiencing a noticeable degree of fragmentation were at first free floating in atmosphere, allowing Hilary to express fragmented thoughts and perceived fears. Astute nursing assessment of current or recurrent stressors was a primary concentration for the therapist. High anxiety associated with job performance and self-expectations accompanied by increased isolation seemed to be recurrent themes. Medication continued to be taken as prescribed. The catharsis that nurse psychotherapy offered appeared to provide relief. No confrontation of the suspected thought disorder was initiated. No judgments were offered, but the therapist proceeded to review Hilary's present and long-range accomplishments, her positive responsible coping with daily living requirements and self-growth, all the while focusing on her positive mental health and actual reality. This method of intervening appeared to relieve the transient self-disintegration episodes and to restore her needed level of self-control and functioning, Renewed efforts by the therapist to institute new coping patterns for stress were again emphasized during ensuing visits.

On the encounter following the first such episode, Hilary appeared uncomfortably anxious. She remained at a secure and remote distance. She appeared to wonder if the therapist would continue to like her when it became known how extremely distressed she was. Trust reestablishment took about an hour. The therapist acknowledged satisfaction at being able to assist her and emphasized that the role of a nurse was to help her cope when she most needed this kind of assistance. To Hilary's questioning, it was acknowledged that others had been given similar assistance and that others had been in equal or in even more turmoil. A climate of trust was again a viable therapy element. The equilibrium of the relationship returned, and its durability was proved.

One might question the value of employing nursing diagnosis as a pivot for nursing intervention. At the termination of this nurse-client relationship, evaluation indicated that all nursing diagnoses remained as problems, although in an altered state. Too often, one adopts a term such as ''diagnosis'' and believes that all the

identified problem behaviors must be removed if nursing intervention is to be considered successful. In reality this is not so, especially when one's focus is on behaviors of long duration and on established pathological behavior patterns and coping mechanisms chosen consciously or unconsciously to protect self-integration.

A parallel might be found in a physician's intervention for the treatment of a diagnosed malignant biological growth. The intervention of choice might be surgical, radiological, chemical, a combination of these choices, or still another choice not mentioned. The physician's goal is to promote life or health and to eradicate, decrease, or contain the identified disease process. Nursing diagnosis of a long-term, emotionally disabled client is the pivot for modification of behavior, personal healing, or pathological process alteration. Psychopathological behavior is rarely removed altogether. Negative behavior patterns and ineffective coping styles can be contained. They can be decreased in the number of times or the manner in which the client employs them. Hilary's thought disorder was contained by medication, reinforcement of a controlled environment, a realistic time structure, and the promotion of insight and significant relationships. Intellectualization became a behavior strength employed to increase health rather than a limitation used to cover pathology or to create an umbrella-like protection for Hilary, blocking healthy person-to-person encounters.

Knowledge, expectations, adequate time durations, support, and experiences allowing emotional and intellectual involvement were necessary variables in effecting nursing intervention and promoting social-emotional-personal healing and growth for Hilary. Nursing diagnosis may be the springboard for intervention, but it is the astute assessment of the client, allowing for both the nurse's and the client's perception, that facilitates the continuous implementation of the nursing process (plan and action) to bring about a new or renewed level of social-emotional-personal healing and growth. It is the client who is the nucleus of the nursing process. It is not the process itself that is important but how skillfully it is employed by the nurse for promotion, establishment and/or reestablishment, or maintenance of the health of one's client that is of primary consequence.

SUMMARY PERSONAL PROFILE
Social adjustment

S   ". . . came for a coke after tennis." "I don't know how to be a friend. I guess I've never had one." "I talk to Mary at coffee breaks . . ." "I ate lunch with . . ." "I enjoy my new room."

O   Invited tennis partner into her home. Insight gains, emotional unburdening, and interpersonal expansion progressively allowing increased psychic equilibrium accompanied by new coping skills, successful communication patterns, and an expanded reality base. Ability to become involved in therapy and develop insight. Joined activity-centered gatherings. Increased circle of acquaintances. Less time alone. More frequent interaction with fellow employees. Home redecorating to meet needs.

Emotional health status

S   ". . . came for a coke after tennis." "I feel . . ." "It's hard for me to do . . ." "I try so hard." "I don't know how to be a friend. I guess I've never had one." "What do you think about . . ." "You mean I don't have to . . ."

O   Initiative to begin and execute project, that is, home redecorating, sewing class, tennis. Self-disclosure. Insight gains, emotional unburdening, and interpersonal expansion progressively allowing increased psychic equilibrium accompanied by new coping skills, successful communication patterns, and an expanded reality base. Ability to become involved in therapy and develop insight.

Physical health status

S   "I feel better when I get more exercise." "I've been less tired lately and sleeping well." "I'm less sluggish feeling."

O   Dull, lusterless eyes. Rigid gait. Limited extrapyramidal syndrome from continuous large dosage of phenothiazine preparations. Photosensitivity. Increased exercise programs, for example, tennis, bicycling. Decreased problem from side effects of medication such as constipation.

Spiritual dimension

S ⎫
O ⎭ No acknowledged or observable change.

Daily living skill performance

S   "Yes, I like my work." "I would like to be able to work more hours." "This house is less work than it used to be." "I like to get things in order every day."

O   Personal appearance neat, well kept, and stylish. Slow, deliberate structured work pace, yielding quality output. Ordered financial management. Less rigidity in structure of life and environment but thorough completion of tasks of living.

Coping skill repertoire

S   "I feel . . ." "I ate lunch with . . ." "I'm uncomfortable in that group, but I'll go back." ". . . came for a coke after tennis." "I enjoy my new room."

O   Limited intellectualization of emotions. Initiative to undertake uncertain tasks and reach out into relationships. Self-disclosure. Involvement in therapy goals and relationship. Increased social interaction skills.

Maturational struggle according to Erikson's developmental stages

S   ". . . came for a coke after tennis." "I ate lunch with . . ."

O   Basic trust vs. basic mistrust—beginning limited drive and hope.

Dependence vs. independence—increasing autonomy.

Intimacy vs. isolation—beginning limited affiliation.

Self-integration

S   "I forgot our appointment. I don't know what's wrong with me." "I can't seem to remember what I was saying." "I feel . . ." "I try so hard."

O   Forgotten appointment. Disheveled appearance. Darkened room. Fragmented thinking. Increased time structure. Rigidly controlled speech, manner, and posture. Recurrent, frequent break in train of thought. These identified behaviors are increasingly infrequent. Ability to allow therapist to enter personal space when distressed. Ability to become involved in therapy and develop insight.

Quality of life

S   ". . . came for a coke." "I ate lunch with . . ." "I enjoy my new room."

O   Expanded interpersonal relationships. Less restrictive with self-indulgence, that is, comfort in home setting. Productive, satisfactory job performance on a reduced time schedule.

SUGGESTED READINGS

American Nurses' Association: Standards of psychiatric mental-health nursing practice, Kansas City. Mo. 1973, The Association.

Baker, C., and Huff, B., editors: Physician's desk reference, ed. 30, Oradell, N.J., 1976, Medical Economics, Inc.

Carruth, B.: Modifying behavior through social learning, American Journal of Nursing **76:**1804-1806, Nov. 1976.

Cline, F. W., editor: Psychotropic medication, Nurse Practitioner **3:**35, March/April, 1978.

Dixon, B.: Interviewing when the patient is delusional, Journal of Psychiatric Nursing **69:**25-34, 1969.

Erikson, E. H.: Identity and the life cycle, New York, 1959, International Universities Press, Inc.

Kerr, N.: Anxiety: theoretical considerations, Perspectives in Psychiatric Care **16:**36-40, Jan./Feb., 1978.

Kline, N., and Davis, J.: Psychotropic drugs. American Journal of Nursing **73:**54-63, 1973.

Kloes, K.: The suicidal patient in the community: a challenge for nurses. In American Nurses' Association clinical sessions, New York, 1968, Appleton-Century-Crofts.

Kolb, L.: Modern clinical psychiatry, Philadelphia, 1977, W. B. Saunders Co.

Millon, T., editor: Modern psychopathology, Philadelphia, 1969, W. B. Saunders Co.

Prentice, G.: Evaluating suicide potential, Nurse Practitioner **2:**30-31, May/June, 1977.

Ray, O.: Drugs, society, and human behavior, ed. 2, St. Louis, 1978, The C. V. Mosby Co.

Sloboda, S.: Understanding patient behavior, Nursing '77 **7:**74-77, Sept., 1977.

Stillman, M.: Territoriality and personal space, American Journal of Nursing **78:**1670-1672, 1978.

Swearingen, D., et al.: Improving patient care through measurement: goal importance and achievement scaling, Journal of Psychiatric Nursing **15:**30-61, Sept., 1977.

Uhley, G.: What is realistic emotional support? American Journal of Nursing **68:**758-762, April, 1968.

Woolstone, A. S.: Stress—a call for a humane approach. Nursing Times **74:**599-600, April 6, 1978.

Yoder, J.: Alienation as a way of life, Perspectives in Psychiatric Care **15**(2):66-71, 1977.

CHAPTER 5

APRIL A *manifests*

PROBLEMATIC LIFE CONDUCT

evidenced by

ABERRANT SELF-DEVELOPMENT AND POOR PROBLEM-SOLVING METHODS

INTRODUCTORY PERSONAL PROFILE
Social adjustment

S   "We'll join a church when Megan is older!" "I enjoy talking to you (nurse) when you come." "I don't get out much. Sometimes I feel I just have to get out."

O   Disheveled home environment. Limited social activities and unexpanded medium for socialization. Communication breakdown within the marital relationship.

Emotional health status

S   "I love babies. They are cuddly and warm." "I'm OK. I don't have any problems anymore." "I don't get out much. Sometimes I feel I just have to get out. I wish Allen would let me . . ." "I like being a mother but . . ."

O   Disheveled home environment. Avoidance of therapy encounters. Unkempt appearance. Living tasks disorganized. Communication breakdown within the marital relationship.

Physical health status

S   "I'm not going to worry about being fat until I've had my last baby."

O   Obese; height 5 feet 3 inches, and weight 150 pounds.

Spiritual dimension

S   "We'll join a church when Megan is older." "I wish we had had a church wedding."

O   No present church affiliation.

Daily living skill performance

S   "This place is a mess today. No one with a 2-year-old has a neat home."

O   Disheveled home environment. Undisciplined 2-year-old child. Unkempt appearance. Prepared nourishing, tasty, economical meals.

Coping skill repertoire

S   "I'm not going to worry about being fat until I've had my last baby." "We'll join a church when Megan is older." "This place is a mess today. No one with a 2-year-old has a neat home." "I'm OK. I don't have any problems anymore." "I wish Allen would let me . . . ." "I like being a mother but . . ."

O   No decision about family size or family planning. No attempt to organize household tasks. Unable to discipline child.

Maturational struggle according to Erikson's developmental stages

S   "I wish Allen would let me . . . ." "We never talk anymore . . . ." "I like being a mother but . . . ." "I love babies. They are cuddly and warm."

O   Autonomy vs. shame and doubt.
Identity vs. role confusion.
Intimacy vs. isolation.

Self-integration

S   "I'm OK. I don't have any problems anymore." "I don't get out much. Sometimes I feel I just have to get out." "I wish Allen would let me . . . ." "I like being a mother but . . ."

O   Environmental disorganization. Living tasks disorganized. Unkempt personal appearance. Avoidance of therapy encounters.

Quality of life

S   "This place is a mess . . ."
O   Environmental disorganization. Living tasks disorganized. Unkempt personal appearance. Communication breakdown within the marital relationship. Strained financial resources.

Time span: 3 years

The A family, consisting of Allen and April and their 2-year-old daughter Megan, live in a recently purchased small, older house. The monthly mortgage payments tax the comfort of their lower middle-class life-style, causing other stressors and unresolved conflicts to come into focus and multiply. Often this couple ponders the question of the correctness of their decision to purchase a home, and they wonder if the purchase should have been delayed. If a more substantial down payment could have been made, the financial strain of their relatively large, monthly mortgage payments could have been eased.

Allen is 32 years old, tall, blond, and boyishly handsome. His frequent smile and his apparently easygoing manner enable him to have many friends, who describe him as having charisma. Allen is not a high achiever and avoids hard work and difficult situations, but he dreams of being successful in the business world. He seems to expect that his smile, winning ways, and charm will get him through life's problems with relative ease and comfort. At home, Allen is demanding and grouchy, and he remains uninvolved in family life or in home responsibilities. His smile has stopped winning April's constant approval for his questionable conduct. Although not verbally acknowledged by April, Allen's behavior is difficult to live with on a day-to-day basis, and her ineffective coping with their relationship problems only exacerbates the difficulties.

April, 5 feet, 3 inches in height, weighs 150 pounds. She expresses concern about being overweight but states that she will not worry about "being fat" until she has completed her family. April would like to have several more children, but Allen is noncommittal and ambivalent on this subject. At the beginning of April's therapy, they both expressed their concern about family size but made no permanent decision about the issue or related birth control question.

April has skillful command of social conversation but is evasive when she perceives the situation to be pressuring her intimate, elusive, fragile self. April is rather nondescript in appearance; her features are not remarkable. She rarely wears makeup, her hair often needs shampooing, and her frequently worn green pants and large plaid over-shirt are generally unclean and seem to be worn to camouflage her protruding abdomen and spreading hips. As April became comfortable with other people, her warm smile, giving manner, and shy presence became increasingly evident. She is very engaging and attractive in personality when she allows one into her intimate space.

April was a poor housekeeper. As a rule, this family's modest home needed to be vacuumed and dusted, and the kitchen floor was almost always sticky, food stained, and cluttered. The kitchen sink was full of used dishes, and the counters and table tops were strained and dusted with crumbs. The soiled laundry was stacked in the kitchen corner. To her credit, April prepared meals that pleased her thin, hungry husband—meals that also did not tax their already precarious financial resources.

The entire house announced that the couple had a 2-year-old. Megan was still wearing diapers. Toys as well as pots, pans, papers, magazines, and snack foods were scattered all over the living room. Megan, an active toddler, had written on the kitchen wall with purple crayon. She was often a whiny child, undisciplined by either parent. April longed for the return of the time when Megan was an infant. "I love babies. They are cuddly and warm." Her frequent unspoken implications were that a small, quiet infant to cuddle made her feel good about herself, loved, warm, and worthwhile. April's shallow relationships, stormy marital situation, and self-deprecating stance rarely allow her to have positive feelings about herself.

April was the identified client in this family. She had received psychiatric care in a confined setting at 16 years of age, at 20 years following the loss of a child, and again at 22 years, 4 weeks after Megan's birth. Each of these hospitalizations was for a 3-month period, and in both the second and third episodes of care, she was treated with electroshock therapy and major tranquilizers. These decompensation episodes were intense, marked by gross reality disorientation and self-disintegration. Discharge plans included outpatient psychotherapy, but April regularly canceled her scheduled appointments and consequently made little progress in therapy. Her position toward psychotherapy was negative. She rationalized dislike for several therapists, most treatment requirements, and treatment goals.

Historical data about April revealed that she was from a divorced nuclear family, that she had little if any recollection of her father, and that she and her mother for the past decade had maintained a distant relationship of fluctuating quality. April was an average to below-average student in high school; she stated that she disliked school and her studies. She had several jobs from 15 years of age until her marriage to Allen, ranging from babysitting to waitress work. At 14 years of age she became sexually active. She recalled feeling little emotional closeness in her various intimate heterosexual relationships and was pregnant at the time of her marriage. Her baby was born with multiple physical defects and died within several hours of his birth. Neither Allen nor April wished to talk about this crisis event. The quality and quantity of their grief work remained a matter of question and professional concern for the stability of their marriage relationship. Megan, born within 2 years of their first child, continued to be physically healthy and active, progressing satisfactorily within accepted norms of growth and development.

It is significant to note that April agreed to nurse psychotherapy as an alternate to other therapy because she perceived nursing home visits as a social occasion. All her previous therapists had been men, and April felt a conflict in male-female relationships beginning with her father and the conflicting male image perpetuated by Allen. In her lack of personally satisfying relationships, April viewed the nursing relationship as a source of need gratification and comfort. At first she did not perceive the relationship as a source of emotional healing, growth, life modification, and health. Visits were almost always accompanied by coffee and cookies or cake amid the clutter of her living room or kitchen. These first sessions were pleasant occasions for her. They were also data-gathering sessions for the nurse-clinician and the arena for professional relationship bonding.

After *several* initial nursing visits, collaboration with her psychiatrist, and a record review and evaluation, nursing judgment resulted in the following nursing diagnosis:

Anxiety

Dependence/independence struggle

Low self-concept

Family disruption

Difficulty in adjustment to parenting

Financial stress

Inability to perform required tasks of daily living

Communication disturbances within the marital relationship

Unkempt environment

Denial

Passive resistance

An idealistic and realistic approach to this case would have been to secure both the involvement and the commitment of this couple to the needed therapy. Allen's involvement was limited to allowing April this kind of treatment, since she was "the sick one." On a few rare occasions, Allen did, on the nurse's request and insistence, join in the therapy hour, but this sporadic effort was restricted to high stress peaks for April and only after the crisis had disturbed Allen's comfortable life-style. Part of Allen's coping style depended on scapegoating his wife for all of their problems as well as for his negative life circumstances.

During one crisis situation, Allen agreed to a marriage counseling effort with a male therapist, which continued irregularly for several years. Nurse psychotherapy was continued

with April as a foundation for her self-integration, emotional healing, and growth. The couple gave written consent for collaborative planning efforts between their marriage counselor and April's nurse. This joint planning and evaluation helped provide a supportive and correlated effort to promote growth and health for April and to decrease the marital conflict experienced by both parties.

April remained elusive and evasive during the early months of nurse psychotherapy. She excelled in the ability to remain on superficial social topics of conversation. She continually evaded any verbal goal setting. She rationalized persuasively with verbal barriers of how good she felt or how well she really was. Gradually, she gained a level of trust as the bonds of the professional relationship were cemented with the therapist's acceptance of the reality of her existence. A mainstay of emotional sustenance for April was through this helping relationship, which provided a medium for "good" feelings, positive emotions, and a new sense of security to her fragile psyche.

Regular nursing evaluation of the sessions and continual assessment of April and her environment finally led to some mutually agreed-on goals. The therapy situation must be paced to the client's readiness. April needed time to feel secure in any relationship, particularly in a situation that asked her to acknowledge that she *did* have problems, actual life dilemmas. Problems that are denied do not have to be mastered or resolved. Goal setting was a mark of growth for April. Acknowledging areas needing assistance rather than concealing their perplexity is the first step to changed or renewed coping and to possible resolution of the behavior in question.

PROCESS IMPLEMENTATION

1—Evaluation

N.D.   *Anxiety*

    S   "I made cookies this morning for your visit." "You dress so well. Where do you buy your clothes?" "I have a new recipe I'll make for your next visit."

O Skillful command of social conversation but evasive when interaction perceived as perilous. Initial nursing visits structured by client to remain on a social interaction level.

N.D. *Low self-concept*

S "I'm not going to worry about being fat until I've had my last baby." "I love babies. They are cuddly and warm." "The house is a mess, but what can you do with a toddler?"

O Rarely wears makeup. Hair often needs shampooing. Frequently worn, unclean green pants and large plaid over-blouse. As a rule the family home needs to be vacuumed and dusted. Kitchen floor is sticky, food stained, and cluttered. Kitchen sink full of unwashed dishes. Table tops stained and dusted with crumbs. Soiled laundry stacked in kitchen corner.

N.D. *Inability to perform required tasks of daily living*

S "The house is a mess, but what can you do with a toddler?" "I don't like to keep house."

O As a rule the family home needs to be vacuumed and dusted. Kitchen floor is sticky, food stained, and cluttered. Kitchen sink full of unwashed dishes. Table tops stained and dusted with crumbs. Soiled laundry stacked in kitchen corner. Rarely wears makeup. Hair often needs shampooing. Frequently worn, unclean green pants and large plaid over-blouse.

N.D. *Unkempt environment*

S "The house is a mess, but what can you do with a toddler?" "I don't like to keep house."

O As a rule the family home needs to be vacuumed and dusted. Kitchen floor is sticky, food stained, and cluttered. Kitchen sink full of unwashed dishes. Table tops stained and dusted with crumbs. Soiled laundry stacked in kitchen corner.

N.D. *Difficulty in adjustment to parenting*

S "The house is a mess, but what can you do with a toddler?"

O Toys, pots, pans, papers, magazines, and snack food scattered over living room. Megan had written on the kitchen wall with purple crayon.

Actual outcome

Basic relationship bonding between client and nurse.

2A—Assessment

N.D. *Difficulty in adjustment to parenting*

S "I just don't know what to do." "I've tried everything."

O No baseline agreements on child-rearing tasks. Recurrent and extensive diaper rash. Examination of Megan showed red, elevated sore areas on buttocks, labia, and inner thighs. Several

areas open and draining. Child whiny and irritable.

N.D. *Inability to perform required tasks of daily living*

S "I just don't know what to do." "I've tried everything."

O Recurrent and extensive diaper rash. Examination of Megan showed red, elevated sore areas on buttocks, labia, and inner thighs. Several areas open and draining. Child whiny and irritable.

N.D. *Low self-concept*

S "I just don't know what to do." "I've tried everything." "I am a good mother." "I want Megan to like me."

O Avoidance of discipline and its ramifications of rejection, hostility, and lack of love.

N.D. *Communication disturbance within the marital relationship*

S "He's too strict." "She shouldn't always . . ."

O No baseline agreements on child-rearing tasks.

N.D. *Unkempt environment*

S "The house is a mess, but what can you do with a toddler?"

O Megan carried and ate food throughout the house.

3—Additional nursing diagnosis

None

4A—Variables

Reality timing	+3
Relationships	−3
Stressors and/or crisis	0
Coping resources	+2
Significant emotional strength	+2
Significant emotional limitations	−2
Therapy relationship	+2
Physical health status	0
Physical and emotional readiness dimension	+2
Available support system	+2
Meaning significance	+4
Values and belief impact	+4
Other	
BALANCE	+

Additional specific knowledge

See case material.

Analysis and synthesis

N.D. *Difficulty in adjustment to parenting.* The insecurity of both parties and inability to reach a common decision regarding values, tasks, and responsibilities of child rearing accompanied by the guilt and grief over the death of the first child create a hostile, uncompromising environment.

N.D. *Inability to perform required tasks of daily living.* Disinterest, lack of organizational skills, anger, and the perceived over-whelming nature of the task prevent April from beginning it. Problem-solving skills are needed.

N.D. *Low self-concept.* Past perceived failures and lack of affirmation and positive feedback decrease self-esteem and initiative and increase fatigue. One parenting task that is objective in nature and can be completed would reinforce a positive "good" mother feeling.

N.D. *Communication disturbance within the marital relationship.* Scapegoating, self-centeredness, hostility, and low self-concept further block open communications within the marriage.

N.D. *Unkempt environment.* The disheveled state of the home encourages further chaos and disruption. Beginning environmental order is a must when client is ready to accept the task.

4B — Design of action

N.D. Difficulty in adjustment to parenting, inability to perform required tasks of daily living, low self-concept, communication disturbance within the marital relationship, unkempt environment.

1. Plan
   a. Assist client with remedial measures to alleviate child's diaper rash.
   b. Assess area of child discipline.
   c. Begin client dialogue on discipline and initiate action to facilitate necessary restrictive behavior.

2. Strategy
   a. Introduce remedial measures to alleviate diaper rash, discussing procedure and rationale.
   b. Role model application of various remedial procedures.
   c. Facilitate discussion of child discipline by April and Allen.
   d. Encourage and expect follow-through of agreed-on, baseline disciplinary tasks.

3. Expected outcomes
   a. Implementation of measures to heal diaper rash.
   b. Discussion and decisions between April and Allen of child discipline principles and techniques.
   c. Implementation of agreed-on disciplinary action at appropriate times.

4. Criteria
   a. Observation of the implementation of remedial measures.
   b. Healing of Megan's tissue inflammation.

c. Clear statements by both parties concerning validating agreed-on child discipline principles and techniques.
d. Observation of April's implementation of agreed-on disciplinary action.

The initial problem areas identified by April were broadly based. Those dealing with child-rearing tasks and the complex daily living task of housekeeping and household responsibilities were labeled as targets for intervention. One would usually begin with the unemotional task of environmental manipulation, but household maintenance was a task closely entwined with April's already fragile self-concept. In addition, the environment was so extremely untidy that it would have been difficult to find a viable positive feedback medium. On the reverse side, observations of this mother-child relationship demonstrated positive verbal and nonverbal interchanges. April spoke lovingly of her child, warmly fondled her, and had specific child-rearing problem areas defined.

Megan had a persistent diaper rash that April had not been able to relieve. A physical examination of Megan showed red, elevated sore areas on the buttocks, labia, and inner thighs. Several small areas were open and draining. Megan had reason to be whiny and irritable in her need for relief from this tissue inflammation.

In a matter-of-fact, objective manner examination and curative procedures designed for Megan's comfort were instituted. April responded knowledgeably concerning the measures to be implemented. She agreed to read material on the subject. She began to bathe Megan and then was assisted in exposing the inflamed areas to the air to promote healing. Proper technique for cleaning and wiping while diapering a baby girl was demonstrated for her. This cleansing technique and the proper inspection of the involved area to ensure cleanliness had not been routinely or thoroughly done by April during regular diapering, or was there an established bathing routine. Several bathtub toys were found, and the therapeutic effort of soaking was transformed into a enjoyable play time for Megan. April laughed and observably enjoyed this time with Megan as she soaked and played in the bathtub. Routine child-caring tasks need not be perceived as chores, but with thoughtful preplanning they can become times of pleasure and enjoyment for both mother and child.

Megan's fluid intake seemed limited so that fluids were added to her diet at regularly scheduled intervals. Megan drank well from a cup when fluids were offered to her and was delighted to exhibit this new achievement. Until this time, she had been bottle fed, since this method was less complicated for April. In April's inner insecurity, beginning a new task was uncertain and was perceived as an impending disaster rather than as a natural transition in her daughter's childhood growth.

April's diaper laundering technique was reviewed. Washing products were changed, diapers were presoaked, and an additional rinse cycle was added to the procedure. This, along with increased fluid intake, cleanliness, and regular exposure of affected areas to the air promoted healing. Megan became an obviously happier and more outgoing child. April received positive reinforcement from the therapist and a significant feeling of achievement from the task accomplishment itself. She was pleased that her child was again comfortable. Increased play time with Megan rewarded her emotional need to be a "good," nurturing mother.

When stress increased for April, Megan's diaper rash recurred. April would need the support of a task review of precisely what to do and how to do it. She needed encouragement to renew her efforts. When the stressors were numerous, April frequently became disorganized in thought and action, resulting in loss of recently gained self-confidence in her abilities to perform routine daily tasks which she knew.

Discipline, with its ramifications of rejection, hostility, and lack of love was a difficult issue for April. She loved her child and *wished to be loved in return*. Allen was a strict, inconsistent, and harsh disciplinarian on the rare occasions when he became involved with disciplinary action. April avoided reproaching Megan at all cost. Frequently, Allen's punishment did not relate to the weight of the act, and April ran to protect her child. Agreement on the tasks of child rearing was dealt with in marriage counseling. The couple was directed to reach some baseline agreements. Consistency in agreed areas was encouraged by her therapists. April was given encouragement to follow through on needed action, and she was mandated to comply with methods of child discipline during nurse psychotherapy.

One such area where April was encouraged to set limits with Megan was in her exploration of the environment. Megan crawled up onto everything, often standing on the table or on top of the back of a chair or couch. She suffered a new bump, scratch, or bruise every week. April was shown how to remove her child quickly and firmly from a dangerous position without hurting the youngster and was directed to comply with similar action the next time this kind of incident occurred. April had no role model in her own childhood experience from which to compare corrective practices of child development and from which to learn self-control. Intellectually, April understood the reasoning for such disciplinary action. Emotionally, she did not always accept the execution of the procedure itself or the need for what she termed "such drastic action." This emotional stance was reinforced by Megan's resistance to any restraint on her exploring self.

During an interview while April and the therapist were conversing, Megan crawled up on a kitchen counter and took a paring knife out of a drawer. This tiny 2-year-old cut herself and provided a graphic answer to the reasoning behind discipline from her mother. Safety is a basic need of human beings, and April had to accept the responsibility for the safety of her dependent child.

Megan carried and ate food throughout the

house, increasing housekeeping tasks. Allen and April were directed to define the limits of where Megan would be allowed to eat. They decided she could eat in the kitchen, at the dining area table, or in her chair, although Megan belligerently resisted. With encouragement, April remained firm in the couple's decision. Allen complained less about the "mess" all over the house, and April had fewer pick-up and clean-up tasks.

PROCESS IMPLEMENTATION

1—Evaluation

N.D.   *Difficulty in adjustment to parenting*
  S   "Your daddy says you can't eat there." "We have to do what daddy says." "Let's sail this boat in the bathtub." "Mommy likes it when you're feeling better."
  O   Read subject material on the defined area. Bathing and proper cleansing routinely done. Increased fluid intake. Revised laundering technique. Increased play time with Megan. Limited, necessary discipline enforced.

N.D.   *Inability to perform required tasks of daily living*
  S   "Your daddy says you can't eat there." "We have to do what daddy says."
  O   Read subject material on the defined area. Bathing and proper cleansing routinely done. Increased fluid intake. Revised laundering technique implemented. Increased play time with Megan. Limited, necessary discipline enforced.

N.D.   *Low self-concept*
  S   "Your daddy says you can't eat there." "We have to do what daddy says."
  O   Achievement from task accomplishment, indicating she was a "good" mother.

N.D.   *Communication disturbance within the marital relationship*
  S   "Your daddy says you can't eat there." "We have to do what daddy says."
  O   Mutually defined the limits where Megan could eat. Remained true to the mutually agreed-on decision.

N.D.   *Unkempt environment*
  S   "There is not as much to clean up now that Megan can't have food all over the house."
  O   Restricting Megan's eating to defined area decreased the disordered environment.

Actual outcome
  Remedial measures implemented by April to arrest diaper rash. Megan's inflamed area restored to a healthy state. Baseline agreement reached on child

discipline measures. April reluctantly implements the required child discipline.

2A—Assessment

N.D.   *Unkempt environment*
  S   "I just can't do it." "When Megan's older, I'll clean up." "Allen won't help." "I'm too tired." "We don't have the money for a new vacuum."
  O   Unable or unwilling to plan or organize task. Disliked housekeeping tasks. Unsafe environment for children.

N.D.   *Passive resistance*
  S   "I just can't do it." "When Megan's older, I'll clean up." "Allen won't help." "I'm too tired." "We don't have the money for a new vacuum."
  O   Unwilling to accept responsibility or blame. Unable or unwilling to plan or organize tasks.

N.D.   *Dependence/independence struggle*
  S   "I just can't do it." "When Megan's older, I'll clean up." "Allen won't help." "I'm too tired." "We don't have the money for a new vacuum."
  O   Unwilling to accept responsibility or blame. Unable or unwilling to plan or organize task. Disliked housekeeping tasks.

N.D.   *Low self-concept*
  S   "I just can't do it." "I'm too tired."
  O   Acknowledged feeling unhappy and disorganized.

3—Additional nursing diagnosis
None

4A—Variables

Reality timing	−1
Relationships	−2
Stressors and/or crisis	0
Coping resources	+1
Significant emotional strength	+2
Significant emotional limitations	−2
Therapy relationship	+3
Physical health status	0
Physical and emotional readiness dimension	0
Available support system	0
Meaning significance	−1
Values and belief impact	−1
Other	
BALANCE	−

Additional specific knowledge
See case material.

Analysis and synthesis

N.D.   *Unkempt environment*. Correlated to inner feelings of disorganization and low self-concept.

N.D. *Passive resistance.* Unable to risk the possible negative reaction of significant others. This external nonresistive stance is a protective shield for April's fragile psyche.

N.D. *Dependence/independence struggle.* This is a continually unresolved dilemma for April. She does not want to choose either dependence or independence but tries to remain safe in the ambivalence, indifference, apathy, and neutrality of the conflict.

N.D. *Low self-concept.* Low self-esteem, disorganization, chronic life chaos, and few supportive relationship or role models have not allowed April's self-development and have encouraged pathological and passive coping methods and a negative life stance.

4B—Design of action
N.D. Unkempt environment, passive resistance, dependence/independence struggle, low self-concept
1. Plan
   a. Discussion, organization, and implementation of elementary household tasks.
2. Strategy
   a. Discussion and assessment of defined tasks.
   b. Schedule elementary defined tasks.
   c. Expect defined task completion.
   d. Positive and corrective feedback and affirmation for compliance with schedule and task completion.
3. Expected outcomes
   a. Adherence to the agreed-on schedule.
   b. Decreased time spent in worry work and indecision.
   c. Noticeable environmental modification.
   d. Reinforcement from Allen for environmental modification.
4. Criteria
   a. Involvement in discussion concerning defined schedule and task organization.
   b. Observable environmental modification.
   c. Satisfaction expressed by April and Allen concerning task completion and environmental modification.

The disordered home environment was distressing to everyone in the household and to the immediate community. Relatives and neighbors found visiting troublesome and uncomfortable. It increased April's person disorganization. It was cause for Allen's complaint and for his seeking outside refuge. It was not conducive to Megan's growth, development, health, or safety.

April acknowledged disliking housekeeping tasks. She also acknowledged feeling unhappy and being unable to get herself organized. She wanted things to look better, but she just "couldn't manage." Frantically and desperately, she put the blame on Megan's age, on Allen's unwillingness to help, on her own fatigue level, and on their shaky financial situation. In reality the unkempt environment was one hostile method of passively expressing her resistance toward Allen's behavior. Some inroads in therapy could be accomplished in the environmental setting, but communication reconciliation and baseline agreements within the marriage would have to be developed to decrease the negativism and aggression of passive resistance.

Housekeeping tasks were discussed with a focus on organization, simple schedules, and a breakdown of elementary task functions. April was encouraged to choose a time for each task each day, every other day, or weekly, depending on the nature of the task. She was direct to do housework for just 2 hours each day, no matter what the task. Scheduling decreased the energy consumed in worrying and procrastination and freed energy potential for the daily assignment. If the living room was given individual attention once a week instead of every 2 or 3 months, the entire task did not loom as overpowering. The home looked better, and both Allen and April were pleased with the progress. As April felt better about herself, it was reflected in the appearance of her home. A good barometer of April's emotional well-being and the stability of the marriage was the observable home environment.

PROCESS IMPLEMENTATION
1—Evaluation
N.D. *Unkempt environment*
   S "I'm pleased you think the house looks better. Allen thinks so too." "The schedule does help. I don't spend so much time deciding what to do."

O Housekeeping tasks were broken down into elementary task functions. Encouraged to choose a time for each task each day, every other day, or weekly. Directed to do housework just 2 hours each day no matter what the task.

N.D. *Passive resistance*

S "Sometimes I give myself a day off from the schedule." "If only Allen would . . ." "If only Megan would . . ." "If only I could have help."

O Actual task performance and task completion decrease the amount of energy to direct in aggression.

N.D. *Dependence/independence struggle*

S "I'm pleased you think the house looks better. Allen thinks so too." "The schedule does help. I don't spend so much time deciding what to do." "If only I could have help."

O Allen expressed pleasure at the increased tidiness of their home.

N.D. *Low self-concept*

S "I'm pleased you think the house looks better. Allen thinks so too." "The schedule does help. I don't spend so much time deciding what to do."

O Increased self-esteem as reflected in the appearance of her home. Increased appropriate affect.

Actual outcome

Involvement in schedule organization and implementation. *Limited* but observable environmental modification. Expressed satisfaction by April and Allen with the increased organization and completion of household tasks.

2A—Assessment

N.D. *Low self-concept*

S "If only Allen would . . ." "I can't." "It won't work anyway."

O Allen refused to babysit on the evenings he was home. Unstated grief, grievances, concerns, and other hostile and self-centered feelings had multiplied over time. Scapegoating of April for being ill. Fault finding a frequent destructive pastime.

N.D. *Communication disturbance within the marital relationship*

S "If only Allen would . . ." "I try to talk to him but he won't listen."

O Allen refused to babysit on the evenings he was home. Unstated grief, grievances, concerns, and other hostile and self-centered feelings had multiplied over time. Discussion of the marital problems led to subject change and circular communication without resolution or increasing

understanding. Scapegoating of April for being ill. Fault finding a frequent destructive pastime.

N.D. *Denial*

S "I don't really have any problems." "When Megan is older, things will be better." "I want to tell you about . . ."

O Unstated grief, grievances, concerns, and other hostile and self-centered feelings had multiplied over time. Discussion of the marital problems led to subject change and circular communication without resolution or increasing understanding. Scapegoating of April for being ill. Fault finding a frequent destructive pastime.

N.D. *Anxiety*

S "If only Allen would . . ." "I can't . . ." "I want to tell you about . . ." "It won't work anyway."

O Allen refused to babysit on the evenings he was home. Discussion of the marital problems led to subject change and circular communication without resolution or increasing understanding. Scapegoating of April for being ill. Fault finding a frequent destructive pastime.

N.D. *Financial stress*

S "If only Allen would babysit" "I can't because we have no money."

O Allen refused to babysit on the evenings he was home. Limited finances encourage social withdrawal for April. Scapegoating of April for being ill. Fault findings a frequent destructive pastime.

3—Additional nursing diagnosis
None

4A—Variables

Reality timing	+3
Relationships	−3
Stressors and/or crisis	−2
Coping resources	+2
Significant emotional strength	0
Significant emotional limitations	−2
Therapy relationship	+4
Physical health status	0
Physical and emotional readiness dimension	+2
Available support system	−2
Meaning significance	+1
Values and belief impact	+1
Other	
BALANCE	+

Additional specific knowledge
See case material.

Analysis and synthesis

N.D. *Low self-concept.* Absence of positive relationships fosters integration of negative messages. Inability to cope effectively with stress is another factor decreasing feelings of self-worth.

N.D. *Communication disturbance within the marital relationship.* Open communication is perceived as threatening by both parties. Retreat into protective behaviors seems to be a pattern of action when the issue or response is uncertain.

N.D. *Denial.* This tight protective mechanism prevents the resolution of any problem or issue. Confronting the behavior only seems to encourage its use. When the timing is correct, an intellectual approach to the behavior may help.

N.D. *Anxiety.* Constant stress and disorganization seem to increase the anxiety and decrease April's ability to cope effectively.

N.D. *Financial stress.* The reality limits of the already strained budget encourage withdrawal and lack of needed relationships. At some points the financial management of this family must be examined for alternatives.

4B—Design of action

N.D. Low self-concept, communication disturbance within the marital relationship, denial, anxiety, financial stress.

1. Plan
   a. Research and guide April to integrate low-cost social activities into her life-style.
   b. Encourage self-disclosure in therapy.
   c. Assess the strengths and limitations of the marriage relationship and encourage open communication.

2. Strategy
   a. Foster self-disclosure in therapy and self-development activities.
   b. Increase feedback, affirmation, and nurturance.
   c. Confront destructive behaviors within the marriage.

3. Expected outcomes
   a. Increased self-disclosure in the therapy hour.
   b. Social task-centered involvement.
   c. Decreased destructive behaviors within the marriage.

4. Criteria
   a. Discussion of several troublesome issues or conflicting situation.
   b. Active involvement in one social task-centered group.
   c. Decreased tension and stress within the marriage relationship.

Allen's and April's budget did not allow for needed socialization. Allen refused to babysit on the evenings he was home. The occasions when April impelled Allen to care for Megan so that she could attend an activity of her choice usually led to bitter fighting, tears, and increased hostility. April needed some outside activity to affirm herself. Removal from the pressures of the sameness, responsibility, and discomforts of her environment would encourage improved emotional health.

In the warm weather and even in the tolerable cold weather, April and Megan walked for several blocks each day. April often walked farther, pulling Megan in a sled or wagon. April needed some time alone. Community activities were studied. The library had a weekly story hour for Megan, which freed April to have a walk alone, to read, to shop, or to do an activity of her own choosing. She stated she enjoyed the alone activity and freedom of choice, and she became a regular patron of the children's story hour.

Visits with the therapist began to be considered ''her time.'' As she found a sense of safety, stimulation, and refreshment in this relationship, she began to unburden herself and drop her social facade. Gradually, she began intellectually to accept the value of acknowledging her concealed problems and directing her energy toward resolution. Her denial consistently remained a tight mental defense. The acknowledgment of problems is seldom easy, nor is the adaptation of dependable coping behavior a rapid process.

The YWCA offered programs of interest for April at a reasonable fee with a provided babysitting service. April participated in activities sporadically and attended programs of her choice. It was positive for her to encounter other young mothers and share some common child-rearing experiences. April received a sense of being a good mother from these encounters—a needed affirmation and an important element in April's self-concept. When stressors were fewer, April did take time to play with Megan. They both enjoyed these happy times of feeling good and an emotional togetherness. When she followed through with positive discipline. April was complimented on how well she did at mothering tasks.

To become a more nurturing person, April needed to experience *nurturance* and self-growth for herself. Nurturance can be provided in a nurse-client relationship by providing a medium in which to foster client growth and sufficient reality-oriented, supportive, and corrective feedback to foster self-confidence and a renewed self-worth. Nurturance must always be measured in sufficient quantity and quality to foster growth as opposed to abundant, randomly selected nurturance effort that can cripple emotional growth or smother the emerging person. Confidence in the client's ability to change and gentle pushing to try new roles are nurturing measures that are helpful in promoting growth and health. To nurture and become a nurturing person one must have received sufficient healthy nurturance oneself. April's "nurturing parent" was in an embryonic stage of development.

April was very concerned about choosing a toilet-training procedure for Megan, and for several weeks these methods were discussed. April read reams of material on the subject and finally decided that neither she nor Megan was ready to attempt this task. Megan became trained easily at about 3 years old when both mother and child were ready and family stress was relatively low. Timing is important in many of life's tasks. It can become complex when one must look at more than one person as well as at the instability of a family system. Correct timing can make the difference between satisfactory accomplishment of life's tasks and increased frustration related to difficult or incomplete task completion.

Honest and clear couple communication was difficult if not impossible for both April and Allen. Trust was a missing element. Unstated grief, grievances, concerns, and other hostile and self-centered feelings had multiplied over time. These factors, fostered by lack of resolution, caused communication breakdown that seemed irreparable.

Allen and April talked, but not on a feeling level. In their dialogue they expressed a need for change in their marriage. Both expressed the wish to remain in the marriage, but neither could define the reasons for his or her decision. Discussion of their marital problems led to subject change, circular communication without resolution, or increased misunderstanding between the couple. Frequently, one or both clients sought direct answers from the therapist. This occurred both with the nurse and with the marriage counselor functioning as the identified therapist.

Fault finding was a frequent destructive pastime for this couple. Resolution or modification did not occur in the marriage relationship. The most frequent solution to fault finding was to scapegoat April as being ill; therefore anything and everything was her fault or error. Often April accepted the role of the "guilty party," since she had little feedback concerning her growth and healthy behavior except from professional encounters. In reality, April could not have been defined as emotionally healthy, and her ambivalence about acceptance versus rejection of the sick role was not conducive to her emotional growth or health status.

Role reversal was attempted in marriage counseling, but neither party *could* or *would* assume the role and feelings of the other party. Tension pervading stressors remained unresolved, and disagreements remained a constant factor in their relationship. The variables were the degree, duration, and number of each unresolved or persistent disagreement.

PROCESS IMPLEMENTATION

1—Evaluation

N.D. *Low self-concept*

S "I do worry about . . ." "What should I do?" "I need to get out sometimes." "He makes me so angry."

O Taking Megan to children's story hour to free time for herself. Attended YWCA programs. Read, discussed, and decided to avoid toilet training until readiness was present.

N.D. *Communication disturbance within the marital relationship*

S "Yes, we need to make some changes." "You tell her what to do." "What should we do?"

O Honest, clear couple communication was difficult if not impossible. Seeking answers from the therapist. Role reversal unsuccessful. Allen refused to babysit on the evenings he was home.

N.D. *Denial*

S "She is ill, that's the problem." "It's all her fault." "If only I could . . ." "He makes me so angry." "I don't really have so many problems."

O Frequent scapegoating and fault finding of the other spouse.

N.D. *Anxiety*

S "It helps to talk to you." "I know you won't tell anybody." "I don't really have so many problems."

O Allen refused to babysit on the evenings he was home. Discussion of the marital problems led to subject change and circular communication without resolution or increasing understanding. Better eye-to-eye contact. Can sit quietly for longer periods of time. Posture more noticeably relaxed.

N.D. *Financial stress*

S "I can't because we have no money." "I'm so glad story hour is free."

O Allen refused to babysit on the evenings he was home. Limited finances encourage social withdrawal for April. Allen unwilling to explore financial problems.

Actual outcome

Involvement in YWCA activities. Regular attendance at library children's story hour. Long walks alone or with children. Unburdening of stress in therapy and intellectual acceptance of previously concealed problems. No positive change in the marital relationship.

2A—Assessment

N.D. *Passive resistance*

S "Everything will take care of itself." "Don't talk about problems, everything is just fine now."

O Refused to cope with the impending future. No problems discussed.

N.D. *Difficulty in adjustment to parenting*

S "Everything will take care of itself." "Don't talk about problems, everything is just fine now."

O Allen remained uninvolved in the childbirth preparations. Mother and daughter spent hours discussing the coming birth. Limited preparation for the birth.

N.D. *Communication disturbance within the marital relationship*

S "Everything will take care of itself." "Everything is just fine now."

O The couple did not assume the responsibility to practice any birth control method. Allen remained uninvolved in the childbirth preparations.

N.D. *Denial*

S "Everything will take care of itself." "Everything is just fine now."

O Refusal to cope with the impending future. No problems discussed.

3—Additional nursing diagnosis

Pregnancy, depression, decompensation episode

Assessment of additional nursing diagnosis

N.D. *Pregnancy*

S "I feel so good when I'm pregnant." "Don't talk about problems, everything is just fine now." Everything will take care of itself." "I just want to hold my new baby."

O Normal pregnancy. Weight gain of 50 pounds. Short labor. Delivered 6-pound, 2-ounce healthy boy without aid of medication.

N.D. *Depression*

S "I must breastfeed my son." (Repeated four times.) "I'm so tired and I can't seem to sleep."

O Weepy. Sad affect. Frequent tears. Fatigue. Dark circles under her eyes. Sleep disturbance. Appetite disturbance. Long silences.

N.D. *Decompensation episode*

S "I must breastfeed my son." (Repeated four times.) "I'm so tired and I can't seem to sleep." "What did you say?" "How long have I been in the hospital?" "Did I ask you that before?"

O Flat affect. Short concentration span. Increased

disorganization. Reality disorientation. Memory gaps. Fragmented thought and speech. Sleep disturbance. Appetite disturbance. Crying. Long silences.

4A — Variables

Reality timing	−4
Relationships	−4
Stressors and/or crisis	−5
Coping resources	−5
Significant emotional strength	−4
Significant emotional limitations	−4
Therapy relationship	+2
Physical health status	−2
Physical and emotional readiness dimension	−4
Available support system	+1
Meaning significance	+3
Values and belief impact	+3
Other	
BALANCE	−

Additional specific knowledge
See case material.

Analysis and synthesis

N.D.   *Passive resistance.* Transient episode of "feeling good" and decreased tension only increased energy to channel into passivity and avoidance of effective coping. Direct verbal expression limited and usually employed to protect denial mechanism.

N.D.   *Difficulty in adjustment to parenting.* Mother and daughter relationship strengthened by shared time and enjoyment.

N.D.   *Communication disturbance within the marital relationship.* Avoidance, denial, and transient euphoria further separate and divide the mutuality of the marital relationship.

N.D.   *Denial.* Client seemed to believe denial would protect her for an indefinite time. The use of this mechanism only increased her intrinsic stress level to a point of nonfunctional behavior.

N.D.   *Pregnancy.* Physically uneventful pregnancy, labor, and birth. Avoidance of coping with reality during this time only entrenched negative behaviors and decreased the client's ability to cope effectively with her life situation.

N.D.   *Depression.* Limited period of depression and sad feelings following childbirth is usual. The intensity and duration of this client's behavior is significant and evidences psychopathology.

N.D.   *Decompensation episode.* Denial, the lack of preparatory work for the entrance of a new family member, fluctuating hormone balance, lack of necessary support, ineffective coping behaviors, and multiple intrinsic stress culminated in a nonfunctional state.

4B — Design of action

N.D.   Passive resistance, difficulty in adjustment to parenting, communication disturbance within the marital relationship, denial, pregnancy, depression, decompensation episode.

1. Plan
   a. Guide client to discuss and plan for the birth of her child.
   b. Assess, plan, and intervene as problems emerge.
2. Strategy
   a. Involve April and Megan in preparation for new family member.
   b. Confront April with the necessity for preparation for the newborn's arrival.
   c. Support reality orientation.
   d. Attempt to prevent impending crisis by guiding client to prepare, plan, and effectively cope with emerging or predictable problems.
3. Expected outcomes
   a. Discussion between April and Megan concerning the arrival of a new child into the family.
   b. Acceptance of the need to prepare for the arrival of the new child.
   c. Preparatory activities for the newborn's arrival.
   d. Prevention of impending crisis.
4. Criteria
   a. Reading and talking about the arrival of the child.
   b. Intellectual acceptance of the need for planning.
   c. Observation of actual preparatory activities.
   d. No crisis.

Based on her history of postpartum instability and the ensuing decompensation episodes, April had been advised not to become pregnant. At some future time, enlarging the family could be possible with increased emotional, social, and financial family stability. April longed to be pregnant again because she liked the feeling of being with child. The couple did not assume the responsibility to practice any birth control method. When Megan was 38 months old, April became pregnant and she was delighted.

Allen was verbally noncommittal on the subject but postured an oppressed position.

The pregnancy was medically noneventful except for a weight gain of 50 pounds. After a short labor without medication, April delivered a 6-pound, 2-ounce healthy son, Allen, Jr. During her son's gestation, April "bloomed" emotionally. She appeared happy, content, and relaxed, and increased stability reigned in the family. Megan became increasingly autonomous, her vocabulary and muscle dexterity accelerated, and she became more affectionate to her mother. April's euphoria and increased feelings of well-being and happiness decreased her negative emotions and behavior toward Allen. This decreased his perceived strain and helped him to feel better about himself, resulting in his being less critical and demanding of April. This family floated along in this superficial state for the duration of her pregnancy. No problems were discussed, and the very existence of problems was repressed and denied.

April did little planning for the time after the birth of her son. Her attitude and words were that "everything will take care of itself." She just wanted to hold her new baby. The therapist could not invalidate a constant "praecox feeling" concerning an imminent emotional disaster for April. April would not cope with the future but held tight to the transient emotional comfort experience.

One area confronted in nurse psychotherapy was the preparation of Megan for the additional family member. Again April was encouraged to read some "how to" manuals on preparing children within a family for the birth of a new baby. Mother and daughter enjoyed hours talking about the event. They felt the baby together and expressed "good" feelings about their own relationship and the coming event in their family. Megan gave up her crib for the new baby and moved into a big bed of her own. Her toilet training was completed satisfactorily and uneventfully during this time. Megan was delighted to tell anyone who would listen about her "new baby brother-baby sister." Allen remained uninvolved in their preparation and this child-rearing family activity.

In her 5 days of postpartum hospitalization, April was noticeably depressed and weepy. She expressed satisfaction for giving birth to a healthy baby boy when she was asked, but her affect was alternately flat or sad, and tears were frequent. Although her physical condition was stable and without complication except for some transient tenderness at the episiotomy site, April expressed fatigue and appeared tired, and there were dark circles under her eyes. She showed sleep disturbances and appetite fluctuation. She successfully began to breastfeed her son, significant since she had not been able to breastfeed Megan. Breastfeeding held a powerful meaning for her, and successful completion of this task was tightly linked to April's self-concept as a "good" mother. Allen visited for a short period daily, but he appeared passive and unobservant of his wife's culminating emotional distress.

Precipitated by the combination of her rapidly changing hormone balance, her lack of emotional support and task assistance from Allen, and her lack of preparation for the responsibility of a totally dependent newborn infant, April began to show signs of self-disintegration, increased disorganization and reality disorientation, memory gaps, fragmented thought and speech expression, continued sleep disturbance, appetite disturbance, and frequent episodes of crying. Her flat affect increased. At 3 weeks' postpartum, April refused to begin psychotropic medication because it would necessitate the cessation of breastfeeding. Discussion of beginning drug treatment with trifluoperazine, 2 mg bid, a previously effective drug of choice, prescribed by her physician, only increased her agitation. The therapist attempted unsuccessfully to pursuade her to take the preparation as prescribed. Such attempts were met with open hostility and increased agitation, despite a previously comfortable therapeutic relationship.

April felt very threatened, uncertain, and unable to cope effectively.

PROCESS IMPLEMENTATION

1—Evaluation

N.D. *Passive resistance*
S "Everything will take care of itself." "Don't talk about problems, everything is just fine now."
O Refusal to cope with the impending future. No problems discussed.

N.D. *Difficulty in adjustment to parenting*
S "Everything will take care of itself." "Don't talk about problems, everything is just fine now."
O Allen remained uninvolved in the childbirth preparations. Mother and daughter spent hours discussing the coming birth. Limited preparation for the birth. Allen visited daily but appeared passive and unobservant of his wife's culminating emotional distress.

N.D. *Communication disturbance within the marital relationship*
S "Everything will take care of itself." "Everything is just fine now."
O The couple did not assume the responsibility to practice any birth-control method. Allen remained uninvolved in the childbirth preparations. He visited daily but appeared passive and unobservant of his wife's culminating emotional distress.

N.D. *Denial*
S "Everything will take care of itself." "Everything is just fine now."
O Refusal to cope with the impending future. No problems discussed.

N.D. *Pregnancy*
S "Yes, I'm happy with my baby."
O Gave birth to a healthy 6-pound, 2-ounce son.

N.D. *Depression*
S "I must breastfeed my son." (Repeated four times.) "I'm so tired and I can't seem to sleep."
O Weepy. Sad affect. Frequent tears. Fatigue. Dark circles under her eyes. Sleep disturbance. Appetite disturbance. Long silences.

N.D. *Decompensation episode*
S "I must breastfeed my son." (Repeated four times.) "I'm so tired and I can't seem to sleep." "What did you say?" "Did I ask you that before?" "How long have I been in the hospital?" "I won't." "Don't tell me what to do." "I'm fine."

O Flat affect. Short concentration span. Increased disorganization. Reality disorientation. Memory gaps. Fragmented thought and speech. Sleep disturbance. Appetite disturbance. Crying. Long silences. Refused prescribed psychotropic drug. Increased hostility and agitation.

Actual outcome
April and Megan spent many happy hours talking about the arrival of a new family member. Megan moved to an adult-size bed, readying the crib for the new child. April did not intellectually or emotionally prepare for the birth and presence of a new family member. Crisis occurred in the immediate postpartum days as evidenced by depression and decompensation.

2A—Assessment

N.D. *Anxiety*
S "No, I won't take those pills." "Megan, be quiet, Mommy is tired." "I don't know when she ate last time." "Is the baby crying?" "I wonder what's wrong with him?"
O Severe agitation. Increased hostility. Refused medication.

N.D. *Decompensation episode*
S "No, I won't take those pills." "Megan, be quiet, Mommy is tired." "I don't know when she ate last time." "Is the baby crying?" "I wonder what's wrong with him?"
O Severe agitation. Increased hostility. Refused medication. Unable to function or meet the demands of life.

N.D. *Family disruption*
S "Megan, be quiet, Mommy is tired." "I don't know when she ate last time." "Is the baby crying?" "I wonder what's wrong with him?"
O Severe agitation. Increased hostility. Refused medication. Unable to function or meet the demands of life. Allen concerned, distressed, passive. Megan frightened, lost bladder and bowel control, whined, slept fitfully, and had many psychogenic complaints.

3—Additional nursing diagnosis
None

4A—Variables
Reality timing	−5
Relationships	−5
Stressors and/or crisis	−5
Coping resources	−5
Significant emotional strength	−5
Significant emotional limitations	−5
Therapy relationship	+1

Physical health status	−2
Physical and emotional readiness dimension	−2
Available support system	−2
Meaning significance	0
Values and belief impact	0
Other	

BALANCE —

Additional specific knowledge
See case material.

Analysis and synthesis

N.D. *Anxiety.* Intrinsic and extrinsic stress reached a point of panic, fragmented thinking, and an increasingly nonfunctional state.

N.D. *Decompensation episode.* April is unable to function or cope effectively and is unsafe as a mother. The protected environment of a hospital setting is needed for the security of both April and her family. Intense treatment with stressors removed will aid the healing process.

N.D. *Family disruption.* April's behavior and functional state spilled over all family members, increasing the disorganization and stress.

4B — Design of action

N.D. *Anxiety, decompensation episode, family disruption*
1. Plan
   a. Assess and collaborate with April's psychiatrist.
   b. Hospitalize client.
   c. Support client and family through crisis period.
2. Strategy
   a. Attempt to persuade client to take prescribed medication.
   b. Assume necessary child-care duties.
   c. Explain definitively to client what is happening in a step-by-step manner. Do not negotiate with client.
   d. Support Allen and direct him to assume necessary family responsibilities.
3. Expected outcomes
   a. Ingestion of medication.
   b. Decreased agitation as children become nurtured and comfortable.
   c. Acceptance of the need for hospitalization.
   d. Assumption by Allen of responsible tasks to aid in the transition period.
4. Criteria
   a. Ingestion of medication.
   b. Decreased agitation and hostility.
   c. Decreased resistance.
   d. Allen will be supportive during hospitalization process.

e. Allen will assume or delegate child-care and house-hold responsibilities.

Increased home nursing visits were helpful but not sufficient support for April to maintain her self-integration and reality orientation. Allen was passive but obviously distressed, and he expressed what was seemingly genuine concern. Megan, puzzled and frightened, lost bladder and bowel control, whined, slept fitfully, and had many psychogenic complaints. House-keeping tasks remained at a standstill.

Psychiatric hospitalization occurred for April 6 weeks postpartum. Allen telephoned for the therapist, requesting an immediate visit when the crisis peaked for both. Neither husband nor wife was coping effectively, and it was extremely obvious that April's decompensation was becoming more severe daily. She was not able to function or meet the demands of her life situation. After the therapist collaborated with April's psychiatrist and because April continued to forcefully refuse medication, she was hospitalized for 4 weeks' duration, receiving both electroshock therapy and antipsychotic drugs.

On the day of her hospitalization, April was severely agitated, openly hostile, and highly distressed. She could not remember when she had last fed her son, who was wet and fussy. April passively watched while the therapist bathed, weighed, and cuddled Allen, Jr., and began supplemental feeding. April seemed to be reassured by her son's normal weight and average weight gain, indicating to her that she was a good mother. She held her sleeping son and appeared less agitated. The therapist held Megan and comforted her as matter-of-fact conversation that April was to be hospitalized was initiated. April was not given the opportunity to question this decision. She remained nonverbal and became less resistive and restless during these hours of intervention. The reassurance about her children seemed to penetrate the maze of her distressed psyche.

Allen mustered his strength and found a

neighbor to babysit and an aunt to care for the children in the following weeks. Allen and the therapist took April to the hospital without further incident. On the return trip the therapist offered to make home visits for the sake of the children while April was hospitalized and to support the aunt if need be.

PROCESS IMPLEMENTATION

1—Evaluation
N.D.   *Anxiety*
 S   Client remained nonverbal.
 O   Refused medication. Became less agitated as therapist assumed parenting role. Held her son.
N.D.   *Decompensation episode*
 S   Client remained nonverbal.
 O   Refused medication. Became less agitated as therapist assumed parenting role. Held her son.
N.D.   *Family disruption*
 S   Client remained nonverbal. Children became calm and quiet. Allen: "Mrs. J will take care of you while Mommy and I are gone." Allen: "I'll be back for supper, Mommy is sick and will be gone for a while."
 O   Children became comfortable as basic needs were met. Allen assumed responsibility for children and household. April was less agitated.

Actual outcome
 April refused medication but became less hostile and resistive as the therapist assumed immediate child-care responsibilities. Hospitalization proceeded without incident. Allen contacted a babysitter and was supportive to his wife and children.

2A—Assessment
N.D.   *Denial*
 S   "I forgot." "Oh, was I supposed to be doing that?" "No one told me."
 O   Verbal agreement but quickly forgetting, changing her mind, or not following through with the agreed-on action. Self-discernments quickly forgotten.
N.D.   *Dependence/independence struggle*
 S   "I forgot." "Oh, was I supposed to be doing that?" "No one told me." "You make me think too hard in our talks."
 O   Verbal agreement but quickly forgetting, changing her mind, or not following through with the agreed-on action. Ambivalence concerning therapy relationship.
N.D.   *Low self-concept*
 S   "I enjoy my children." "You make me think too hard in our talks."

 O   Allowing time for herself. Increased self-disclosure. Self-discernments quickly forgotten.
N.D.   *Passive resistance*
 S   "I forgot." "Oh, was I supposed to be doing that?" "No one told me." "You make me think too hard in our talks."
 O   Verbal agreement but quickly forgetting, changing her mind, or not following through with the agreed-on action.
N.D.   *Difficulty in adjustment to parenting*
 S   "I enjoy my children."
 O   Allen built limited affectionate bond with children. April smiled, laughed. April played and read to Megan. Sharing responsibilities. Mutual problem solving.
N.D.   *Financial stress*
 S   "Allen's second job helps to pay the bills." "We even went to a movie last week."
 O   Allen secured a second job on a part-time basis. Mutual problem solving.
N.D.   *Inability to perform required tasks of daily living*
 S   "Yes, the schedule helps." "Allen is helping, too." "I just don't know what to do."
 O   Allen assisted with household and child-rearing tasks. Household cleaned and reorganized. Return to the housekeeping schedule.
N.D.   *Communication disturbances within the marital relationship*
 S   "Yes, the schedule helps." "Allen is helping, too." "I just don't know what to do." "Allen's second job helps to pay the bills." "We even went to a movie last week."
 O   Forgot old hostilities. Less guarded manner. Sharing responsibilities. Mutual problem solving.

2B—Validation by assessment
N.D.   *Passive resistance*
 S   "I forgot." "Oh, was I supposed to be doing that?" "No one told me." "You make me think too hard in our talks." (Comments repeated four times in four consecutive visits.)
 O   Verbal agreement but quickly forgetting, changing her mind, or not following through with the agreed-on action. Pattern of action observed in four consecutive visits.

3—Additional nursing diagnosis
N.D.   *Lack of insight*
 S   "I just don't know what to do." "If you say so, but . . ." "Did I really tell you that?"
 O   Increased self-disclosure. Self-discernments quickly forgotten.

4A—Variables

Reality timing	+4
Relationships	+3
Stressors and/or crisis	0
Coping resources	+2
Significant emotional strength	+2
Significant emotional limitations	−2
Therapy relationship	+2
Physical health status	0
Physical and emotional readiness dimension	0
Available support system	+1
Meaning significance	+3
Values and belief impact	+3
Other	
BALANCE	+

Additional specific knowledge
See case material.

Analysis and synthesis
N.D. *Denial.* This protective mechanism is less prevalent in behavior. The client's increased comfort with reality allows for more effective coping with life problems and issues. Self-disclosure should be encouraged in therapy.

N.D. *Dependence/independence struggle.* Decreased anxiety and increased effective coping behavior allow this struggle to be a more active process. The struggle itself rather than a state of apathy will eventually culminate in a decision. Therapy efforts will guide the client to independence.

N.D. *Low self-concept.* A broadened environment allowing for positive feedback and person affirmation will promote self-esteem and personal growth.

N.D. *Passive resistance.* This method of coping with stress remains part of April's life stance. Although less prominent and less destructive, it continues to inhibit growth.

N.D. *Difficulty in adjusting to parenting.* Sharing of child-care responsibilities and increased satisfaction from mothering ease the perceived stress of child care.

N.D. *Financial stress.* This factor relieved by Allen's efforts at a part-time job and by his earned promotion.

N.D. *Inability to perform required tasks of daily living.* Renewed order and structure of the household decrease the overwhelming nature of the tasks. Scheduled duties assist in maintaining a limited organization and task completion.

N.D. *Communication disturbance within the marital relationship.* Resolution and compromise on troublesome areas increased trust and promoted new level of open communication and mutual problem solving. Increased fondness bonds paved the way for growth.

N.D. *Lack of insight.* Self-revelations remained painful and were frequently denied after disclosure, but limited insights can be viewed as progress.

4B—Design of action
N.D. Denial, dependence/independence struggle, low self-concept, passive resistance, difficulty in adjustment to parenting, financial stress, inability to perform required tasks of daily living, communication disturbance within the marital relationship, lack of insight.

1. Plan
   a. Support and guide client and family to a functioning restorative state.
2. Strategy
   a. Offer guidance to solve problems of daily living tasks and personal adjustment.
   b. Encourage time to meet personal needs and accomplish couple-related activities and activities outside the family scope.
   c. Offer supportive and correct feedback and person affirmation.
   d. Encourage more open couple communication and mutual problem solving.
3. Expected outcomes
   a. Organization and realignment of child-rearing tasks and household duties.
   b. Maintenance of prescribed drug regimen.
   c. Grappling with mutual dilemmas within the marriage relationship and mutual resolution of defined areas of concern, such as birth control.
   d. Renewed self-disclosure and insight gains through therapy.
   e. Involvement for April and the couple in social activities outside the home.
4. Criteria
   a. Limited but observable organization of household tasks. Shared duties. Shared child-rearing tasks. Expressions of enjoyment related to children.
   b. Intellectual and emotional acceptance of the need for a maintenance drug regimen.
   c. Open discussion and resolution by the couple of the birth control issue. Implementation of decision.
   d. Limited self-disclosure and insights revealed in therapy dialogue.

e. Actual involvement in activity of choice outside the scope of the family.

For his part, Allen agreed to see the marriage counselor weekly. The shock value of the trauma of this hospitalization and the support and confrontation of his therapist spurred Allen to secure a second job on a part-time basis to help relieve the additional financial stress of hospitalization and unpaid bills. He also assumed some task-centered family chores such as removing trash, mowing the lawn, doing kitchen clean-up duties, and grocery shopping. With encouragement from the marriage counselor and pressured by the realities of his life circumstance, Allen began to build some affectionate bonds with his children, although his manner remained aloof. His aunt did an efficient and thorough housecleaning and began to organize the essential housekeeping and basic child-rearing tasks. At the time of April's discharge, both the emotional environment and household milieu had a new and increased climate of security and order. Allen was trying, and April's confused sensorium allowed her to forget old hostilities and become open to change in a less guarded manner.

In the following weeks, April's emotional responses became more appropriate. She could laugh and smile with her children. Her ambivalence seemed less prominent. The reorganized environment supported her associative process. Broad therapy goals were focused on enabling her psyche to remain intact as her sensorium cleared, to maintain the restored balance in the environment, and to buttress the sensitive equilibrium of the family system.

April's previous associative disturbance, as manifested in her personal and environmental disorganization, was an intervention target. Verbal assistance to work out daily tasks slowly and carefully was encouraged. Prime learning time for new thinking behaviors occurs in the immediate period following a course of electroshock therapy, when memory loss for old coping styles can be replaced with new and healthy coping methods.

The combination of isolation and enforced aloneness of this young mother compounded by the perceived multiple stimuli of child rearing and daily living tasks complicated her associative disturbance. This pathological process needed to be contained to restore a relative balance. Disruptive environment and a stressed life-style foster dormant thinking disturbances. Stressor bombardment from within and without yield associative breakdown, culminating in poor problem-solving methods and coping method choices.

April continued a maintenance dosage of trifluoperazine, 2 mg b.i.d., and she demonstrated no negative, drug-related side effects. Periodically, she attempted to bargain for medication reduction or withdrawal. Sometimes she forgot to take her drugs as prescribed. Kindly but firmly with no bargaining allowed in this issue, April was told the expected, predictable outcome of her failure to continue the regimen. For several years this was to remain a nonnegotiable area of treatment.

April had a limited degree of insight, and her discernment was painful. These distressing self-perceptions were quickly denied, thus stunting personal growth in therapy. Her passive resistance style of coping returned as her sensorium cleared. Although April did want the support of therapy, and the dependency need satisfaction, she could or would not grapple with some of the realities of her life-style and personhood. Her passive resistance led to verbal agreement in therapy, but she soon forgot, changed her mind, or did not have time to follow through with the action agreed upon. One must accept the actuality of the client's situation. A desire for emotional stability versus the attainment of becoming relatively stable or symptom free may present an unresolvable dilemma. One can often tilt the balance to the negative by pushing the client too forcefully rather than by accepting the client in his present state. Reality orientation and timing are essential components of growth, insight, and goal achievement in therapy.

The decision for emotional health or emotional illness is always the choice of the client. The responsibility of the therapist is to employ persuasive communication efforts skillfully to throw the balance toward a decision of positive choice and action. A prime factor to remember is that the resolution must be determined by and lived by the client. The client's judgment for or against emotional stability in no way reflects on the competence of the therapist.

In a combined effort of nurse psychotherapy, marriage counseling, and psychiatrist intervention, Allen and April chose a birth control method. April was fitted for a diaphragm, and the couple was educated by the nurse-clinician in its use and effectiveness. They expressed no resistance to the idea of birth control based on religious belief or personal values. They both expressed no desire or need to discuss their sexual relationship, and they showed relief when the subject of sex and birth control was set aside.

Periodically, April was asked by the clinician if she was having problems using her diaphragm. She denied experiencing any problems and quickly changed the subject. The therapist took time to impart information matter-of-factly before moving on to another topic. April did not become pregnant again.

Child-rearing tasks proved to be more satisfying to April after hospitalization. She was encouraged to spend time with her children, doing things they would enjoy. Efforts were made to decrease the environmental stimuli, and Megan continued to nap each afternoon for several hours. During this time, April bathed, fed, and played with her son. Sometimes she expressed guilt at not caring for him during her illness, but expressed delight in caring for him now. When she settled him for sleep, she had time to devote to herself, often taking a nap until Megan woke. Sometimes April read or showered and shampooed her hair. The therapist verbally reinforced this relaxed time for April's personal needs. One cannot expect a client to relax without helping to provide both a time and method to facilitate the tension reduction and relaxed feeling needed for a climate of growth.

Megan enjoyed being read to, and April enjoyed reading to her. They read together each morning while Allen, Jr., napped. April bathed and played with Megan each evening after dinner, and sometimes Allen loaded the dishwasher during this time. He also continued with his other newly assumed, family housekeeping tasks.

April was encouraged to purchase and use a second-hand playpen. April reluctantly made the purchase through a newspaper advertisement. She was directed to begin placing Allen, Jr., in the playpen to accustom him to it. Restraining her son as he began to explore and toddle would decrease the stimuli and activity for April. Allen, Jr., adjusted to being confined. His relative comfort and minimal resistance helped April to tolerate this device for her own benefit and comfort.

Housekeeping tasks were difficult and perceived as a weighty chore. Allen's assistance with some routines did help. The contract agreed on before the hospitalization, that April would work for 2 hours each morning on planned tasks, was reinstituted. In addition, each day she would prepare the meals, a task that she enjoyed, and she would wash three loads of clothes. Allen agreed not to complain about the housekeeping as long as she completed her contracted time allotment. He had previously stated that if he was not satisfied, he would open the issue up in therapy and be willing to assume increased burdens himself. This method was effective, although on days when stressors were high, it was difficult to see that 2 hours of actual work had been completed. Task assignments were not completed within the allotted time span. All parties, clients and therapists, came to accept some disorder in the home. Allen and April agreed to compromise on their differences in values, and each had to adapt to their life responsibilities and duties. Renegotiation of house-keeping expectations was possible as the children matured. As finances improved, increased help with household tasks could be secured from within the family and from outside as well.

Although action-oriented demonstrative change was not visible in all areas of April's life, she did begin to disclose emotion more freely. Catharsis and self-revelation seemed to expand her sense of self. By the time Allen, Jr., reached his first birthday, April emerged as a stronger person. She became involved in two projects of her choosing. She joined a weight-control group, which delighted Allen, and he was free with his compliments on her weight loss, to April's surprise. She joined a community fund-raising project that was recruiting new volunteers. Association with other young women of similar interest was a positive encounter for her. In addition, mother and children returned to a YWCA group weekly. Having time for pursuing her own interest and being away from the confining boundaries of her home decreased April's emotional dependency on Allen and nurtured her developing self. April was gaining insight by sharing with her therapist her feelings, her concerns, her decisions, her actions, and her growth. Equilibrium was precarious but in relative balance.

The marriage and family system were less stressed, and a new sense of unfolding happiness was evident. Allen had received an employment promotion with a substantial accompanying raise in salary, enabling him to stop his moonlighting. Some couple social associations evolved. They both enjoyed the treat of an occasional evening together away from home and children. Couple communication was less direct and honest than ideal, but it had improved.

April chose to terminate nurse psychotherapy. She reasoned this choice in an elusive but decided manner. With some prodding she expressed restrained grief for the dissolution of the nurse/client relationship. Expressions of loss were new to April and very healthy for her. However, marriage counseling on a monthly basis was continued by the couple.

Home-based nurse psychotherapy was the treatment of choice for April. Her last episode of confined care was short. The length of hospitalization was influenced by the availability of concentrated, goal-directed, posthospitalization care within the family system. Nursing offered the needed experience and expertise in child growth and development, psychopathology, and communication to promote health within the family system and also the skilled relationship for April as the identified client. Coordination and collaboration with other health-care professionals were the pivots for holistic client-centered treatment. Knowledgeable nursing intervention established on nursing process skill can be the central treatment in long-term client situations that indicate a need for emotional growth, support, and adaptation as a constant therapy element. This treatment occurs within a solid, professional interpersonal relationship offering a climate of trust, care and concern, compassion, and acceptance as the constant variables in the overall restorative process.

SUMMARY PERSONAL PROFILE
Social adjustment

S "I do my work as I agreed." "It's good to know Allen will help sometimes." "We had dinner out on Friday." "I like my weight-control group."

O Acceptance of some disorder within the A's home. Contract to complete 2 hours of housework daily, prepare meals, and wash three loads of laundry. Husband assistance with household tasks. Involvement in weight-control group, community fund-raising project, and YWCA. Couple social association. Occasional evening for couple away from home. Improved couple communication.

Emotional health status

S "I don't like to take pills, but I do it." "The diaphragm doesn't present any problems." "I played with the baby." "Megan likes me to read to her." "I feel . . ." "I don't really like to . . ." "I had a good time at . . ."

O Maintenance dosage of trifluoperazine, 2 mg b.i.d. Taking time for personal needs such as rest, shower, shampoo. Giving adequate physical and emotional child care. Choice of a birth control method. Decreased ambivalence. Improved couple communication.

Physical health status

S "I don't like to take pills, but I do it." "The diaphragm doesn't present any problems." "I like my weight-control group."

O Maintenance dosage of trifluoperazine, 2 mg b.i.d. Choice of a birth control method. Weight-loss program initiated.

Spiritual dimension

S ⎫
O ⎭ No acknowledged or observable change.

Daily living skill performance

S "It's good to know Allen will help sometimes." "I do my work as I agreed." "I played with the baby." "Megan likes me to read to her." "I had my hair cut last week."

O Contract to complete 2 hours of housework daily, prepare meals, and wash three loads of laundry. Taking time for personal needs such as rest, shower, shampoo. Giving adequate physical and emotional child care.

Coping skill repertoire

S "I do my work as I agreed." "I like my weight-control group." "I played with the

baby." "Megan likes me to read to her." "It's good to know Allen will help."

O Maintaining contracted task agreements. Choice of a birth control method. Taking time for personal needs such as rest, shower, shampoo. Giving adequate physical and emotional child care. Involvement in weight-control group, community fund-raising project, and YWCA. Limited but operable child discipline and control methods.

Maturational struggle according to Erikson's developmental stages

S "I do my work as I agreed." "I had a good time at . . ." "We decided I should be fitted for a diaphragm." "I decided to . . ."

O Autonomy versus shame and doubt struggle—developing self-control and willpower.
Identity versus role confusion struggle—developing limited affiliation.
Intimacy versus isolation struggle—developing limited fidelity.

Self-integration

S "I like getting out among other people." "I do my work as I agreed." "I don't worry about the baby when he's in the playpen." "I feel . . ." "I don't really like to . . ." "I had a good time at . . ." "I decided to . . ."

O Maintenance dosage of trifluoperazine, 2 mg b.i.d. Decreased ambivalence. Improved couple communication. Couple social association. Involvement in weight-control group, community fund-raising project, and YWCA. Increased self-disclosure.

Quality of life

S "The house does look better." "I like getting out among other people." "I like my weight-control group."

O Less environmental disorganization. Involvement in weight-control group, community fund-raising project, and YWCA. Couple social association. Occasional evening for couple away from home. Taking time for personal needs such as rest, shower, shampoo. Improved couple communication. Increased financial resources.

SUGGESTED READINGS

Ackerman, N.; The psychodynamics of family life, New York, 1958, Basic Books, Inc; Publishers.

Aguilera, D., and Messick, J.: Crisis intervention: theory and methodology, St. Louis, 1978, The C. V. Mosby Co.

American Nurses' Association: Standards of psychiatric mental-health nursing practice, Kansas City, 1973, The Association.

Bates, B.: A guide to physical examination, Philadelphia, 1974, J. B. Lippincott Co.

Bell, J.: Stressful life events and coping methods in mental-illness and wellness behaviors, Nursing Research 26:136-141, March/April, 1977.

Blair, C., and Salerno, E.: The expanding family: child-bearing, Boston, 1976, Little, Brown & Co., Inc.

Dixon, B.: Interviewing when the patient is delusional, Journal of Psychiatric Nursing 69:25-34, Jan.-Feb., 1969.

Eichel, E.: Assessment with a family focus, Journal of Psychiatric Nursing 16:11-14, Jan. 1978.

Fiegenheimer, W. V.: The patient therapist relationship in crisis intervention, Journal of Clinical Psychiatry 39:348-350, April, 1978.

Finkelman, A. W.: The nurse therapist: outpatient crisis intervention with the chronic psychiatric patient, Journal of Psychiatric Nursing 15:27-32, Aug. 1977.

Johnson-Soderberg, S.: Theory and practice of scapegoating, Perspectives in Psychiatric Care 15(4): 153-159, 1977.

Jourard, S.: Roles that sicken and transactions that heal, The Canadian Nurse 57:628-634, July, 1961.

Kleinman, C. S.: Psychological processes during pregnancy, Perspectives in Psychiatric Care 15(4):175-178, 1977.

Kline, N., and Davis, J.: Psychotropic drugs, American Journal of Nursing 73:54-63, Jan., 1973.

Knapp, M.: Non-verbal communication in human interaction, New York, 1972, Holt, Rinehart & Winston, Inc.

Kolb, L.: Modern clinical psychiatry, Philadelphia, 1977, W. B. Saunders Co.

Levine, M.: Adaptation and assessment: a rationale for nursing intervention, American Journal of Nursing 66:2450-2453, Nov., 1966.

Mitchell, H., et al.: Nutrition in health and disease, Philadelphia, 1976, J. B. Lippincott Co.

Morgan, S., et al.: Three assessment tools for family therapy, Journal of Psychiatric Nursing 16:39-42, March, 1978.

Ray, O.: Drugs, society, and human behavior, ed. 2, St. Louis, 1978, The C. V. Mosby Co.

Rubin, T.: The angry book, New York, 1969, Collier Books.

Sparling, S. L., et al.: Setting: a contextual variable associated with empathy, Journal of Psychiatric Nursing 15: 9-12, April, 1977.

CHAPTER 6

KARL Z *manifests*

PROBLEMATIC LIFE CONDUCT

evidenced by

WITHDRAWAL AND ISOLATION

INTRODUCTORY PERSONAL PROFILE
Social adjustment

S   "Girls still make me nervous. Never did like them (girls)." "I don't talk much." "Don't got nothin' to say."

O   No documented family of record. Acknowledges no living relatives. Verbal communication restricted to short sentences and phrases.

Emotional health status

S   "Girls still make me nervous. Never did like them (girls)." "Don't got nothin' to say."

O   Avoided eye-to-eye contact. Flat expression. Speech slow and deliberate in monosyllables and monotone.

Physical health status

S   "I'm too fat." "I need to sit after walking them stairs." "I take those pills." "Polish sausage and sauerkraut is my favorite lunch." "I walked to church on Sunday. Had to stop to rest four times."

O   Short (5 feet, 5 inches), muscular frame. Weighs 205 pounds. Edematous hands and ankles. Labored breathing on exertion. Flared nostrils and barrelled chest. Slow, rigid, shuffling gait. Moderate dosage of prescribed phenothiazine preparation. Inadequate diet to meet health needs.

Spiritual dimension

S   "I walked to church on Sunday. Had to stop to rest four times." "I'm going to church dinner next Sunday." "Always went to the same church."

O   Regular church attendance. Special attire for church services. Conversation frequently focuses on church attendance or church-related activity.

Daily living skill performance

S   "Always did it this way." "I have a good lunch at noon." "I make my money last all month."

O   Unable to be gainfully employed because of physical health problems. Responsible management of home and finances within acknowledged personal, social, educational, and financial limitations.

Coping skill repertoire

S "Girls still make me nervous. Never did like them (girls)." "I walked to church on Sunday. Had to stop to rest four times." "I don't talk much." "Don't got nothin' to say." "Always did it this way." "I make my money last all month."

O Ineffective behavior to sustain personal integration. Limited by current life-style; number of years of hospitalization; and personal, social, educational, and financial resources. Maintains a fluctuating degree of functional life requirements. Long silences in therapy.

Maturational struggle according to Erikson's developmental stages

S "Girls still make me nervous. Never did like them (girls)." "I don't talk much." "Don't got nothin' to say."

O Basic trust vs. basic mistrust.
Autonomy vs shame and doubt.
Intimacy vs. isolation.

Self-integration

S *

O Associative disturbance evidenced by blocking, slow speech, fragmented thoughts, and concentration difficulties. High ambivalence indicated by indecision and anxiety within an interpersonal relationship. Emotional disturbance evidenced by flat affect and responses inappropriate to stimuli. Autism used as a mental activity to achieve gratification. A joyless posture indicative of anhedonia.

---

*Absence of subjective data indicates limited verbal exchange, extended periods of silence in therapy, or lack of comment to the clinician's queries.

Quality of life

S *

O Environment deprived of intimate person encounters and necessary social-emotional stimuli. Extremely limited financial resources.

Time span: 5 years

Karl Z, as a person, is elementary and uncomplex to describe. An unsophisticated eye would describe Karl as a plain person with an unvarnished life-style. A trained clinical eye would quickly diagnose him as schizophrenic.

Karl is 55 years old and single. There is no documented family of record for Karl and he acknowledges no living relatives. He has never been married. He stated, "Girls still make me nervous. Never did like them (girls)."

Karl's verbal communication was restricted to short sentences and phrases. When he did speak, it was slowly and deliberately, in monosyllables and in a monotone. He avoided eye-to-eye contact, and a flatness of expression made it difficult to establish a contact base to form an interpersonal relationship. It remained a laborious task to evaluate the impact of another person on Karl.

In describing Karl, one easily resorts to the use of a negative cliché: "He looks like a typical state hospital patient of the 1950s." In resisting the impulse to label Karl, one can be more accurate in describing the man. Karl is 5 feet, 5 inches tall and has grey, sparse hair and a ruddy complexion. He shaves only on Saturday and Wednesday and on special occasions. He carries 205 pounds on his short, muscular frame. His hands and ankles are edematous, his breathing is labored on exertion, his nostrils are flared, and his chest is barrelled. Karl walks with a slow, rigid shuffling gait, partially attributed to a moderate dosage of phenothiazine medication to control his thought disorder. Karl's usual attire is khaki cotton trousers, a dark muted plaid flannel shirt, heavy long flannel underwear, and a worn dark grey sweater. On special outings and for Sunday church services, Karl wears an old tweed sport jacket.

Karl lives in a small room measuring about 10 by 12 feet with one small uncurtained window overlooking an alley. The room contains a single bed covered with greyish sheets and two olive-drab army blankets. This room contains a chest of drawers, a small table with a one burner hot plate, a straight wooden chair, and a wicker rocker in need of repair. The walls of the room are a sooty grey in need of fresh paint, and there are no pictures on them. One corner contains a curtained-off closet. The ceiling light is a dim light bulb. One floor lamp minus a shade sits next to the often-used rocker adjacent to a small table. Two green pillows, placed solely for comfort in the rocker, brighten the room.

Bathroom facilities are at the end of the hall and are shared by four other roomers, as is a community refrigerator standing in the dark hall. Karl's room is reached by way of a steep flight of twenty-one stairs over a merchandise store. The stairs exit outside, over the room and down to the alley. The rent for the room is paid from Karl's supplemental security allowance.

Karl's life is extremely routinized. He rises at 4 A.M., fixes breakfast on his hot plate, has a morning walk and a nap, lunches on the daily special of a nearby bar and grill, watches T.V. in this establishment for several hours, has an afternoon walk and nap, fixes an evening meal of soup and sandwiches, and retires early. Once a week Karl grocery shops. Once a month, Karl visits his physician, and once a month he visits his mental health professional. On Sunday he attends church services.

Karl's sparse history shows that he was hospitalized initially at the age of 24 years after several years of employment as a transient farm worker. He completed school through Grade 4. Little data are available concerning his family or early life. At 27 years of age Karl contracted tuberculosis, which necessitated several hospital transfers within the state mental hospital system and several years of enforced, supervised bed rest and other standard treatment for tuberculosis current in 1940. Annals of treatment for tuberculosis at that time establish that the long-term restorative process of isolation encouraged a sense of aloneness and emotional deprivation, often stimulating fantasy and thought disorder. Lack of stimulus and interrelationships are detrimental to emotional and social growth and to person integration. The absence of notations in Karl's records leads one to conclude that he was cooperative and quiet. The records do state that his tuberculosis was arrested after several years of treatment.

Karl remained a rather anonymous being until the community-focused mental health movement of the 1960s. He quickly became a prime candidate for discharge. Karl settled into community life in a pattern of living similar to his years of hospitalization. He ordered his life-style according to the hospital routine. Karl was unaware of other adjustments one might choose in life.

Approximately 2 years after discharge, Karl was referred for therapy to assess his life routine and adjustment and encourage further socialization. After an initial interview and a record review, the following nursing diagnosis was concluded:

Anxicty
Dependence/independence struggle
Low self-concept
Thought disorder
Emotional deprivation
Environmental deprivation
Difficulty in life adjustment after long-term hospitalization
Interpersonal relationship disturbance
Short concentration span
Limited physical energy
Obesity
High blood pressure
Edema
Breathing difficulties
Faulty support system

Clinically, it was readily apparent that Karl had long been labeled chronic schizophrenic. Eugen Bleuler's four A's—(1) associative disturbance, (2) ambivalence, (3) affective disturbance, and (4) autism, as well as anhedonia— were readily apparent.

Associative disturbance was evidenced by blocking, slow speech, infrequent fragmented thoughts, and short attention span. Withdrawal and isolation protected Karl from the embarrassment of spontaneous crossing up of his associations.

Ambivalence was indicated by indecision and difficulty in life adjustments. High initial anxiety was present in his relationships and correlated with a vagueness and ambiguity about interpersonal relationship per se and about his position in a person-to-person encounter.

Affective disturbance was evidenced by a flat facial expression and a grinning smile without observable stimuli. The low or reduced stimuli in his environment and life-style protected his dormant pathology.

Autism resulted from the extensive time spent alone in an environment enhancing fantasy, day dreaming, and boredom. Gratification from this mental activity fostered withdrawal, isolation, and aloneness.

Additionally, anhedonia was demonstrated by a posture of joylessness. Lack of significant other persons in Karl's life and the absence of ongoing, quality interpersonal relationships resulted in a protective wall, insulating him from the pleasures of personal encounters and diminishing his capacity to take part in interpersonal experiences.

This knowledge is essential to the implementation of the nursing process for Karl's future health. The nurturance and maturation of Karl as a person are best served without the label of schizophrenia and all the negative associations the term entails. The applied nursing diagnoses are less intimidating and more appropriate to facilitate goal-directed health care.

With Karl's reluctant consent and the support of his physician, a nurse was assigned to become his primary therapist. A succession of several nurses was engaged in this capacity over the 5-year span of nurse psychotherapy. No relationship was longer than 6 months. Karl needed an increase in the number of his relationships as well as in the quality and quantity of these relationships. Had Karl ever learned to relate to another human being on a person-to-person level? Was a relationship involving intensity and duration possible for him? What would the stress of the risk of a person-to-person relationship precipitate for Karl? These were crucial questions to the formation and evolution of this relationship.

The succession of therapists was designed to provide several interpersonal relationships for Karl that would yield care, concern, and goal-directed, nonthreatening activities. A rotation of relationships would decrease the uncertainty of involvement for Karl and provide a medium for him to learn how to relate to another person. The planning and evaluation of the nursing process interventions and the relationship evaluations were supervised by the initial therapist to provide a cohesive approach and therapy effort.

In beginning any nursing activity, one must view the behavior patterns and situational variables to establish and pursue goals. Karl's behavior patterns had a static but ordered quality. Sameness seemed to create a degree of security in his existence. The observable variables in his life were limited. In a crisis situation intervention to reduce the interacting variables is routine action. Chronic care of the emotionally disabled often mandates the reverse of this approach. Karl's behavior patterns of living needed an increase in the number and kinds of variables to broaden his human contacts and the quality of his life.

Initially, the environmental setting for the beginning of nurse psychotherapy provided problems. Sessions began in the bar and grill where Karl had his noon meal. With growth and ease in the relationship, sessions were moved to

Karl's room. The milieu for the therapy visits provided comfort for Karl but demanded adjustment for the nurse. One is often more comfortable in traditional therapy settings. Community-based therapy calls for adaptability— a quality often tested through the development of increased flexibility within a therapeutic encounter.

Security within the relationship was developed through rapport, the climate of trust, and the routine format of the visits with stress placed on physical nursing measures done with skill and precision. Karl's history of hypertension required that his blood pressure be checked and recorded during each visit. This monitoring of a physical health problem offered a degree of reality-based reassurance. His blood pressure remained elevated but stable. Karl received this positive feedback and accepted the physical nursing task as an acceptable "thing" for a nurse to do. With the same objective, quiet, competent approach, his medication regimen was evaluated each month. Karl took his prescribed drugs as directed and again received positive reinforcement for his accurate task performance. Acceptable task-centered physical nursing care can often create a needed security and validate the integrity base of the caregiver. This trust and honesty can form the base for building and binding a growth-centered relationship.

Initial sessions with Karl were largely nonverbal. Karl took little or no initiative. His face would flush with embarrassment. His foot would begin to swing, and he would sit uneasily in his booth or rocker. Karl was agreeable, almost eager, to please. Talking for him was difficult, but he learned to play pastime activities, enabling him to interact with less emphasis on talking.

For the client, with the passage of time, it was necessary to set a minimum of 2 contact hours of therapy a week, 1 hour for interaction, self-expression, and personal growth and 1 hour for structured pastime activities. The choice of activities such as checkers, monopoly, cribbage, chess, and card games provided both comfort and supportive "thereness" of the therapist. They also provided intellectual stimuli for Karl and a competence in a social activity that could assist in fostering other future relationships. Karl's task achievement would provide a skill to help facilitate other-person interaction. Therapy interaction would expand his emotional self.

At first the learning of these activities was slow. Checkers was Karl's first choice. His short concentration span, limited physical energy, anxiety, and interpersonal relationship disturbance created learning problems. At the same time these activities created therapeutic media to intervene in the identified areas with nonthreatening feedback. Emotional deprivation was also countered as Karl gained skill in the activities.

In his usual slow, deliberate manner, Karl mastered checkers in several months and moved on to cribbage. During this activity he began to sit more comfortably and for longer periods of time. His periods of concentration lengthened. His previously hidden wittiness emerged. He became comfortable with a female nurse-visitor in his territorial space. He was acquiring new social skills. Often he had his small table moved, the chairs positioned, and the checker board ready to be used on her arrival. He related that he practiced his game during his alone hours. He was enjoying the positive feedback from his accomplishment. He was acquiring a level of self-discipline and filling a previous void in his long, empty day.

Although Karl never responded verbally to comments such as, "You won again," "Good game, Karl," "You aren't a match for me anymore, Karl," or "I enjoy playing checkers with you, Karl, even if I do lose so often lately," his body relaxed, his eyes sparkled, and his task refinement continued. At times he even smiled in a very appropriate manner.

PROCESS IMPLEMENTATION

1—Evaluation

N.D. *Anxiety*
    S   *
    O   Sessions moved from bar and grill to his room. Less foot swinging, more relaxed posture. Extremely limited verbal exchange. Eyes sparkled. Task refinement continued.

N.D. *Interpersonal relationship disturbance*
    S   *
    O   Small table moved, chairs positioned, and checker board ready for nurse. Extremely limited verbal exchange. In his slow deliberate manner, client mastered checkers over several months. Concentration period lengthened. Task refinement continued.

N.D. *Short concentration span*
    S   *
    O   In his slow deliberate manner, client mastered checkers over several months. Concentration period lengthened. Task refinement continued.

N.D. *High blood pressure*
    S   *
    O   Elevated but stable. Medication taken as prescribed.

N.D. *Difficulty in life adjustment after long-term hospitalization*
    S   *
    O   Small table moved, chair positioned, and checker board ready for nurse. Extremely limited verbal exchange. In his slow deliberate manner, client mastered checkers over several months. Concentration period lengthened. Task refinement continued.

N.D. *Limited physical energy*
    S   *
    O   In his slow, deliberate manner, client mastered checkers over several months. Extremely limited verbal exchange. Less foot swinging, more relaxed posture.

N.D. *Emotional deprivation*
    S   *
    O   Small table moved, chairs positioned, and checker board ready for nurse. Extremely limited verbal exchange. In his slow deliberate manner, client mastered checkers over several months. Concentration period lengthened. Task refinement continued.

Actual outcome
    Basic relationship bonding developed between client and nurse. Limited verbal exchange. Acquired pastime activity skills.

2A—Assessment

N.D. *Interpersonal relationship disturbance*
    S   "I'm worried about my friend."*
    O   Voice soft, almost inaudible, and client looking away from therapist. Concerns slipped out during pastime activities. Unable to find a method to contact his friend Joe or gather information about his state of health.

N.D. *Faulty support system*
    S   "I'm worried about my friend."*
    O   Significant other person dependent on Karl for daily tasks as well as mutual companionship. Unable to find a method to contact his friend or gather information about his state of health.

N.D. *Emotional deprivation*
    S   "I'm worried about my friend."*
    O   Voice soft, almost inaudible, and client looking away from therapist. Concerns slipped out during pastime activities. Unable to find a method to contact his friend or gather information about his state of health.

N.D. *Dependence/independence struggle*
    S   "I'm worried about my friend."*
    O   Unable to find a method to contact his friend or gather information about his state of health.

N.D. *Low self-concept*
    S   "I'm worried about my friend."*
    O   Unable to find a method to contact his friend or gather information about his state of health.

3—Additional nursing diagnosis
None

4A—Variables

Reality timing	+2
Relationships	−2
Stressors and/or crisis	0
Coping resources	−2
Significant emotional strength	0
Significant emotional limitation	−3
Therapy relationship	+3
Physical health status	−3
Physical and emotional readiness dimension	+3
Available support system	−2
Meaning significance	+2
Values and belief impact	+2
Other	
BALANCE	0

---

*Absence of subjective data indicates limited verbal exchange, extended periods of silence in therapy, or lack of comment to the clinician's queries.

Additional specific knowledge

See case material.

Analysis and synthesis

N.D. *Interpersonal relationship disturbance.* Few healthy relationships over a lifetime as a basis in which to test and develop relationship skills. Poor problem-solving methods prevent the client from searching out resources and finding adequate answers.

N.D. *Faulty support system.* Assessment seems to validate a lack of positive support system other than from professional caregivers.

N.D. *Emotional deprivation.* A lifelong emotional void does not encourage feelings or need expression or the tools or skills to initiate and express them.

N.D. *Dependence/independence struggle.* An insecure and falsely autonomous life stance continues the struggle between the opposing forces. Karl, presently, has insufficient life skills to reach a true autonomous resolution.

N.D. *Low self-concept.* Uncertainty and difficulty expressing self often elicits further negative reinforcement of the already faulty self-concept. Dehumanization from years of institutional living further complicates the self-development.

4B — Design of action

N.D. Interpersonal relationship disturbance, faulty support system, emotional deprivation, dependence/independence struggle, low self-concept.

1. Plan
   a. Investigate Joe's health status.
   b. Encourage relationship.
   c. Foster new sources of relationship.
2. Strategy
   a. Relay facts concerning Joe and guide client's problem solving to explore methods of maintaining the significant relationship.
   b. Support Karl's efforts no matter how minimal.
   c. Explore the impact and tenuous nature of the relationship between Karl and Joe.
   d. Encourage new relationships.
3. Expected outcomes
   a. Visiting Joe in the hospital and making telephone contacts.
   b. Resumption of the relationship when Joe returns home.
   c. Coping with Joe's illness and preparing for the impact of the dissolution of the relationship by death.
   d. Initiation of group therapy.
4. Criteria
   a. Visiting Joe in the hospital and making telephone contacts.
   b. Resuming the relationship when Joe returns home.
   c. Expressing grief during therapy.
   d. Expressing reactions to group therapy.

As Karl became relatively assured in his relationships with "my nurse," he became equally more conversive. It was apparent that there were few or no significant others in his life. He had things he wished to share, and he had worries. His sharing had a simplistic quality—what he had for lunch, the weather, the sales at the grocery store, his impression of his neighbors, the kindness of his landlord, a T.V. story he had seen, something new from the church bulletin, something he remembered from his childhood, or an article he read in the local newspaper. Karl's worries were not shared easily, but they became less uncertain topics as he found that there were resolutions to some of his concerns, such as weight reduction, which could be solved through sharing and resultant action in therapy.

As his self-confidence and feelings of accomplishment increased, Karl began to take the risk of restrained self-disclosure during nursing visits. He verbalized his concerns and worries. At first, his efforts were soft-spoken, almost inaudible, and he was always looking down and away from the therapist. His concerns usually slipped out during a pause in the current pastime activity. Acute listening abilities and readiness to focus on the voiced stress helped Karl to increase his level of trust within the therapy relationship, and he continued to risk voicing matters of personal concern.

One of his concerns was for a significant other person in his life. Karl had a friend named Joe who lived about eight blocks distant from Karl's home. Joe was physically disabled and used a wheelchair. He was about 70 years old and a friend from Karl's youth. It seemed that Joe depended on Karl for many daily tasks as well as for their mutual need for companionship.

Joe was currently hospitalized for an evaluation of an exacerbation of his disability. Karl's worry was other centered. He was interested in the well-being of his friend. Joe had been hospitalized for 2 weeks with no communication between the two men when Karl first voiced his concern.

The therapist was able to check on Joe's condition and found that he was in stable condition but would require further care in a confined setting. Karl was told this news and was encouraged to telephone his friend, using the pay phone in a nearby store. The two men had short conversations several days each week. Karl expressed less anxiety and began to relate incidents to the nurse concerning his relationship with Joe. Karl was encouraged to use public transportation to visit his hospitalized friend. This venture seemed impossible and confusing to Karl, who felt he would be unable to ''catch a bus.'' Karl, accompanied by ''his nurse,'' made one bus trip to the hospital. Encouraged by the therapist he made a second visit the following week on his own initiative, an achievement he recounted with pride.

After several more weeks Joe's return home was met with Karl's muted enthusiasm. Karl resumed his grocery and errand shopping for Joe. He again had a significant friend whom he could visit almost daily. With a new level of involvement, Karl taught Joe checkers and then new card games. This was a renewed interpersonal relationship for both men. It was anticipated that Joe's illness and the impact of the dissolution of this relationship by death or distance would create new trauma for Karl. He resisted discussion of Joe's health and was not open to formation of any new relationship other than with his rotating nurse-therapists.

An evaluation of Karl's progress indicated he was likely candidate for a group therapy program. Karl was resistive to this idea. Talking among groups of more than two or three people and involvements with other people continued to be perceived as an overwhelming experience

by Karl. In his accessible community, small group therapy sessions or support groups were not available and needed group therapy was discounted as a viable tool to promote healthy encounters for Karl.

PROCESS IMPLEMENTATION

1—Evaluation

N.D.   *Interpersonal relationship disturbance*

S   ''I took the bus to the hospital.'' ''I called Joe three times this week.'' ''I don't like groups.''

O   Visit to Joe in hospital accompanied by nurse. Ensuing visit made independently. Telephone conversations with Joe. Taught Joe card games and checkers. Resistance to group activity. Resistant to acknowledge Joe's ill health.

N.D.   *Faulty support system*

S ⎫ Joe and nurse therapist only viable support
O ⎭ system in Karl's world.

N.D.   *Emotional deprivation*

S   ''I took the bus to the hospital.'' ''I called Joe three times this week.'' ''I don't like groups.'' ''I can't . . .'' ''I don't know how to . . .'' ''I never did it.''

O   Visit to Joe in hospital accompanied by nurse. Ensuing visit made independently. Telephone conversations with Joe. Taught Joe card games and checkers. Resistance to group activity. Resistant to acknowledge Joe's ill health.

N.D.   *Dependence/independence struggle*

S   ''I took the bus to the hospital.'' ''I called Joe three times this week.'' ''I don't like groups.''

O   Visit to Joe in hospital accompanied by nurse. Ensuing visit made independently. Telephone conversations with Joe. Taught Joe card games and checkers. Resistance to group activity. Resistant to acknowledge Joe's ill health.

N.D.   *Low self-concept*

S   ''I took the bus to the hospital.'' ''I called Joe three times this week.'' ''I don't like groups.'' ''I can't . . .'' ''I don't know how to . . .'' ''I never did it.''

O   Visit to Joe in hospital accompanied by nurse. Ensuing visit made independently. Telephone conversations with Joe. Taught Joe card games and checkers. Resistance to group activity. Resistant to acknowledge Joe's ill health.

Actual outcome

Karl visited Joe accompanied by the therapist. He made a visit to Joe in the hospital alone. Telephone contacts were made by Karl to Joe during his hospitalization. Karl resumed the relationship and tasks when Joe returned home. In addition, Karl taught Joe new pastime activities. Karl refused to cope with the implications of Joe's ill health. Karl refused to participate in any group activities.

2A—Assessment

N.D. *Obesity*
S "My doctor wants me to lose weight and I can't."
O Client 5 feet, 5 inches tall; weight 205 pounds.

N.D. *High blood pressure*
S "Yes, sometimes I have headaches."
O Stable blood pressure, controlled by medication but remains elevated.

N.D. *Edema*
S "My feet and hands are fat."
O Pitting edema in both ankles and edematous hands.

N.D. *Breathing difficulty*
S "Sometimes I have to sit down halfway up the stairs."
O Rapid and labored breathing during and after exertion such as climbing stairs.

N.D. *Low self-concept*
S "My doctor wants me to lose weight and I can't."
O Client 5 feet, 5 inches tall. Weight 205 pounds. Pitting edema in both ankles and edematous hands. Rapid and labored breathing during and after exertion such as climbing stairs.

3—Additional nursing diagnosis

None

4A—Variables

Reality timing	+2
Relationships	−2
Stressors and/or crisis	0
Coping resources	−2
Significant emotional strength	−2
Significant emotional limitations	−2
Therapy relationship	+3
Physical health status	−3
Physical and emotional readiness dimension	+3
Available support system	−2
Meaning significance	+3
Values and belief impact	+1
Other	
BALANCE	−

Additional specific knowledge

See case material.

Analysis and synthesis

N.D. *Obesity.* Obesity is a central problem that is intricate to the client's life-style. All inter-

vention must be carefully examined so as not to alter his already delicate emotional balance.

N.D. *High blood pressure.* Significant weight loss and dietary regimen may alter imbalance positively.

N.D. *Edema.* Significant weight loss and dietary regimen may alter imbalance positively.

N.D. *Breathing difficulty.* Significant weight loss and dietary regimen may alter imbalance positively.

N.D. *Low self-concept.* Decrease in distress from identified physical problems will promote an increase in self-esteem. Excessive weight validates negative perception of body image and detracts from positive self-feelings.

4B—Design of action

N.D. Obesity, high blood pressure, edema, breathing difficulty, low self-concept.
1. Plan
   a. Compile and assess a food record.
   b. Examine variables of exercise, income, food likes and dislikes, and meaning of food.
   c. Initiate dietary changes.
2. Strategy
   a. Initiate client food record maintenance. Assume a nonjudgmental stance.
   b. Discuss food record and life-style associated with food.
   c. Validate meaning and willingness to adapt taste.
   d. Initiate dietary changes slowly with feedback, support, and affirmation.
3. Expected outcomes
   a. Assessment and evaluation of an available adequate food record.
   b. Increased task interaction between client and nurse.
   c. Involvement by client in food project.
   d. Decreased weight will elicit positive feedback and affirmation from significant others.
4. Criteria
   a. Written food record covering at least 2 weeks.
   b. Discussion and disclosure of information relevant to the task.
   c. Adherence to the diet program with consistent weight loss.
   d. Pride expressed related to weight loss.

Karl's physical health problems were a realistic concern for him and "his nurse." Karl had

had a severe myocardial infarction. He received daily medication to control high blood pressure. He had arrested tuberculosis. He was obese. He had pitting edema in both ankles and edematous hands. His breathing was rapid and labored during and after exertion such as climbing stairs. Karl voiced concern about his weight. "My doctor wants me to lose weight and I can't."

In the many months that followed, a valiant attempt was made to monitor Karl's diet, in view of his low economic status and eating routine. Karl was on an extremely low fixed income. He managed to subsist without complaint, but foods were chosen for *low price* and *taste*. Karl's palate was tuned to Polish sausage, sauerkraut, pickles, weiners, gravy, sandwich meats, and excess breads and potatoes. Most foods that he enjoyed were high in sodium and/or calorie content, often supporting his fluid retention. Because of his income, a low-calorie, low-cholesterol, low-sodium prescribed diet was difficult to implement. Several consultations were held between nurse and dietitian to promote Karl's health.

An important variable in monitoring and changing Karl's diet was the fact that Karl truly enjoyed food. Eating seemed to be his only pleasurable experience in life. Time was measured from one meal to the next. Food was luxury or treat. Unhappily, foods that he most enjoyed were from the forbidden food list on his prescribed diet regimen. He did not lose weight. Instead he gradually gained weight, yet he voiced frequent worry about his physician's warning to reduce. He felt a sense of security in his relationship with "his nurse" and was open to having his diet monitored. The therapist slowly began by attempting to get him involved in a dietary-weight-loss project.

The first step was to have Karl keep a diary or record of all the food consumed each day and the times during a day when he ate. The duration of the first record-keeping task was 2 weeks. Previous diet discussions had been vague and had led to little concrete information.

To discuss diet was like speaking a foreign language to him. It caused confusion and created distance and communication breakdown within the nurse-client relationship. The structure of a food record would give Karl a task that could provide actual data to be evaluated. Karl worked diligently at the maintenance of this document. During the initial 2 week period of data gathering, therapy hours focused on the diet diary and how to judge actual amounts of foods. No judgments or opinions about Karl's eating habits were offered during this period.

The focus on the diet diary gathered other meaningful information. Karl's routine of eating his main noon meal at a local eating establishment offered more than simply a meal. Karl walked to and from this eating establishment, approximately ten blocks. He often added several blocks to his jaunt on the return home before his afternoon nap. The noon special at reasonable price ranged from $1.25 to $1.60 a meal, falling within the mean of Karl's budget. This meal was also served in generous amounts and was food that Karl favored.

A sample noon lunch consisted of the following: 8 ounces breaded and fried pork steak, 1 cup cabbage salad, 2 cups whipped potatoes consisting of a generous portion of gravy, $3/4$ cup buttered peas, 2 buttered rolls, and occasionally a pudding type of dessert.

Another sample meal consisted of 3 Polish sausages, 3 cups sauerkraut, 2 cups whipped potatoes and a generous portion of gravy, $3/4$ cup cream-style corn, 2 pieces buttered bread, and an ice cream or pudding type of dessert. When he recalled the contents of a typical lunch, Karl's eyes sparkled as they did when he received a warm compliment. This noon meal was the focus and high point of many of Karl's otherwise uneventful days.

In reviewing this dietary diary with Karl, it was discovered that he spent 3 hours—from 11 A.M. to 2 P.M. daily—at the restaurant. The therapist found that Karl's routine had been the same as described for several years, and he had made several acquaintances during this time. While he was at the restaurant, many people spoke to Karl and he replied. These acquaintances remained in Karl's distant social space but offered a stroking and human contact that were otherwise missing in his life. This variable would hold considerable weight in monitoring Karl's diet.

In reviewing the food record and associated life habits, the therapist was surprised to hear Karl say that he no longer drank. This was followed with a quick defense, ''That was no good for me. On some hot days I'd sure like a beer, but I don't.''

Karl offered no more comments and did not answer the therapist's questions for further data. A return to the available but inadequate historical data did not validate a history of chemical dependency. The physician of record recalled verbal mention of the arrested problem when Karl was discharged to the community. No evidence of chemically dependent behavior had been noted by community caregivers. The nurse-clinician noted the information on the current record. Awareness of potential limitations can aid astute assessment.

Evaluation of a 2-week food record and the variables in Karl's continuous emotional deprivation made this a precarious intervention when one looked at Karl's total health needs. It was decided that Karl's noon routine could not be altered. The first focus would be on breakfast and then on dinner, considering the variable of budget and limited cooking facilities, the hot plate being the only method of heating foods. Morning meal gradually became fruit, cereal, and coffee instead of bread and coffee, and evening meals became fresh or water-packed fruit, tea, vegetables, sometimes lean meat, and limited dairy products instead of sandwich meat, breads, and canned soups.

Karl gradually became involved and cooperated in this project. He probably increased his quantity of food above set limits several times each week because he did not lose weight at first. He just stopped gaining weight. Then weight loss was slow and erratic, often measured in quarter pounds and time durations of a month rather than a week.

Structured group weight-loss programs were a consideration that was quickly discarded. Karl remained firm in his resistance to group encounters of any kind. Realistically, Karl did not have the financial resources to allow him to participate in the program of any readily available weight-loss group. Group activity as a nursing intervention measure was again aborted.

Karl's total weight loss over 4 years was 10 pounds, but his weight loss did gain some praise from his physician, an important and needed support for his change efforts and reinforcement to continue in his dieting regimen.

During the initial diet regimen, grocery shopping became a topic of discussion during therapy. Shopping occupied an increased number of hours a month for Karl. He needed new and different foods that would fit into his budget. Slow-paced walking to shop at several food markets increased Karl's exercise, another important factor in his diet-health regimen. He seemed to trudge slowly about his task as he made new decisions. He appeared to be more alert in dialogue with ''his nurse,'' and he became keen in his observations and playing skills at pastime games. Healthier eating habits were having a holistic effect on his well-being.

PROCESS IMPLEMENTATION

1—Evaluation

N.D. *Obesity*

S ''It's hard to lose weight.'' ''I try to stay on the diet.'' ''She offered me a fourth Polish sausage and I said no.'' ''My doctor is pleased with me.''

O Sample diet: 8 ounces breaded and fried pork steak, 1 cup cabbage salad, 2 cups whipped potatoes consisting of a generous portion of gravy, $^3/_4$ cup buttered peas, 2 buttered rolls, and occasionally a pudding type of dessert *or* 3 Polish sausages, 3 cups sauerkraut, 2 cups whipped potatoes and a generous portion of gravy, $^3/_4$ cup cream-style corn, 2 pieces of buttered bread, and an ice cream or pudding type of dessert. Focus was on breakfast and then dinner, considering budget and cooking facilities. Morning meals became fruit, cereal, and coffee instead of bread and coffee, and evening meals became fresh or water-packed fruit, tea, vegetables, sometimes lean meat, and limited dairy products instead of sandwich meat, breads, and canned soups. Exercise gained from walking to restaurant ten or more blocks. Grocery shopping to adapt to dietary changes increased amount of exercise.

N.D. *High blood pressure*
  S "I don't have many headaches."
  O No change in blood pressure readings.

N.D. *Edema*
  S
  O } No acknowledged or observable change.

N.D. *Breathing difficulty*
  S
  O } No acknowledged or observable change.

N.D. *Low self-concept*
  S "It's hard to lose weight." "I try to stay on the diet." "She offered me a fourth Polish sausage and I said no." "My doctor is pleased with me."
  O Enjoyed food. Time measured from one meal to the next. Diligently maintained a food record. Noon meal was focus of Karl's day. More alert dialogue with nurse. Increasingly became more keen in observations and pastime activities.

Actual outcome
  Two-week written food record to evaluate. Information on food and relevant life-style freely given. Weight loss of 10 pounds over 4 years. Affirmation for task achievement from nurse and physician.

2A—Assessment
N.D. *Environmental deprivation*
  S "This place is OK for me."
  O Living quarters a small 10- by 12-foot room with one window overlooking the alley. Room contains a single bed with greyish sheets and two olive-drab army blankets. This room contains a chest of drawers, a small table with a one-burner hot plate, a straight wooden chair, and a wicker rocker in need of repair. The walls are sooty grey. There are no pictures on the wall. One corner contains a curtained-off closet. The ceiling light is a dim light bulb. The floor lamp is minus a shade.

N.D. *Difficulty in life adjustment after long-term hospitalization*
  S "This place is OK for me."

O Living quarters a small 10- by 12-foot room with one window overlooking the alley. Room contains a single bed with greyish sheets and two olive-drab army blankets. This room contains a chest of drawers, a small table with a one-burner hot plate, a straight wooden chair, and a wicker rocker in need of repair. The walls are sooty grey. There are no pictures on the wall. One corner contains a curtained-off closet. The ceiling light is a dim light bulb. The floor lamp is minus a shade.

N.D. *Thought disorder*
  S "This place is OK for me." "I close my eyes and think."
  O Spent hours in the environment of his room devoid of stimuli, comfort, and human interaction.

3—Additional nursing diagnosis
None

4A—Variables
Reality timing	0
Relationships	0
Stressors and/or crisis	0
Coping resources	0
Significant emotional strength	0
Significant emotional limitations	0
Therapy relationship	+4
Physical health status	−2
Physical and emotional readiness dimension	+2
Available support system	0
Meaning significance	−1
Values and belief impact	−1
Other	
BALANCE	+

Additional specific knowledge
See case material.

Analysis and synthesis
N.D. *Environmental deprivation.* Encourages thought disorder and feelings of aloneness. Authentic stimuli help to focus on the real world of person-centered relationships and decrease the void in one's life.

N.D. *Difficulty in life adjustment after long-term hospitalization.* The years of routine and sameness do not encourage adaptation even if the direction is positive. Security is perceived in maintenance of long-standing habits. Change is perceived as disruptive and uncertain.

N.D. *Thought disorder.* Long hours of aloneness encourage daydreaming, autism, and affect disturbance. Entrance of real-world stimuli promote an authentic focus to life and help to encourage interpersonal relationship skills.

4B — Design of action

N.D. Environmental deprivation, difficulty in life adjustment after long-term hospitalization, thought disorder.

    1. Plan
        a. Gradually modify environment with paint and comfort measures.
    2. Strategy
        a. Involve Karl in the decisions.
        b. Secure community volunteers to do the physical work.
        c. Pace the changes to Karl's level of adaptability.
    3. Expected outcomes
        a. Room will be clean and comfortable according to Karl's standards.
    4. Criteria
        a. Involvement in projects.
        b. Expressions of satisfaction regarding the changes.

The environmental deprivation of Karl's living arrangements was an area of great concern. He spent many hours in his surroundings, where the absence of stimuli could only add to his thought disorder, self-involvement, and degree of depression. Karl was initially resistant to change. He had no financial assets and little physical strength. During the third year into the nursing relationship, Karl allowed the pursuit of environmental manipulation. His landlord provided paint; Karl chose a pale green color, and community volunteers painted the walls. Karl was quietly pleased, but he wanted no further modification in his environment. The following year a nurse to whom Karl became particularly close brought him a picture at the termination of their relationship. The scene, which depicted a country summer day with children fishing in a creek, was reminiscent of Karl's childhood memories. Karl was pleased and showed the picture to anyone who came into his room. Toward the end of the 5-year relationship with Karl, the therapist assisted in purchasing for him a colorful bedspread and curtains at a church rummage sale. This improved room was probably the most comfortable surrounding Karl had ever lived in. He had acquired a small radio to listen to the local news and sports broadcasts, and he began to listen to country-western music. Karl's room no longer had the effect of smothering one in dark drabness. Karl smiled appropriately more frequently and created less physical distance. His environment was not rich, but it contained pleasant, positive stimuli, increased warmth, and realism. Other changes could have been made, but it was Karl's home, and his expressed perception was that "It's better than I've ever had it." Years of hospitalization had a dehumanizing effect, providing less privacy, solace and coziness for Karl. He now considered himself most fortunate.

Intimacy within a relationship has a humanizing effect. This emotional closeness provides a degree of "stroking" or need satisfaction essential to feeling level growth. Some clients need to talk and share innermost emotions, conflicts, desires, and opinions. A noticeable reticence followed by withdrawal was usual when the clinician directed conversation to the nurse-client relationship or to matters requiring self-disclosure. Karl's capacity for intimacy was relatively superficial and encompassed his need to share "things" that he had experienced.

PROCESS IMPLEMENTATION

1 — Evaluation

N.D. *Environmental deprivation*
    S "It's better than I've ever had it." "See the picture Mrs. L gave me." "The ball game was good last night."
    O Walls painted green. Picture on wall depicting a country summer day with children fishing. Colorful curtains and bedspread. Acquired a radio and listened to news, sports, and country-western music.

N.D. *Difficulty in life adjustment after long-term hospitalization*
    S "It's better than I've ever had it."
    O Walls painted green. Picture on wall depicting a country summer day with children fishing. Colorful curtains and bedspread. Acquired a radio and listened to news, sports, and country-

western music. Smiled appropriately and more frequently and created less physical distance.

N.D. *Thought disorder*

S "It's better than I've ever had it." "See the picture Mrs. L gave me." "The ball game was good last night."

O Smiled appropriately and more frequently and created less physical distance.

Actual outcome

Karl chose the color of the paint. Volunteers painted his room. Gradually a picture, curtains, bedspread, and radio were added. Karl expressed satisfaction verbally and nonverbally.

2A — Assessment

N.D. *Anxiety*

S "Boo!" "My room rent went up to $5.00." "Joe's goin' to the nursing home."

O Inappropriate grin and disheveled appearance. Long silences. Swinging foot.

N.D. *Dependence/independence struggle*

S "Joe's goin' to the nursing home." "I gained 2 pounds and my doctor yelled at me."

O Game choice checkers, a regressive behavior.

N.D. *Low self-concept*

S "Boo!" "I gained 2 pounds and my doctor yelled at me."

O Inappropriate grin and disheveled appearance. Game choice checkers, a regressive behavior. Long silences. Swinging foot. Mumbling inaudibly.

N.D. *Thought disorder*

S "Boo!"

O Inappropriate grin and disheveled appearance. Game choice checkers, a regressive behavior. Long silences. Swinging foot. Mumbling inaudibly.

N.D. *Interpersonal relationship disturbance*

S "Boo!" "Joe's goin' to the nursing home." "My room rent went up $5.00."

O Inappropriate grin and disheveled appearance. Game choice checkers, a regressive behavior. Long silences. Swinging foot. Mumbling inaudibly.

N.D. *Faulty support system*

S "My room rent went up $5.00." "Joe's goin' to the nursing home." "I gained 2 pounds and my doctor yelled at me."

O Absence of person supports. Absence of problem-solving skills.

3 — Additional nursing diagnosis

None

4A — Variables

Reality timing	+5
Relationships	−5
Stressors and/or crisis	−5
Coping resources	−3
Significant emotional strength	−3
Significant emotional limitations	−3
Therapy relationship	+5
Physical health status	−2
Physical and emotional readiness dimension	+2
Available support system	−2
Meaning significance	+2
Values and belief impact	0
Other	
BALANCE	−

Additional specific knowledge

See case material.

Analysis and synthesis

N.D. *Anxiety.* Multiple stressors, poor problem-solving abilities, and absence of an adequate support multiply the perceived stress in a negative manner.

N.D. *Dependence/independence struggle.* Feelings of inadequacy and ambivalence increase stress of the unresolved struggle. Resolving the episode should promote increased ability to take more autonomous stance.

N.D. *Low self-concept.* Lifelong reinforced belief of inadequacy promotes ineffectual behavior under stress. A positive resolving of the episode should promote new feelings of self-esteem and self-sufficiency.

N.D. *Thought disorder.* A previous ineffective method of coping is resorted to under extreme stress. Despite its negative connotations, these behaviors do draw help and attention of caregivers.

N.D. *Interpersonal relationship disturbance.* Ineffective coping creates distance in existing relationships or association. Attention is drawn to the hurting self, but it only encourages withdrawal and isolation.

N.D. *Faulty support system.* Problem solving and guiding through such an episode should promote adaptation of new coping techniques at times of stress that encourage rather than discourage other support systems.

4B — Design of action

N.D. Anxiety, dependence/independence struggle, low self-concept, thought disorder, interpersonal relationship disturbance, faulty support system.

1. Plan
    a. Find solution to the issue.
    b. Guide client to cope and resolve the episode.
2. Strategy
    a. Active listening and assessment.
    b. Guide client through verbal problem solving.
    c. Support and encourage decision making and actions to resolution.
3. Expected outcomes
    a. Verbal expression of grief in transition of relationship with Joe.
    b. Method of continuing the limited relationship with Joe.
    c. Reestablishment of diet pattern.
    d. Negotiation of room rent with landlord.
4. Criteria
    a. Expression of feelings of loss.
    b. A viable plan for visiting Joe.
    c. Loss of regained weight.
    d. Compromise on rental fee increase.

One such sharing concerned an incident in his residence. Karl routinely spoke with the other four boarders, but this entailed only "Hello," "Good morning," "How are you?" "Goodbye," and other accepted social interactions.

One warm summer night at about 2 A.M., Karl heard repeated loud noises at the other end of the hall. After a lengthy period he began to investigate the continuous commotion. He found an intoxicated roomer, who had fallen out of his bed and was physically injured. Karl, unable to assist the injured man and unsure of what to do, walked two blocks to a telephone and called the landlord, who summoned the proper authority, leading to the hospitalization of the injured man.

This was an exciting yet disturbing incident in Karl's life. He received relief and support for his actions by verbalizing the incident as he relayed the night's events to "his nurse." There are those who would have laughed or even ridiculed Karl's slowness of action and indecisiveness during the actual incident. The sense of security and relative degree of intimacy in the nurse-client relationship allowed Karl to disclose himself and to reveal his feelings and ac-

tions without threat of ridicule. There was affirmation for the outcome from this incident, which was directly correlated to Karl's responsible actions. Others might have done better than Karl in such a situation, but he did gain the needed assistance as well as he could at that point. Positive support allowing for one's limitation without negative judgment can often foster growth.

On one dark, cold, rainy spring day a noteworthy and unforgettable incident took place. The therapist was late for an appointment—a negative reinforcer for trust and caring. As she entered the hall from the outside entrance leading to Karl's room, Karl jumped out of a dark corner, yelling, "Boo!"

Startled but not frightened, the therapist proceeded in her usual manner. Karl's inappropriate grin and disheveled appearance indicated that stressors must be operating to influence his now strange and inappropriate behavior. The nurse said "Hello," while walking into Karl's room where he had the checker board already set up.

The usual pastime activity now was chess, and this game choice seemed to be regressive behavior. Quietly, the two played checkers. Karl's concentration abilities were decreased, his game skill was impaired, and his anxious body movements were obvious.

About 30 minutes into the game and supported by the therapist's quiet "thereness," Karl began letting his worries slip out verbally as he had in the early days of the relationship. It seems that Karl's room rent had been raised by $5.00. This was a significant stressor for Karl. In addition, Karl's friend Joe had decided he could not manage living alone any longer, even with Karl's assistance, and he was about to move into a convalescent care center. This was an added significant stressor. Joe would be within a reasonable distance to allow Karl to visit him, although the visits could not be made daily. The cost of public transportation would tax Karl's already strained financial resources. Furthermore, Karl had gained 2 pounds and had received what he perceived as criticism from his physician. These multiple stressors interacted and led to behavior demonstrating emotional distress. If one defines mental illness as noticeable behavioral deviations that indicate a degree of self-disintegration accompanied by functioning impairment within the culturally accepted norm of a community, Karl's behavior demonstrated this disorganization.

This transient episode of poor coping or decompensation passed in a 10-day period. Nurse therapy sessions increased to daily contact for 3 days, then to sessions every other day until a new equilibrium was gained. Ventilation helped Karl to reevaluate his available effective coping mechanisms. With carefully thought-out support, Karl reluctantly took the initiative to talk to his landlord, who compromisingly agreed to raise Karl's rent by only $3 instead of the original $5.

Karl began some healthy grieving for the loss of visiting frequency in his friendship with Joe, and nursing visits were used to facilitate this process slowly but realistically. A community volunteer service agreed to provide Karl with transportation six times a month. This would afford him the combined supportive service of transportation for medical maintenance care and for regular scheduled visits to Joe.

These solutions allowed Karl to reestablish an equilibrium as stress decreased. There was decreased observable anxiety, allowing Karl to return to a more healthy diet. The regained weight was slowly lost by quarter pounds, again producing needed positive feedback from his physician. A sense of inner security returned and was demonstrated by lengthened concentration periods, more appropriate affect, greater physical energy, increased decision-making abilities, some flexibility in his living style, and new and expanded healthy coping mechanisms.

Karl's striking simplicity and the repetition of nursing interventions could open to criticism the

"core" pathology he demonstrated, the amount of progress in the relationship, or the value of written space given to such a seemingly nondynamic, nonimpelling person. There are many Karls in every community who receive little or no attention until they create a disturbance. Only then are they returned to the hospital for psychological first aid and a new equilibrium.

The only sense of equilibrium available for Karl and others like him is in the stability of a relationship that invites entry and participation in the real world. The process of chronicity of the illness for many emotionally disabled individuals is disrupted through a goal-directed relationship that provides care, concern, positive human encounters, learning, relearning, space for growth, adaptation and change, and a degree of security and comfort. Karl became a nursing client because this profession was the most qualified discipline to intervene in the defined problem areas.

Long-term emotionally distressed persons are a special target group for nursing expertise. Often they have physical health problems, and routine physical health care can break the initial relationship barrier and facilitate interpersonal relating by demonstrating caring. Nursing process has unending potential as a tool for touching the total individual. Knowledgeable deciphering of minute areas of behavior allows one to begin to focus on the problems of another human being within the safe climate and rapport of a professional relationship.

After his initial discharge, Karl never returned to the mental hospital, his abode of 30 years. By all standards his adjustment would be described as marginal. Karl speaks to people today, creates distant social relationships, smiles pleasantly and appropriately when he talks about "my nurse," has good and bad days, is often in a compromised physical status, and can ask for help at times of emotional stress. This may be optimum health for Karl at a maintenance level that was reestablished and maintained primarily by nursing.

SUMMARY PERSONAL PROFILE
Social adjustment

S   "I don't know if I can." "It's better than I have ever had it." "Joe learned my new card game." "Don't got nothin' to say.''*

O   Proficiency in pastime activities and related social and interaction skills. Care, concern, other-centered involvement with friend.

Emotional health status

S   "I don't know if I can." "It's better than I have ever had it." "Don't got nothin' to say.''*

O   Increased concentration and involvement in pastime activities. Body visibly relaxed. Eyes sparkle in reaction to positive feedback. Involvement and cooperation with diet project.

Physical health status

S   "I'm too fat." "I need to sit after walking them stairs." "I take those pills." "Polish sausage and sauerkraut is my favorite lunch." "I walked to church on Sunday. Had to stop to rest four times." "I did lose 1 pound this month." "The diet ain't too bad. Sometimes I sneak what I want."

O   Involvement and cooperation with diet project. Weight loss over 4 years was 10 pounds (195 pounds). Slow but regular exercise pattern.

Spiritual dimension

S ⎱ No noticeable change. Behavior remains
O ⎰ constant.

Daily living skill performance

S   "Always did it this way." "I have a good lunch at noon." "I make my money last all

---

month." "Yesterday I walked six blocks to buy fresh oranges.''*

O   Unable to be gainfully employed because of physical health problems. Responsible management of person, home, and finances within acknowledged personal, social, educational and financial limitations.

Coping skill repertoire

S   "Don't got nothin' to say," "Always did it this way." "I don't know if I can." "Yesterday I walked six blocks to buy fresh oranges.''*

O   Disclosed concerns during a pastime activity. Disclosed troubling life events to clinician.

Maturational struggle according to Erikson's development stages

S   "I don't know if I can." "I decided to buy a radio." "It's the best place I've ever had.''*

O   Basic trust vs. basic mistrust—limited hope.
Autonomy vs. shame and doubt—limited developing self-control.
Intimacy vs. isolation—basic isolation.

Self-integration

S   "It's nice." "It's better than I've ever had it." "I decided to buy a radio." "I like to listen to the ball games.''*

O   Care-concern, other-centered involvement with friend. Ability to disclose concerns and troubling life events to the clinician. Increased appropriate affect. Increased concentration span. Time structure interfering with autistic thinking. Occasional statements indicating a relative degree of enjoyment.

Quality of life

S   "It's nice." "Best place I've ever lived." "I'm comfortable now." "It's better than I've ever had it.''*

O Environmental manipulation, that is, painted walls, pictures, curtains, bedspread, radio, fan, new box spring and mattress. Finances remained limited.

SUGGESTED READINGS

American Nurses' Association: Standards of psychiatric mental-health nursing practice, Kansas City, 1973, The Association.

Bachinsky, M.: Geriatric medications: how psychotropic drugs can go astray, RN **41**:50-55, Feb., 1978.

Beland, I.: Clinical nursing, ed. 2, New York, 1970, The Macmillan Co.

Cancro, R., editor: Annual review of schizophrenic syndrome, New York, 1967, Brunner/Mazel, Inc.

Coburn, D.: The experience of schizophrenia, Journal of Psychiatric Nursing **15**:9-13, Dec., 1977.

Craig, A., and Hyatt, B.: Chronicity in mental illness: a theory on the role of change, Perspectives in Psychiatric Care **16**:139-154, May/June, 1978.

Dixon, B.: Interviewing when the patient is delusional, Journal of Psychiatric Nursing **69**:25-34, Jan.-Feb., 1969.

Hall, E.: The hidden dimension, Garden City, N.Y., 1966, Doubleday & Co., Inc.

Kline, N., and Davis, J.: Psychotropic drugs, American Journal of Nursing **73**:54-63, Jan. 1973.

Kolb, L.: Modern clinical psychiatry, Philadelphia, 1977, W. B. Saunders Co.

Lewis, C.: Body image and obesity, Journal of Psychiatric Nursing **16**:22-24, Jan., 1978.

Ludwig, A. M.: Chronic schizophrenia: clinical and therapeutic issues, American Journal of Psychotherapy **24**:380-399, 1970.

Ludwig, A. M., and Farrelly, F.: The code of chronicity, Archives of General Psychiatry **15**:562-658, 1966.

Mitchell, H., et al.: Nutrition in health and disease, Philadelphia, 1976, J. B. Lippincott Co.

Parent, L. H.: Effects of low stimulus environment on behavior, American Journal of Occupational Therapy **32**:19-25, Jan., 1978.

Ray, O.: Drugs, society, and human behavior, ed. 2, St. Louis, 1978, The C. V. Mosby Co.

Roberts, S.: Territoriality: space and the schizophrenic patient, Perspectives in Psychiatric Care **7**(1):28-33, 1969.

Rodman, M., and Smith, D.: Pharmacology and drug therapy in nursing, Philadelphia, 1968, J. B. Lippincott Co.

Rowan, F. P., Theurer, L. S., and Welch, M. R.; Psychosocial nursing skills, Winona, Minn., 1976, Nursing Consultation, Inc.

Schaefer, K.: The effect of restricted manipulative experience on problem-solving, American Journal of Occupational Therapy **32**:165-170, March, 1978.

Sencicle, L.: Taking the labels off, Nursing Times **74**:52, Jan. 12, 1978.

Stillman, M.: Territoriality and personal space, American Journal of Nursing, **78**:1670-1672, Oct., 1978.

Thurmott, P.: The elderly: a challenge to nursing . . . isolation and loneliness, Nursing Times **73**:1884-1886, Dec. 1, 1977.

Topalis, M., and Aguilera, D.: Psychiatric nursing, ed. 7, St. Louis, 1978, The C. V. Mosby Co.

CHAPTER 7

BETTY L *manifests*
PROBLEMATIC LIFE CONDUCT
evidenced by
SELF-ABSORPTION, INNER CONFLICT, AND A NONAUTONOMOUS STANCE

INTRODUCTORY PERSONAL PROFILE
Social adjustment

S "Hello, yes, I'm Betty." "This is my room. We can be alone." "I have terrible headaches." "It's pleasant here but . . ." "Oh, I can't go out, my legs hurt."

O Self-imposed isolation from social contact. Shares room with an elderly woman in a board-and-care facility.

Emotional health status

S "I have terrible headaches. They last for days." "It's pleasant here but . . ." "Oh, I can't go out, my legs hurt." "Mother and I used to go to church. Now it's too far to walk." "You live alone, who cooks for you?"

O Many psychophysiological reactions such as migraine headaches, hypertension, various menstrual difficulties, musculoskeletal complaints, and chronic gastrointestinal distress. Self-imposed isolation from social contact.

Physical health status

S "I have terrible headaches. They last for days." "Oh, I can't go out, my legs hurt." "Look, I take all these pills, and sometimes they don't help."

O Height 5 feet, 6 inches; weight 135 pounds. Protruding abdomen. Many psychophysiological reactions such as migraine headaches, hypertension, various menstrual difficulties, musculoskeletal complaints, and chronic gastrointestinal distress. Elevated blood pressure familial in nature and controlled by daily medication. Takes barbiturates and narcotics for headaches. At times eyes dull, lusterless, and blood streaked; eyelids edematous.

Spiritual dimension

S "Mother and I used to go to church. Now it's too far to walk."

O Professes to be a Protestant but does not attend church services or any church-centered activities.

Daily living skill performance

S   "I have terrible headaches. They last for days." "It's pleasant here but . . ." "Oh, I can't go out, my legs hurt." "Mother and I used to go to church. Now it's too far to walk." "You live alone, who cooks for you?" "Look, I take all of these pills, and sometimes they don't help."

O   Lost job position. A legal guardian was appointed by the court because of functional incompetence. Cannot prepare a meal or manage a home or finances. Presents a neat, clean person. Self-imposed isolation from social contacts. Professes to be a Protestant but does not attend church services or any church-centered activities.

Coping skill repertoire

S   "I have terrible headaches. They last for days." "It's pleasant here but . . ." "Oh, I can't go out, my legs hurt." "Mother and I used to go to church. Now it's too far to walk." "You live alone, who cooks for you?" "Look, I take all of these pills, and sometimes they don't help."

O   Many psychophysiological reactions such as migraine headaches, hypertension, various menstrual difficulties, musculoskeletal complaints, and chronic gastrointestinal distress. Self-imposed isolation from social contact. Lost job position. A legal guardian was appointed by the court because of functional incompetence. Cannot prepare a meal or manage a home or finances. Presents a neat, clean person. Professes to be a Protestant but does not attend church services or any church-centered activities.

Maturational struggle according to Erikson's developmental stages

S   "Oh, I can't go out, my legs hurt." "It's pleasant here but . . ." "Look, I take all these pills and sometimes they don't help."

O   Basic trust vs. basic mistrust.
Dependence vs. independence.

Self-integration

S   "I have terrible headaches. They last for days." "It's pleasant here but . . ." "Oh, I can't go out, my legs hurt." "Mother and I used to go to church. Now it's too far to walk." "You live alone, who cooks for you?" "Look, I take all of these pills, and sometimes they don't help."

O   Many psychophysiological reactions such as migraine headaches, hypertension, various menstrual difficulties, musculoskeletal complaints, and chronic gastrointestinal distress. Self-imposed isolation from social contact. Lost job position. A legal guardian was appointed by the court because of functional incompetence. Cannot prepare a meal or manage a home of finances. Presents a neat, clean person. Professes to be a Protestant but does not attend church services or any church-centered activities.

Quality of life

S   "I have terrible headaches. They last for days." "Oh, I can't go out, my legs hurt." "Look, I take all these pills, and sometimes they don't help."

O   Many psychophysiological reactions such as migraine headaches, hypertension, various menstrual difficulties, musculoskeletal complaints, and chronic gastrointestinal distress. Self-imposed isolation from social contact. Lost job position. A legal guardian was appointed by the court because of functional incompetence. Cannot prepare a meal or manage a home or finances. Presents a neat, clean person. Professes to be a Protestant but does not attend church services or any church-centered activities.

Time span: 3 years

Betty L is a 38-year-old unemployed, single woman. At the onset of nurse psychotherapy, she lived in a board-and-care home, sharing a double room with an elderly woman who demonstrated transient confused behavior. Ms.

L's living expenses, medical expenses, and personal needs are paid for by an allotment from a social service agency.

Ms. L has one living relative, a brother, Edward, who is severely disabled with arthritis and lives in a nursing home 10 miles from his sister's residence. These siblings have had little communication in the years since their parents' deaths. Betty talks frequently of Edward, usually in the past tense. She plans to visit him but rarely does so. Infrequently, they telephoned one another, but these contacts were acknowledged as unsatisfactory encounters by both individuals when they were questioned about the calls.

Edward's physical handicap is severe. He is dependent on others for his physical needs. Psychologically and socially, he appears withdrawn, uncommunicative, short tempered, and self-centered. At first, the encounters by the therapist attempting to bridge the gap between Betty and her brother were met with verbal resistance and stated disinterest. Edward was more emphatic about his negative tolerance for his sister than she was for him.

Betty and Edward have no living relatives. Their parents' deaths 10 years ago occurred within 6 months of each other. Betty was unprepared for the death of her parents, on whom she depended for nurturance, decision making, friendship, and guidance. She possessed no coping skills to deal effectively with the sudden ensuing grief. Betty worked as a typist for a small insurance office at the critical time of her parents' deaths, but she lived with her parents and lacked the necessary autonomy for independent living. Her mother provided all the comforts of living, such as good food, clean clothes, interaction, and psychological stroking. She watched Betty walk to and from work *each* day just as she had always watched Betty walk to and return from school as a child and also as an adolescent. Betty's mother laid out clean clothes for her to wear to work each day and even helped her bathe and dress. Betty had no idea how to begin to cope with the demands of the real world when her parents' sudden deaths left her to face reality. She could not manage her life, living needs, home, or finances or prepare a meal. Data about Edward during this loss period were absent from the available records. Over several years of unresolved grief, an inadequate support system, and few financial resources Betty became less functional in the real world. She lost her job, and a legal guardian was appointed by the court because of her functional incompetence. She was placed in a board-and-care home at the age of 32 years. All professional attempts to help this young woman to become more functional, productive, and autonomous in the real world had been aborted because of her resistance, increased psychophysiological problems, lack of minimal goal achievement, or any objectively measurable progress.

Betty is 5 feet, 6 inches tall and large boned with a protruding abdomen. Her face is square, with light-toned pale skin. Her facial features are unremarkable except for deep-set, clear, pale blue eyes. They sparkle except after heavy drug ingestion precipitated by frequent migraine headache attacks. At these times her eyes lose their luster and become dull and blood streaked, and she has noticeably edematous eyelids. Betty has soft brown hair styled in a simple cut resembling a popular hair trend of her childhood years. Her usual attire is a simple cotton "house dress," dark flat oxford-type shoes, and a white cardigan sweater worn for warmth. She wears no makeup. Betty is always clean and neat in appearance, but her style of dress adds years to her appearance and indicates her withdrawal from the mainstream of daily living.

Little documented historical data are available in a record review. Progress notes detail various therapists' unsuccessful efforts as well as their futile feelings about their association with Betty. Medical records validated a detailed list of psychophysiological reactions. Most prominent symptoms were migraine headaches, hypertension, various menstrual difficulties, musculoskeletal complaints, and chronic gastrointestinal distress. Collaboration with her physician documented no etiology for her physical distress. Her elevated blood pressure was familial in nature and was stable and well controlled by daily medication. She had several prescriptions for medication to ease her frequent and severe migraine pain. Some of these drugs contained barbiturates and/or narcotic substances. She took no tranquilizers or mood-controlling drugs.

Betty was referred for nurse psychotherapy as a final attempt at specific psychiatric intervention. She had refused to see a psychiatrist, expressing no need for such treatment and rationalizing that her problems were totally physical in nature. Several scheduled appointments with a psychiatrist were aborted by her refusal to leave her room and were associated with several days of acute migraine headache attacks accompanied by nausea and vomiting. Nurse psychotherapy would be accomplished on a home visit basis. It was hoped that this treatment medium along with presenting nursing in a broad spectrum would decrease the threat of needed psychotherapy for this client.

A telephone call to her with a brief introduction of the nurse-clinician secured an appointment for a first home visit. On the appointed day and hour, Betty graciously greeted the nurse at the front door of her residence. She ushered her visitor to her room, where she had prevailed on her roommate to allow her privacy. There seemed to be a pleasant aura of a new experience surrounding Betty.

The room was clean and bright. Soft flowered wallpaper and white priscilla curtains on two large windows gave a fresh and comfortable air to the room. Twin beds with firm mattresses and green chenille bedspread were standing parallel to one another. A rocker, two straight chairs, two chests of drawers, adequate light, a small mirror, a decorative wall piece, and a green room-size rug completed Betty's home. Community bathroom facilities were two doors down the hall. Women residents shared four

bedrooms on the second floor and men residents shared two bedrooms on the main floor. A community dining room and living room or recreation area were on the first floor.

The first nurse-client encounter was pleasant—superficial but revealing. Betty had not ventured out of her residence except for her physician's appointments for over a year. She read the daily newspaper from cover to cover and could engage in a fluent conversation in matters concerning local events. Her memory of the community and its landmarks was accurate. She frequently focused on and asked questions concerning the therapist and about current affairs. She expressed puzzlement nonverbally as well as verbally on learning that the nurse lived alone, worked full time, and had no immediate family in the community. Betty seemed hungry for the stroking comfort of verbal intercourse. She needed to remain in control of the conversation and was quick to inject a new topic if the clinician asked for her to reveal more of her personal self than was comfortable for her. Betty artfully hid her feelings and emotions as well as camouflaged her life-style. One would always question her insight level. The greater part of her energy was involved in maintenance of this fragile security and life-style. Any move by someone to alter the pattern caused conflicts, disequilibrium, and psychophysiological reactions.

After a complete assessment, nursing judgment concluded with the following nursing diagnosis:

Anxiety
Dependence/independence struggle
Low self-concept
Psychophysiological reaction to stress
Self-centered life focus
Emotional deprivation
Low stress tolerance
Acceptance of the illness role
Passive resistance
Controlling (manipulative) behavior
Interpersonal relationship disturbance

Absent support system

Unrealistic expectations in relationships

Inability to perform required tasks of daily living

High blood pressure

Lack of insight

Financial stress

Early interviews were focused on client strength assessment. This effort seemed futile because, in reality, Betty had few strengths. She continued to attempt to control the conversation with her review and comments on newspaper articles, her physical ailments, her increasing complaints about her living arrangements, and her negative opinions concerning the other residents. The therapist finally concluded that reading was an interest, crossword puzzles were enjoyed, and crocheting was a talent of this client.

Despite many power and control struggles and refusals both directly and indirectly to partake in activities, Betty always welcomed the therapist's return. The therapy hours helped fill the human void in Betty's life. The security of an authority figure lent some stability to the disequilibrium she felt in her existence. The nurturance, structure, defined expectations, and limitations of the therapy relationship added a needed reassurance to her floundering ego strength. Any idea of altering her life-style was not acceptable, but the entrance of a significant other into her personal space was accepted. This person was trusted like her mother but was different in that the nurse-clinician mother figure fostered growth rather than impeded it, as her real-life mother had apparently done.

To create a milieu of growth and abdication of unhealthy control by the client, interviews were strictly structured. At the beginning of each session, actual time limits were stated and the topics to be discussed were agreed on by client and nurse. The first 20 minutes were allotted to Betty's complaints. Release of built-up hostility and catharsis were temporarily helpful, but self-discipline and acceptable social

norms had to be encouraged. Betty's sensitivities focused on self and self-protection; she was not other-person sensitive. There appeared to be a direct correlation between Betty's void of relationships and her hostile, complaintive, psychosomatic conversation. Often at the end of the hour, Betty would attempt to continue the conversation, especially if in her self-sensitive perception she thought she had been resistive or uncooperative. When this happened, a date for the next interview was arranged and Betty was encouraged to remember these concerns and conversation topics for the next visit. The establishment of the authority of the therapist was essential to therapy progress. No goals or progress could be achieved unless the client-therapist power and control struggle was resolved. Lack of resolution in such a power conflict binds all energy to an unproductive end.

During each of the beginning months of therapy, Betty's blood pressure was routinely monitored. She was also asked if she continued to take the antihypertensive medication as prescribed. Her answer was always yes. Her blood pressure remained elevated but controlled and stable. The mode reading was 164/90 mm Hg, varying less than 10 degrees in systolic reading and 6 degrees in diastolic reading. Each time her hypertension supervision was implemented, she was given positive, health-oriented feedback as to the state of her wellness. "Your blood pressure is very good. I can tell you are taking your pills as prescribed. Your blood pressure is very well controlled. That should make you feel good. You look good today, too," were typical therapist messages concerning Betty's condition. If Betty heard 10% of the positive messages about herself, it would have been helpful toward reorienting her faulty self-concept. Health had to be perceived as good, for which Betty received reward in interactions with others. Affirmation from person-to-person contact was a missing element in Betty's existence.

Betty enjoyed reading, but the newspaper

was her only available reading source. The therapist brought her several light novels in paperback form and some women's magazines. Betty seemed pleased. She read and returned the materials. Discussion of a trip to the nearby library or book store for reading material was abruptly terminated by an impending headache that loomed more threateningly as the discussion of leaving her residence continued. The environment did provide a false sense of safety and security, but it was the only protective enclosure Betty could cling to.

A comment about the attractive afghan on Betty's bed encouraged her to produce a second afghan that she was making. Her work was of very fine quality, with delicate and intricate stitching that she had learned in her teen years from her mother. Betty's rigid body seemed to relax for the first time in the therapist's presence as the nurse complimented her on this task. Betty volunteered that she worked on this afghan each afternoon. She pointed to an error in her work of the previous day, but the nurse could not see the faulty stitch. Betty planned to spend the day ripping out the faulty work. "If I make too many mistakes I get a headache," she stated. "I don't work very fast either. I know you can't see it, but it's there. I must take it out." This project would take several years to complete because her goal was a perfect product rather than any joy or relaxation derived from her artistic talent.

PROCESS IMPLEMENTATION

1—Evaluation

N.D. *Anxiety*
    S "Oh, I can't go out." "I like it when you come." "My headaches are so bad." "I had a stomachache all day yesterday." "No one likes me here." "She sat in my chair."
    O Discussion of relationships, activities, environmental changes, or problems was terminated by multiple physiological complaints.

N.D. *Dependence/independence struggle*
    S "Oh, I can't go out." "I like it when you come." "My headaches are so bad." "I had a stomachache all day yesterday." "No one likes me here." "She sat in my chair."

N.D.   O Discussion of relationships, activities, environmental changes, or problems was terminated by multiple physiological complaints.

N.D. *Controlling (manipulative) behavior*
    S "Did you see the new post office building?" "My headaches are so bad." "I had a stomachache all day yesterday." "No one likes me here." "She's confused." "She sat in my chair." "You know, I'll always have high blood pressure so I shouldn't get upset."
    O Discussion of relationships, activities, environmental changes, or problems was terminated by multiple physiological complaints.

N.D. *High blood pressure*
    S "Yes, I take my medicine." "You know, I'll always have high blood pressure so I shouldn't get upset."
    O Blood pressure 164/90 mm Hg varying less than 10 degrees in systolic reading and 6 degrees in diastolic reading.

N.D. *Interpersonal relationship disturbances*
    S "Did you see the new post office building?" "My headaches are so bad." "I had a stomachache all day yesterday." "No one likes me here." "She's confused." "She sat in my chair." "You know, I'll always have high blood pressure so I shouldn't get upset." "Oh, I can't go out." "I like it when you come."
    O Discussion of relationships, activities, environmental changes, or problems was terminated by multiple physiological complaints.

N.D. *Psychophysiological reaction to stress*
    S "Yes, I take my medicine." "You know, I'll always have high blood pressure so I shouldn't get upset." "My headaches are so bad." "I had a stomachache all day yesterday." "No one likes me here." "If I make too many mistakes, I get a headache."
    O Discussion of relationships, activities, environmental changes, or problems was terminated by multiple physiological complaints. Blood pressure 164/90 mm Hg, varying less than 10 degrees in systolic reading and 6 degrees in diastolic reading.

Actual outcome
Limited, initial therapy relationship bonding.

2A—Assessment

N.D. *Interpersonal relationship disturbances*
    S "She is in the room too much, talks too much, sleeps too much, is old, doesn't like me, is never nice to me, gets in my drawers, doesn't make her bed right." "It won't help. I don't want to." ". . . She won't talk to me. You know she doesn't like me."

O Refusal to discuss issue with parties involved.
N.D. *Dependence/independence struggle*
   S "She is in the room too much, talks too much, sleeps too much, is old, doesn't like me, is never nice to me, gets in my drawers, doesn't make her bed right." "It won't help. I don't want to." ". . . She won't talk to me. You know she doesn't like me."
   O Refusal to discuss issue with parties involved.
N.D. *Low stress tolerance*
   S "She is in the room to much, talks too much, sleeps too much, is old, doesn't like me, is never nice to me, gets in my drawers, doesn't make her bed right."
   O Refusal to discuss issue with parties involved.
N.D. *Passive resistance*
   S "It won't help. I don't want to." ". . . She won't talk to me. You know she doesn't like me."
   O Refusal to discuss issue with parties involved.

3—Additional nursing diagnosis
None

4A—Variables
Reality timing	0
Relationships	−5
Stressors and/or crisis	−3
Coping resources	−5
Significant emotional strength	−3
Significant emotional limitations	−3
Therapy relationship	−1
Physical health status	−3
Physical and emotional readiness dimension	−3
Available support system	−5
Meaning significance	−3
Values and belief impact	−3
Other	
BALANCE	−

Additional specific knowledge
See case material.
Analysis and synthesis
N.D. *Interpersonal relationship disturbance.* All interactions and relationships must be carried out by the covert rules of the client. She seems to set up a lose-lose situation where no one can win. A sense of satisfaction is achieved in maintaining the stance.
N.D. *Dependence/independence struggle.* Client portrays an extremely dependent life position. Standing back and viewing her need to control, one must wonder if she is not really potentially autonomous but presently using her strength to a negative end.
N.D. *Low stress tolerance.* Client is unable to

tolerate the idiosyncrasies of her roommate. It is significant to note the lack of positive qualities depicted in this other person.
N.D. *Passive resistance.* Satisfaction seems to be achieved from blaming others and from fault finding. Confrontation of the issue is not an acceptable solution, since the client does not desire a solution but desires the disruption from the conflict.

4B—Design of action
N.D. Interpersonal relationship disturbance, dependence/independence struggle, low stress tolerance, passive resistance.
   1. Plan
      a. Confront the living arrangement problem by encouraging client and her roommate to discuss the issues.
      b. Discuss issues with housemother.
   2. Strategy
      a. Support and guide client to define issue.
      b. Support and guide client to confront issues.
   3. Expected outcomes
      a. Resolution of problematical living arrangement.
   4. Criteria
      a. Expressions of satisfaction.
      b. Decrease or elimination of problematical issues.

Betty had numerous complaints about her roommate. Her litany of laments included that she (her roommate) was "in the room too much, talks too much, sleeps too much, is old, doesn't like me, is never nice to me, gets in my drawers, doesn't make her bed right" and numerous other comments. Betty refused to discuss her dissatisfaction with her roommate even if she was accompanied by the therapist. "It won't help. I don't want to," she would say. After some coercion, she reluctantly agreed to speak with the house-mother. Betty reported later than the housemother "won't talk with me. You know she doesn't like me." With Betty's approval the therapist made an appointment with the housemother, only to learn that "Betty can't get along with anybody." It was disclosed that she had six roommates during her several years' stay, none of whom had been considered satisfactory by Betty.

In a matter-of-fact manner this encounter was discussed with Betty. At the time the house-mother had refused any living arrangement changes. Betty would have to cope as well as she could. On hearing this information, Betty hung her head down like a naughty child and withdrew emotionally from the therapist, who again volunteered to talk with her and her roommate to help negotiate the stated problem. Finally, this session was reluctantly agreed on and arranged for. At the appointed time Betty greeted the therapist with a broad smile and the news that her roommate was hospitalized and so "there is no problem." For Betty this conflict confrontation was a dead issue and would remain so until a new relationship problem became perilous and stressful. She refused to discuss the ramifications of her method of coping or alternatives to her unsuccessful coping style. Entrenchment in avoidance and in passivity was reinforced. Betty rested comfortably in her chance victory over the therapist, over therapy, and over health. One had to question the commitment of this client to her life role of illness.

PROCESS IMPLEMENTATION

1—Evaluation

N.D.   *Interpersonal relationship disturbance*
  S   "I suppose I'll have to talk to her. You have to help me." "There is no problem."
  O   Hung her head down and emotionally withdrew from the therapist. Smiled while telling therapist that roommate was hospitalized.

N.D.   *Dependence/independence struggle*
  S   "I suppose I'll have to talk to her. You have to help me." "There is no problem."
  O   Hung her head down and emotionally withdrew from therapist.

N.D.   *Low stress tolerance*
  S   "I suppose I'll have to talk to her. You have to help me." "There is no problem."
  O   Hung her head down and emotionally withdrew from the therapist. Smiled while telling therapist that roommate was hospitalized.

N.D.   *Passive resistance*
  S   "There is no problem."
  O   Smiled while telling therapist that roommate was hospitalized.

Actual outcome
  Problem resolved not through nursing design but because of exacerbation of roommate's health problem, requiring hospitalization.

2A—Assessment

N.D.   *Self-centered life focus*
  S   "Oh, I can't walk, my legs will hurt." "I have a terrible headache." "I didn't sleep much last night." "My stomach hurts." "I'm too sick to do what you want." "I need rest."
  O   Headache somewhat relieved by cancellation of scheduled walk. Headache worsened when walk scheduled for the next day. Rejection of supportive measures.

N.D.   *Psychophysiological reaction to stress*
  S   "Oh, I can't walk, my legs will hurt." "I have a terrible headache." "I didn't sleep much last night." "My stomach hurts."
  O   Headache somewhat relieved by cancellation of scheduled walk. Headache worsened when walk scheduled for the next day.

N.D.   *Controlling (manipulative) behavior*
  S   "I'm too sick to do what you want." "I need to rest."
  O   Headache somewhat relieved by cancellation of scheduled walk. Headache worsened when walk scheduled for the next day. Rejection of supportive measures.

N.D.   *Acceptance of the illness role*
  S   "I'm too sick to do what you want." "I need to rest."
  O   Headache somewhat relieved by cancellation of scheduled walk. Headache worsened when walk scheduled for the next day. Rejection of supportive measures.

N.D.   *Passive resistance*
  S   "Oh, I can't walk, my legs will hurt." "I have a terrible headache." "I didn't sleep much last night." "My stomach hurts."
  O   Headache somewhat relieved by cancellation of scheduled walk. Headache worsened when walk scheduled for the next day. Rejection of supportive measures.

N.D.   *Low stress tolerance*
  S   "Oh, I can't walk, my legs will hurt." "I have a terrible headache." "I didn't sleep much last night." "My stomach hurts."
  O   Headache somewhat relieved by cancellation of scheduled walk. Headache worsened when walk scheduled for the next day.

N.D.   *Dependence/independence struggle*
  S   "Oh, I can't walk, my legs will hurt." "I have a terrible headache." "I didn't sleep much last

night.'' ''My stomach hurts.'' ''I'm too sick to do what you want.'' ''I need rest.''

O   Headache somewhat relieved by cancellation of scheduled walk. Headache worsened when walk scheduled for the next day. Rejection of supportive measures.

3 — Additional nursing diagnosis
None

4A — Variables

Reality timing	0
Relationships	−4
Stressors and/or crisis	−4
Coping resources	−5
Significant emotional strength	−3
Significant emotional limitations	−3
Therapy relationship	−1
Physical health status	−3
Physical and emotional readiness dimension	−5
Available support system	−5
Meaning significance	−5
Values and belief impact	−5
Other	
BALANCE	−

Additional specific knowledge
See case material.

Analysis and synthesis

N.D.   *Self-centered life focus.* Intense desire for immediate need satisfaction or gratification.

N.D.   *Psychophysiological reaction to stress.* Illness and threats of increasing illness are employed to protect the client from new, uncertain, and threatening situations.

N.D.   *Controlling (manipulative) behavior.* Control of environment is maintained with illness. Rejection of the illness stances only encourages the client's withdrawal and increased symptoms.

N.D.   *Acceptance of the illness role.* An intellectual and emotional acceptance of ''I am sick'' seems to be a primary message this client relays. She strongly rejects any refusal of this message with increased illness behaviors.

N.D.   *Passive resistance.* If confronted with the need for more direct action, client stress increases and calls for behaviors and coping skills for which she is unprepared to initiate.

N.D.   *Low stress tolerance.* Stress is perceived in any new encounter and when familiar, protective coping behaviors are ineffective.

N.D.   *Dependence/independence struggle.* Retreat to bed and somatic behaviors validate for others that this client must be ''taken care of'' or protected because of limitations.

4B — Design of action

N.D.   Self-centered life focus, psychophysiological reaction to stress, controlling (manipulative) behavior, acceptance of the illness role, passive resistance low stress tolerance, dependence/independence struggle.

1. Plan
   a. Expand client environment.
2. Strategy
   a. Firmly encourage and expect participation in planned walk.
   b. Focus interaction on positive aspects of life.
   c. Respond matter-of-factly to psychophysiological complaints.
   d. Affirm positive behaviors.
3. Expected outcomes
   a. Walk outside of residence accompanied by therapist.
   b. Walk outside of residence alone.
4. Criteria
   a. Walk outside of residence accompanied by therapist.
   b. Reporting during therapy regular walks completed by client.

The narrow world that contained Betty's fragile person had to be expanded. Her need to remain in control of her environment and her limited vision beyond the periphery of her person, enclosed her in a narrow and unrealistic world. The therapist first suggested and later required that Betty and she enter the world outside her residence. The presence of the therapist was percieved as a negative pressure and a treatening thrust. In a counter-client move, all supportive measures were rejected. Betty retreated into her world of psychosomatic behavior, despite the intitial expectations being limited, clear, concise, and within the sphere of her familiar existence. Life was viewed with blinders, blocking any peripheral vision or newness and safeguarding sameness.

The first planned outside excursion was to be a walk from her home to the corner and return as part of the usual therapeutic hour. Several weeks of verbal gymnastics of resistance were encountered and overridden by the firmness of the nurse-therapist. On the appointed day when Betty had agreed to walk, the nurse arrived to find her in bed suffering from a migraine attack which seemed somewhat relieved by cancellation of the planned walk. The headache worsened when the walk was scheduled for the next day. The therapist did not stay to visit or listen to Betty's complaints but withheld interpersonal reward by leaving. Four such encounters occurred on four successive days before the therapist found the client up, dressed, and supposedly ready to walk. Ambivalently, Betty neither wanted to walk nor wanted the disapproval of her therapist.

Nurse and client proceeded downstairs and out onto the front porch. The therapist talked about the nice day, how good the fresh air felt, and how well Betty appeared. Betty talked about how she felt when she had walked 2 years ago, how weak her legs now felt, how her head was beginning to hurt, and that she was too cold. Betty stopped abruptly and stated she was "just too cold to walk." The nurse directed her to return to her room for a sweater. Some 20 minutes later Betty returned, wearing her sweater but announcing that she was "sick to my stomach" and would "probably throw up if you make me walk." Slowly, the therapist responded that she knew that Betty was anxious about the walk, but she also knew Betty was all right. The nurse stated in a nonnegotiable manner that they would walk one-half block and return. Surprised, Betty restated, "but I'll throw up." Matter-of-factly, the therapist responded that if she did begin vomiting, they would manage the problem when it happened. Nurse and client walked silently one-half block and returned to the residence. The nurse put her hand on Betty's arm to provide physical and emotional support. Betty, although pale and hesitant, did not begin vomiting. Later in Betty's room, nurse and client enjoyed candy as a reward provided by the therapist. Betty received verbal supportive feedback for her accomplishment, and the therapist listened to

Betty's physical complaints and her conflicts of living.

This was a hard-fought game, challenging the intelligence of both parties and the endurance and care-concern quality of the therapist. In a client-centered situation, no one should have to win or lose, but the relationship with Betty almost always remained a struggle between health and illness; between therapist and client. The nurse-clinician does not have the emotional investment in winning or losing or in the playing of the game itself and cannot allow this negative practice to override client-centered, goal-directed care. In this particular situation the game stakes were high for the client. All of her time and energy and her life itself were directed toward maintaining her position and retaining the perceived rewards of remaining ill. Pathologically, Betty enjoyed the games, often receiving stimuli and challenge from the maneuvers as well as from the outcome. Health was perceived as a new and frightening experience. Unconsciously, Betty must have felt she could never play the game of living as well if she were forced to be honest and if she were stripped of the old game skills and covert rules. The new open and honest rules were uncertain and frightening, and the rewards indistinct in her unstructured, impaired abstract thinking process.

The walks continued twice each month. Although at first encouraged and then directed to walk on other days, Betty did not walk alone. The therapist closed the topic, acknowledging the conflict, and focused on other areas needing intervention. Again Betty portrayed a sense of winning. Precious time was being lost in the struggle rather than in the resolution of problematic areas.

PROCESS IMPLEMENTATION
1—Evaluation
N.D.   *Self-centered life focus.*
    S   "I'm sick to my stomach." "I'll probably throw up if you make me walk." ". . . but I'll

throw up." "My head hurts." "I'm just too cold."

O Four encounters where client took to her bed too ill to walk. Pale and hesitant. Silently walked one-half block with nurse and returned to residence. No vomiting.

N.D. *Psychophysiological reaction to stress*

S "I'm sick to my stomach." "I'll probably throw up if you make me walk." ". . . but I'll throw up." "My head hurts." "I'm just too cold."

O Four encounters where client took to her bed too ill to walk. Pale and hesitant. Silently walked one-half block with nurse and returned to residence. No vomiting.

N.D. *Controlling (manipulative) behavior*

S "I'm sick to my stomach." "I'll probably throw up if you make me walk." ". . . but I'll throw up." "My head hurts." "I'm just too cold."

O Four encounters where client took to her bed too ill to walk. Pale and hesitant. Silently walked one-half block with nurse and returned to residence. No vomiting.

N.D. *Acceptance of the illness role*

S "I'm sick to my stomach." "I'll probably throw up if you make me walk." ". . . but I'll throw up." "My head hurts." "I'm just too cold."

O Four encounters where client took to her bed too ill to walk. Pale and hesitant. Silently walked one-half block with nurse and returned to residence. No vomiting.

N.D. *Passive resistance*

S "I'm sick to my stomach." "I'll probably throw up if you make me walk." ". . . but I'll throw up." "My head hurts." "I'm just too cold."

O Four encounters where client took to her bed too ill to walk. Pale and hesitant. Silently walked one-half block with nurse and returned to residence. No vomiting.

N.D. *Low stress tolerance*

S "I'm sick to my stomach." "I'll probably throw up if you make me walk." ". . . but I'll throw up." "My head hurts." "I'm just too cold."

O Four encounters where client took to her bed too ill to walk. Pale and hesitant. Silently walked one-half block with nurse and returned to residence. No vomiting.

N.D. *Dependence/independence struggle*

S "I'm sick to my stomach." "I'll probably throw up if you make me walk." ". . . but I'll

throw up." "My head hurts." "I'm just too cold."

O Four encounters where client took to her bed too ill to walk. Pale and hesitant. Silently walked one-half block with nurse and returned to residence. No vomiting.

Actual outcome

After considerable resistance the client walked outside of her residence with the nurse. Walks continued twice each month in the company of the therapist. Client refused to walk on other occasions despite ability, support, and encouragement.

2A—Assessment

N.D. *Interpersonal relationship disturbance*

S "I think I'll like being a typist again." "Someone to visit with me each week will be nice." "I like people." "Do you think they'll like me?"

O Rigid body posture. Smiling.

N.D. *Psychophysiological reaction to stress*

S "I've been sick for years." "I have migraines, high blood pressure, a bad stomach, etc., etc. . ."

O Smiling as she relays symptoms.

N.D. *Unrealistic expectations in relationships*

S "I think I'll like being a typist again." "Someone to visit with me each week will be nice." "I like people." "Do you think they'll like me?"

O Rigid body posture. Smiling.

N.D. *Controlling (manipulative) behavior*

S "I think I'll like being a typist again." "Someone to visit with me each week will be nice." "I like people." "Do you think they'll like me?" "Maybe they will do . . ." "Maybe she can help me with . . ."

O Rigid body posture. Smiling.

N.D. *Dependence/independence struggle*

S "I've been sick for years." "I have migraines, high blood pressure, a bad stomach, etc., etc. . ." "Do you think they'll like me?"

O Smiling as she relays symptoms.

N.D. *Low stress tolerance*

S "I've been sick for years." "I have migraines, high blood pressure, a bad stomach, etc., etc. . ." "Do you think they'll like me?"

O Smiling as she relays symptoms.

N.D. *Passive resistance*

S "I've been sick for years." "I have migraines, high blood pressure, a bad stomach, etc., etc. . ." "Do you think they'll like me?"

O Smiling as she relays symptoms.

N.D. *Low self-concept*

S   "I've been sick for years." "I have migraines, high blood pressure, a bad stomach, etc., etc. . ." "Do you think they'll like me?"

O   Smiling as she relays symptoms.

N.D.   *Self-centered life focus*

S   "I think I'll like being a typist again." "Someone to visit with me each week will be nice." "I like people." "Do you think they'll like me?"

O   Rigid body posture. Smiling.

N.D.   *Emotional deprivation*

S   "I think I'll like being a typist again." "Someone to visit with me each week will be nice." "I like people." "Do you think they'll like me?" "I've been sick for years." "I have migraines, high blood pressure, a bad stomach, etc., etc. . ."

O   Smiling as she relays symptoms. Rigid body posture.

3—Additional nursing diagnosis

None

4A—Variables

Reality timing	−1
Relationships	−4
Stressors and/or crisis	−4
Coping resources	−5
Significant emotional strength	−3
Significant emotional limitations	−3
Therapy relationship	0
Physical health status	−2
Physical and emotional readiness dimension	−4
Available support system	−5
Meaning significance	−5
Values and belief impact	−5
Other	
BALANCE	−

Additional specific knowledge

See case material.

Analysis and synthesis

N.D.   *Interpersonal relationship disturbance.* At first client illness stance receives attention and sympathy but when client is unable to adjust to the demands of the situation and unable to interact on adult-to-adult level, withdrawal, anger, and hostility occur.

N.D.   *Psychophysiological reaction to stress.* Client is unable to adjust to the productive and interaction demands of the work situation, and she withdraws into safe, acceptable illness symptoms. Anger and hostility are introjected.

N.D.   *Unrealistic expectations in relationships.*

Client seems to expect that no one should put responsible life demands on her. Her only style of interacting is adult-to-child or child-to-adult.

N.D.   *Controlling (manipulative) behavior.* Illness and withdrawal and prominent ways in which the self is protected.

N.D.   *Dependence/independence struggle.* An "I can't" stance protects this client from entering a situation that would initiate or promote autonomy in a healthy, growth-producing, reality setting.

N.D.   *Low stress tolerance.* New situations and new expectations create a stress level that decreases her already low functioning level.

N.D.   *Passive resistance.* Unable to confront the problems, the client withdraws into the protectiveness of being "too ill" to notify the proper party.

N.D.   *Low self-concept.* This client's self-concept is that of a helpless, incapable, ill person who must be cared for. If the energy she expends in maintaining the concept could be harnessed to growth and health, a great potential would unfold.

N.D.   *Self-centered life focus.* Life in protective environment has allowed a self-centered, "me first" life focus. Life energy has been directed inward.

N.D.   *Emotional deprivation.* A normal growth and development pattern was interrupted early with a stunting of emotional growth and an absence of growth experiences that allow the individual to emerge as an integrated person.

4B—Design of action

N.D.   Interpersonal relationship disturbance, psychophysiological reaction to stress, unrealistic expectations in relationships, controlling (manipulative) behavior, dependence/independence struggle, low stress tolerance, passive resistance, low self-concept, self-centered life focus, emotional deprivation.

1. Plan
   a. Expand client environment through a part-time volunteer typist position and with a volunteer visitor-friend relationship.

2. Strategy
   a. Support and encourage self-growth and positive new behaviors.
   b. Focus on wellness and strengths rather than limitations.
   c. Direct conversation in therapy to positive topics.

3. Expected outcomes
   a. Satisfactory production as a typist.
   b. Increased new interpersonal relationships.
   c. Acceptance of a relationship with the visitor-friend volunteer.
4. Criteria
   a. Expression of satisfaction and achievement by client and supervisor.
   b. A one-to-one visitor relationship of quality and duration.

Betty's dissatisfaction with her living arrangement increased. She wanted to move, but there was no adequate facility that would meet her dependency needs. To broaden her environment, she was informed of a plan to have her volunteer as a typist at a church rectory. Surprisingly, she agreed. Transportation was provided, and two mornings each week she went out to her new job. Her typist skills were rusty, but expectations were paced to meet her production level. Betty regained some speed as a typist, but her output remained low because she redid material until her end product was perfect.

At first all of her new contacts listened sympathetically as she expounded on her ills and her poor living arrangement. But all these people had their own tasks and work demands to fulfill and could not spend endless time with her. Soon Betty began to complain about the pastor, his secretary, her volunteer driver, the typewriter, the amount of work, and how extremely fatigued she was from working two mornings each week. Some mornings, Betty did not go to work or did she call in to notify the responsible party, since she was "too ill to get out of bed." After several months of this erratic behavior, her volunteer positions was terminated to the relief of all parties.

As in past situations, she had a migraine attack when the therapist began to discuss the problematical area. Betty was relieved to have aborted this task and once again received reinforcement for her negative behaviors. "No one likes me," she smilingly told the therapist. It would have been helpful but not honest to be able to respond with "I like you." "Some days

it is difficult to like you, Betty" was the honest response she had to hear. She quickly threatened, "I'll tell my doctor on you." Surprised and struck with the insecurity of this young woman, the therapist gently responded with, "You know I won't go away, Betty. I do want to help you." The therapist was to hear this "I'll tell . . ." threat many times during the course of Betty's treatment. Like a child unable to cope in a threatening situation, who yells, "I'll tell my mom" or "My dad will beat you up" and then runs home for familiar protection, Betty was attempting to cope in the same way. The fallacy in Betty's thinking regarding safeguarding her person and a lack of maturational skill in daily living procedures provided a void and ineffectiveness in the familiar but inadequate technique. It may have provided false security at one time, but now this maneuver produced pain and increased conflict.

Psychophysiological symptoms as such are difficult to encounter. When they are entrenched as a significant operational life factor, the pathology has to be acknowledged but carefully avoided by the therapist as a source of gratification or reward reinforcement for the client. There is real pain experienced as the traumatized and weakened psyche bleeds destruction to vulnerable body sites. The afflicted client does experience pain, hurt, and discomforts. Furthermore, the client lacks adequate resources to cope with the affliction or to make the needed life-style adjustments to promote healing of the wounded psyche and soma.

The principle of secondary gains from illness at first achieves the needed psychophysiological stroking of body and mind as encounters produce sympathy and caregiving to console the afflicted individuals. Unfortunately, this consolation is never sufficient to assist with positive coping toward a healthy end. No matter how much solace is given to mend or aid in the individual's required adjustment, the negative behavior remains constant. The positive response and acceptance of illness-related behavior by others usually has a limited duration of effectiveness. Soon, other people grow weary of the headache, stomachache, backache, the "I would if I could" responses to questions, whiny, demanding interactions, unrealistic expectations, and the entire life-style of the sick individual. Secondary gains from the illness stance are short lived, and when reliance on this sole source of gratification is not fulfilling, frustration, conflict, and psychological illness become more pronounced. The dynamic of this behavior was the core of Betty's existence as a person.

Studies of stress and its effects on the body are abundant in the literature. Effective intervention techniques are thorny issues that many skilled clinicians have grappled with. There is no treatment providing the expected cure panacea. Betty had a phenomenal amount of expertise in acquiring personal need satisfaction through tactful deployment of her physical illness behaviors and her precise manipulative behaviors to life situations. The entire focus of Betty's living had been on the employment of these unhealthy skills to gain her desired end or need achievement. Discernment of the at-least partially subconscious nature of this ploy was mandatory. The skill precision comes with a total person and time commitment to this action or more broadly to this life-style. The therapist is in a position of disadvantage in this maneuver, since even if highly skilled in identifying and confronting this game, or negative controlling behavior, the therapist's entire existence between therapy hours is not a thought process with a focus on the needed intervention for the client. The healthy therapist has neither the time, energy, nor desire to devote every waking hour to engaging in "one-upmanship." The therapist must have the qualities of personal and professional strength and objectivity along with knowledge, insight, skill, care, and concern. To stop the vicious cycle of control, frequently the knowledgeable and healthful intervention skill of the therapist is hallmarked by a refusal to take part in the maneuver unless acknowledged ground rules are

agreed on and *adhered* to *without* exception.

Betty retained her many psychophysiological problems throughout the therapy. For short intervals they were relatively dormant, but the symptoms were never in remission. Betty did hurt and her pain was real, and it limited her living mode. It also protected her from those life stresses perceived as a threat or risk to her vulnerable self. The absence of an adequate support system providing healthy encounters and positive, corrective feedback was an obstacle to new behavior adaptation and new modes of coping.

A succession of volunteer visitor-friend relationships was attempted to supplement nurse psychotherapy and to provide healthy companionship and needed human interaction. College girls, young housewives, retired women, single women, married women, church-affiliated women—all offered Betty friendship in a chain of faltering relationships. Betty had objections to all of these people after the first 3 to 5 weeks of contact. They were too old, too young, not her type, or they possessed unacceptable personal qualities. Sometimes she whispered terse-sounding comments into the therapist's ear about these volunteers. "Do you notice how short her skirt was?" or "She wears awful perfume," or "I think there is something wrong with her," or "She didn't believe I had a headache," or "Do you know she told me I should get a job?" All hushed comments came in sarcastic tones with a scowling face and firmly positioned body. A posture of immovable rejection descended when the therapist did not agree with the harsh judgment and changed the subject. A headache was added to the resolute rejection stance if the therapist made any positive comment about the volunteer under scrutiny. In a year's time all resources for a volunteer companion were depleted. Any suggestion of employing a male visitor was vigorously and emphatically rejected. All personal encounters were threatening to Betty's fragile self, but men were a source of much greater anxiety.

All interpersonal relationships, even professional affiliations, were perceived as a new ground to prove that no one liked Betty. She would not abdicate this perception and eagerly accepted all the personal need satisfaction she could absorb. Ambivalently, her psyche was starved for someone to like her and to take care of her, but no one was acceptable in the role. This destructive pattern would have to occur according to her self-imposed rules. In Betty's twisted sense of reality, she believed that if she had physical ills, the health caregivers of society could not abandon her. If she were always ill, she would always be taken care of. Illness produced a sense of security for Betty, and she was staunch in her commitment to maintain this falsely secure position.

Betty's psychophysiological behavior could be contained for short time spans. "Poor Betty" comments were skillfully elicited and amplified by this client whenever possible.

PROCESS IMPLEMENTATION

1—Evaluation

N.D.   *Interpersonal relationship disturbance*

S   "I'm tired." "No one likes me." "I was too ill to get out of bed." "I'll tell my doctor on you." "Do you notice how short her skirt was?" "She wears awful perfume." "I think there is something wrong with her." "She didn't believe I had a headache." "Do you know she told me I should get a job?"

O   New contacts listened sympathetically, at first, as she expounded on her ills. Absenteeism. Fatigue. Unable to follow work protocol. Migraine attack when therapist began to discuss problematical area.

N.D.   *Psychophysiological reaction to stress*

S   "I'm tired." "I was too ill to get out of bed." "I would if I could but . . ."

O   New contacts listened sympathetically, at first, as she expounded on her ills. Absenteeism. Fatigue. Unable to follow work protocol. Migraine attack when therapist began to discuss problematical area.

N.D.   *Unrealistic expectations in relationships*

S   "I would if I could but . . ." "I was too ill to get out of bed." "Do you notice how short her skirt was?" "She wears awful perfume." "I think there is something wrong with her." "She didn't believe I had a headache." "Do you know she told me I should get a job?"

O   Whiny, demanding interaction. Hushed com-

ments, sarcastic tone, scowling face, and firm body position.

N.D.   *Controlling (manipulative) behavior*

S   "I'm tired." "No one likes me." "I was too ill to get out of bed." "I'll tell my doctor on you." "Do you notice how short her skirt was?" "She wears awful perfume." "I think there is something wrong with her." "She didn't believe I had a headache." "Do you know she told me I should get a job?" "I would if I could but. . ."

O   New contacts listened sympathetically, at first, as she expounded on her ills. Absenteeism. Fatigue. Unable to follow work protocol. Migraine attack when therapist began to discuss problematic area.

N.D.   *Dependence/independence struggle*

S   "I'm tired." "I was too ill to get out of bed." "I would if I could but. . ."

O   New contacts listened sympathetically, at first, as she expounded on her ills. Absenteeism. Fatigue. Unable to follow work protocol. Migraine attack when therapist began to discuss problematical area.

N.D.   *Low stress tolerance*

S   "I would if I could but. . ." "I was too ill to get out of bed." "Do you notice how short her skirt was?" "She wears awful perfume." "I think there is something wrong with her." "She didn't believe I had a headache." "Do you know she told me I should get a job?"

O   Whiny, demanding interaction. Hushed comments, sarcastic tone, scowling face, and firm body position.

N.D.   *Passive resistance*

S   "I would if I could. . ." "I'll tell my doctor on you." "Do you notice how short her skirt was?" "She wears awful perfume." "I think there is something wrong with her." "She didn't believe I had a headache." "Do you know she told me I should get a job?"

O   Whiny, demanding interaction. Hushed comments, sarcastic tone, scowling face, and firm body position.

N.D.   *Low self-concept*

S   "I would if I could. . ." "I'll tell my doctor on you." "I'm tired." "No one likes me." "I was too ill to get out of bed."

O   New contacts listened sympathetically, at first, as she expounded on her ills. Absenteeism. Fatigue. Unable to follow work protocol. Migraine attack when therapist began to discuss problematical area.

N.D.   *Self-centered life focus*

S   "I would if I could. . ." "I'll tell my doctor

on you.'' ''I'm tired.'' ''No one likes me.'' ''I was too ill to get out of bed.'' ''Do you notice how short her skirt was?'' ''She wears awful perfume.'' ''I think there is something wrong with her.'' ''She didn't believe I had a headache.'' ''Do you know she told me I should get a job?''

O Whiny, demanding interaction. Hushed comments, sarcastic tone, scowling face, and firm body position.

N.D. *Emotional deprivation*

S ''I would if I could. . .'' ''No one likes me.''

O New contacts listened sympathetically, at first, as she expounded on her ills. Absenteeism. Fatigue. Unable to follow work protocol. Migraine attack when therapist began to discuss problematical area.

Actual outcome

Initially began typing assignment but quickly lapsed into conflict with fellow workers and absenteeism. No one out of a number of volunteer vistor-friends was acceptable to client.

2A — Assessment

N.D. *Controlling (manipulative) behavior*

S ''I would if I could. . .'' ''I didn't sleep.'' ''My headache is getting worse.'' ''I had a stomachache all day yesterady.'' ''I'll throw up.'' ''I need a pill.''

O New contacts listened sympathetically, at first, as she expounded on her ills. Absenteeism. Fatigue. Unable to follow work protocol. Migraine attack when therapist began to discuss problematical area. Whiny, demanding interaction.

N.D. *Dependence/independence struggle*

S ''I would if I could. . .'' ''I didn't sleep.'' ''My headache is getting worse.'' ''I had a stomachache all day yesterday.'' ''I'll throw up.'' ''I need a pill.''

O New contacts listened sympathetically, at first, as she expounded on her ills. Absenteeism, Fatigue. Unable to follow work protocol. Migraine attack when therapist began to discuss problematical area. Whiny, demanding interaction.

N.D. *Low self-concept*

S ''I would if I could. . .'' ''I didn't sleep.'' ''My headache is getting worse.'' ''I had a stomachache all day yesterday.'' ''I'll throw up.'' ''I need a pill.''

O New contacts listened sympathetically, at first, as she expounded on her ills. Absenteeism. Fatigue. Unable to follow work protocol. Mi-

graine attack when therapist began to discuss problematical area. Whiny, demanding interaction.

N.D. *Absent support system*

S ''I would if I could. . .'' ''I didn't sleep.'' ''My headache is getting worse.'' ''I had a stomachache all day yesterday.'' ''I'll throw up.'' ''I need a pill.''

O New contacts listened sympathetically, at first, as she expounded on her ills. Absenteeism. Fatigue. Unable to follow work protocol. Migraine attack when therapist began to discuss problematical area. Whiny, demanding interaction.

N.D. *Psychophysiological reaction to stress*

S ''I would if I could. . .'' ''I didn't sleep.'' ''My headache is getting worse.'' ''I had a stomachache all day yesterday.'' ''I'll throw up.'' ''I need a pill.''

O New contacts listened sympathetically, at first, as she expounded on her ills. Absenteeism. Fatigue. Unable to follow work protocol. Migraine attack when therapist began to discuss problematical area. Whiny, demanding interaction.

2B — Validation by assessment

N.D. *Controlling (manipulative) behavior*

S ''I would if I could. . .'' ''I didn't sleep.'' ''My headache is getting worse.'' ''I had a stomachache all day yesterday.'' ''I'll throw up.'' ''I need a pill.''*

O New contacts listened sympathetically, at first, as she expounded on her ills. Absenteeism, Fatigue. Unable to follow work protocol. Migraine attack when therapist began to discuss problematical area. Whiny, demanding interaction.*

N.D. *Dependence/independence struggle*

S ''I would if I could. . .'' ''I didn't sleep.'' ''My headache is getting worse.'' ''I had a stomachache all day yesterday.'' ''I'll throw up.'' ''I need a pill.''*

O New contacts listened sympathetically, at first, as she expounded on her ills. Absenteeism. Fatigue. Unable to follow work protocol. Migraine attack when therapist began to discuss problematical area. Whiny, demanding interaction.*

N.D. *Low self-concept*

S ''I would if I could. . .'' ''I didn't sleep.''

---

*Same behaviors observed in several situations over extended time.

"My headache is getting worse." "I had a stomachache all day yesterday." "I'll throw up." "I need a pill."*

O New contacts listened sympathetically, at first, as she expounded on her ills. Absenteeism. Fatigue. Unable to follow work protocol. Migraine attack when therapist began to discuss problematical area. Whiny, demanding interaction.*

N.D. *Absent support system*

S "I would if I could. . ." "I didn't sleep." "My headache is getting worse." "I had a stomachache all day yesterday." "I'll throw up." "I need a pill."*

O New contacts listened sympathetically, at first, as she expounded on her ills. Absenteeism. Fatigue. Unable to follow work protocol. Migraine attack when therapist began to discuss problematical area. Whiny, demanding interaction.*

N.D. *Psychophysiological reaction to stress*

S "I would if I could. . ." "I didn't sleep." "My headache is getting worse." "I had a stomachache all day yesterday." "I'll throw up." "I need a pill."*

O New contacts listened sympathetically, at first, as she expounded on her ills. Absenteeism. Fatigue. Unable to follow work protocol. Migraine attack when therapist began to discuss problematic area. Whiny, demanding interaction.*

3—Additional nursing diagnosis
None

4A—Variables

Reality timing	0
Relationships	0
Stressors and/or crisis	0
Coping resources	+1
Significant emotional strength	0
Significant emotional limitations	−1
Therapy relationship	+4
Physical health status	0
Physical and emotional readiness dimension	0
Available support system	+2
Meaning significance	−3
Values and belief impact	−3
Other	
BALANCE	0

Additional specific knowledge
See case material.

---

*Same behaviors observed in several situations over extended time.

Analysis and synthesis

N.D. *Controlling (manipulative) behavior.* Relinquishing control to an authority monitoring a new life direction is perceived as uncertain and perilous. No positive direction in therapy can be gained until a ground rule restricting somatic conversation is established.

N.D. *Dependence/independence struggle.* Client has experienced a rigid life-style. The task of living with a restricted amount of pain-control substances will initiate new, limited self-discipline and limited autonomous task performance.

N.D. *Low self-concept.* Shelter from real world experiences and encasement in a falsely protective environment have limited experiences that lead to the development of a healthy self-concept. Negative, restrictive, or controlled feedback has circumscribed personal growth.

N.D. *Absent support system.* In reality, the client is alone. Cooperation from the housemother and completing supportive tasks may help the client begin to relinquish negative protective behaviors.

N.D. *Psychophysiological reaction to stress.* Client clings to this learned behavior for a sense of security. It is mandatory to this client's potential for growth that somatic behaviors are gradually replaced with more effective coping behaviors. Learned support measures that relieve pain may begin the process of expanding the client's effective coping behaviors.

4B—Design of action

N.D. Controlling (manipulative) behavior, dependence/independence struggle, low self-concept, absent support system, psychophysiological reaction to stress.

1. Plan
   a. Establish a ground rule of no dialogue concerning physical ills in therapy.
   b. Establish a nonnegotiable limit to the number of pain-control substances allowed the client each month.

2. Strategy
   a. Provide supportive measures to develop self-discipline.
   b. Affirm client growth for remaining within established limits.
   c. Expand diversionary activity.
   d. Maintain a nonnegotiable stance for established limits.

e. Allow time for client to express negative ideas and complaints that do not have a physical focus.
3. Expected outcomes
   a. Exclusion of physical complaints of physical focus from therapy dialogue.
   b. Remain within the confines established regarding pain-control substances.
4. Criteria
   a. Therapy conversation excludes physical complaints or focus.
   b. Client's verbal comments, drug inventory, and druggist records will validate control within established norms.

All health caregivers, especially nursing personnel, are educated to ease pain by responding to symptoms with treatment that includes sympathy and empathy for the afflicted person. The only honest and helpful stance for any professional in Betty's care and nurturance was one of objectivity. One must not consciously respond to illness-related complaints while also consciously maintaining the interaction focus on positive, nonillness-oriented topics. Gradually, a therapy ground rule of no conversation about physical ills was established for Betty. At the same time the initially instituted time of client self-expression for other frustrations was continued. This ground rule of the relationship, once secured, was adhered to by the therapist with various levels of client resistance. It was maintained with considerable effort as a nonnegotiable area of therapy.

After collaboration with Betty's physician, routine blood pressure checks were eliminated from the therapy routine. Her blood pressure remained stable and was monitored monthly by the physician. Betty adhered to her medication maintenance program. The nursing suggestion of psychotropic medication to assist with anxiety control and aid in her level of accessibility to psychotherapy was rejected in this collaborative planning effort. Antidepressants were contraindicated, based on the antagonistic quality of her antihypertension prescription to the drug group of choice. Antianxiety agents were discounted because of Betty's increasing abuse of

pain-control substances for her migraine episodes. A plan to control these pain-abetting drugs was instituted successfully by her physician. She was allowed a limited number of analgesic and barbiturate drugs each month. She had neither financial resources nor the needed person resources to implement physician and pharmacy changes. This control was unhappily but docilely accepted.

The pleasure/pain principle resolved the issue. Betty had a limited quantity of needed medication that she had to ration successfully over each month. No amount of bargaining was allowed to increase the drug quantity or dosage. For a certain number of days each month, Betty had to cope effectively or accept the alternative of pain without the helpful drugs. The nurse-clinician supported and reinforced this medical intervention. Effective control would assist in achieving other health goals needing self-discipline. Hostility abounded, but the plan was effective. Antipsychotic agents might have been helpful, but they would not be instituted until Betty had a face-to-face encounter with a psychiatrist. Even the idea of the availability of a helpful drug could not motivate Betty into the psychiatrist's office. She staunchly maintained her emphatic posture of physical illness being her sole debilitating problem.

Despite the hostile atmosphere precipitated by these controls, the nurse-clinician made several nonverbal interventions to bolster Betty's self-concept. The regulations had the effect of shattering her world of receiving what she wanted through time-tested measures. The therapist offered a hand to hold or placed it on her shoulder, adopting a soft steady tone of voice and a warm supportive presence. Verbally, the therapist supported Betty for remaining within the new limits. Comments such as, "It's great you haven't had a pill in 2 days despite having a headache." "You look better to me since you take fewer pills. Your eyes are brighter and you do have pretty eyes." "I know you only slept 4 hours last night, but you slept only 2 hours one night last week." Later, "It's great you slept 7 hours last night. No, Betty, I don't believe you need 10 hours' sleep every night. You're young. You do little physical work and you're getting healthier all the time.'' Betty did not respond verbally. Her rigid composure portrayed her anger. She did not want to be better.

The nurse-clinician helped with maintenance interventions to ease Betty's discomforts without the need for taking medication. Facilitation of remaining within the established limits was of prime importance to her overall treatment and life adjustment. The housemother's cooperation was secured, and remedial measures were instituted. Betty was directed to make a cup of hot black tea to ease her ''upset stomach.'' Hot milk was to be made by Betty at bedtime or during a restless night. An extra shower or tub bath was prescribed to ease her fatigue feelings and restless behavior. A cold washcloth or ice pack was suggested for her headache relief. She was instructed in relaxation techniques and hypnotherapy. Betty was supplied with sufficient reading material of her choice, and the community sitting room was made available to her during its usually closed hours so that she could read during the night when sleep was difficult. This arrangement would not disturb her sleeping roommate or add fuel to their already conflicting living arrangement. Both Betty and the housemother received the emphatic direction that these remedial measures were to be executed solely by Betty without assistance. New residents fell prey to Betty's demands. Older, more seasoned residents ignored not only her complaints but also, sadly, Betty herself. Facilitation of remedial techniques was established. Inescapable reinforcement and emphatic feedback were given by the therapist for any execution of such measures. Betty was noticeably dismayed, openly hostile, increasingly complaintive but adaptive in a limited degree to these measures. Most importantly, when these steps were taken, she received physical relief in varying degrees and her state of health increased despite her resistive stance.

PROCESS IMPLEMENTATION

1—Evaluation

N.D. *Controlling (manipulative) behavior*
S ''I don't like the food here.'' ''Those exercises you taught me help, sometimes,'' ''I don't know why they don't let me have more pills.'' ''I am sick.''
O Routine blood pressure monitoring absent from therapy hour. Rigid posture. Implementation of remedial measures such as drinking warm milk, reading, showering, or relaxation exercise. Maintained self on drug allotment.

N.D. *Dependence/independence struggle*
S ''The ice packs help my head.'' ''I don't know why they don't let me have more pills.'' ''I am sick.''
O Routine blood pressure monitoring absent from therapy hour. Rigid posture. Implementation of remedial measures such as drinking warm milk, reading, showering, or relaxation exercise. Maintained self on drug allotment.

N.D. *Low self-concept*
S ''I read a good story last night.'' ''The ice packs help my head.'' ''I don't know why they don't let me have more pills.'' ''I am sick.''
O Rigid composure. Maintained self on drug allotment. Implemented remedial measures such as drinking warm milk, reading, showering, or relaxing exercise.

N.D. *Absent support system*
S ''I read a good story last night.'' ''Those exercises you taught me help, sometimes.''
O Implementation of remedial measures such as warm milk, reading, shower, or relaxation exercise.

N.D. *Psychophysiological reaction to stress*
S ''I need more sleep.'' ''I haven't had a pill in 2 days.'' ''I don't know why they don't let me have more pills.'' ''I am sick.''
O Routine blood pressure monitoring absent from therapy hour. Rigid posture. Implementation of remedial measures such as drinking warm milk, reading, showering, or relaxation exercise. Maintained self on drug allotment.

Actual outcome
Norm established and honored in a limited manner within therapy to exclude physical ills from the interaction. Client maintains self on a limited amount of analgesic and barbiturate drugs.

2A—Assessment

N.D. *Dependence/independence struggle*
S ''Maybe I should be moved into his nursing

home.'' ''I'm just too ill to go.'' ''My life would be so much better if I were near my brother.''

O   Plans made to visit Edward, but plans always aborted when the appointed time arrived. Taxicabs and volunteer drivers arrived, but Betty could or would not leave.

N.D.   *Controlling (manipulative) behavior*

S   ''Maybe I should be moved into his nursing home.'' ''I'm just too ill to go.'' ''My life would be so much better if I were near my brother.''

O   Plans made to visit Edward, but plans always aborted when the appointed time arrive. Taxicabs and volunteer drivers arrived, but Betty could or would not leave.

N.D.   *Absent support system*

S   ''Maybe I should be moved into his nursing home.'' ''I'm just too ill to go.'' ''My life would be so much better if I were near my brother.''

O   Plans made to visit Edward, but plans always aborted when the appointed time arrived. Taxicabs and volunteer drivers arrived, but Betty could or would not leave.

N.D.   *Unrealistic expectations in relationships*

S   ''Maybe I should be moved into his nursing home.'' ''I'm just too ill to go.'' ''My life would be so much better if I were near my brother.''

O   Plans made to visit Edward, but plans always aborted when the appointed time arrived. Taxicabs and volunteer drivers arrived, but Betty could or would not leave.

N.D.   *Interpersonal relationship disturbance*

S   ''Maybe I should be moved into his nursing home.'' ''I'm just too ill to go.'' ''My life would be so much better if I were near my brother.''

O   Plans made to visit Edward, but plans always aborted when the appointed time arrived. Taxicabs and volunteer drivers arrived, but Betty could or would not leave.

N.D.   *Low stress tolerance*

S   ''Maybe I should be moved into his nursing home.'' ''I'm just too ill to go.'' ''My life would be so much better if I were near my brother.''

O   Plans made to visit Edward, but plans always aborted when the appointed time arrived. Taxicabs and volunteer drivers arrived, but Betty could or would not leave.

N.D.   *Psychophysiological reaction to stress*

S   ''Maybe I should be moved into his nursing home.'' ''I'm just too ill to go.'' ''My life

would be so much better if I were near my brother.''

O   Plans made to visit Edward, but plans always aborted when the appointed time arrived. Taxicabs and volunteer drivers arrived, but Betty could or would not leave.

N.D.   *Self-centered life focus*

S   ''Maybe I should be moved into his nursing home.'' ''I'm just too ill to go.'' ''My life would be so much better if I were near my brother.''

O   Plans made to visit Edward, but plans always aborted when the appointed time arrived. Taxicabs and volunteer drivers arrived, but Betty could or would not leave.

2B — Validation by assessment

N.D.   *Dependence/independence struggle*

S   ''Maybe I should be moved into his nursing home.'' ''I'm just too ill to go.'' ''My life would be so much better if I were near my brother.'' (Comments repeated during four or more interviews.)

O   Plans made to visit Edward, but plans always aborted when the appointed time arrived. Taxicabs and volunteer drivers arrived, but Betty could or would not leave. Plans to visit brother carried through to this point on three different occasions.

N.D.   *Controlling (manipulative) behavior*

S   ''Maybe I should be moved into his nursing home.'' ''I'm just too ill to go.'' ''My life would be so much better if I were near my brother.'' (Comments repeated during four or more interviews.)

O   Plans made to visit Edward, but plans always aborted when the appointed time arrived. Taxicabs and volunteer drivers arrived, but Betty could or would not leave. Plans to visit brother carried through to this point on three different occasions.

N.D.   *Unrealistic expectations in relationships*

S   ''Maybe I should be moved into his nursing home'' ''I'm just too ill to go.'' ''My life would be so much better if I were near my brother.'' (Comments repeated during four or more interviews.)

O   Plans made to visit Edward, but plans always aborted when the appointed time arrived. Taxicabs and volunteer drivers arrived, but Betty could or would not leave. Plans to visit brother carried through to this point on three different occasions.

N.D.   *Interpersonal relationship disturbance*

S   ''Maybe I should be moved into his nursing

home." "I'm just too ill to go." "My life would be so much better if I were near my brother." (Comments repeated during four or more interviews.)

O   Plans made to visit Edward, but plans always aborted when the appointed time arrived. Taxicabs and volunteer drivers arrived, but Betty could or would not leave. Plans to visit brother carried through to this point on three different occasions.

N.D.   *Low stress tolerance*

S   "Maybe I should be moved into his nursing home." "I'm just too ill to go." "My life would be so much better if I were near my brother." (Comments repeated during four or more interviews.)

O   Plans made to visit Edward, but plans always aborted when the appointed time arrived. Taxicabs and volunteer drivers arrived, but Betty could or would not leave. Plans to visit brother carried through to this point on three different occasions.

N.D.   *Psychophysiological reaction to stress*

S   "Maybe I should be moved into his nursing home." "I'm just too ill to go." "My life would be so much better if I were near my brother." (Comments repeated during four or more interviews.)

O   Plans made to visit Edward, but plans always aborted when the appointed time arrived. Taxicabs and volunteer drivers arrived, but Betty could or would not leave. Plans to visit brother carried through to this point on three different occasions.

N.D.   *Self-centered life focus*

S   "Maybe I should be moved into his nursing home." "I'm just too ill to go." "My life would be so much better if I were near my brother." (Comments repeated during four or more interviews.)

O   Plans made to visit Edward, but plans always aborted when the appointed time arrived. Taxicabs and volunteer drivers arrived, but Betty could or would not leave. Plans to visit brother carried through to this point on three different occasions.

3—Additional nursing diagnosis
None

4A—Variables

Reality timing	0
Relationships	−4
Stressors and/or crisis	−3
Coping resources	−5
Significant emotional strength	−4
Significant emotional limitations	−4
Therapy relationship	0
Physical health status	−3
Physical and emotional readiness dimension	−5
Available support system	−5
Meaning significance	+1
Values and belief impact	+1
Other	
BALANCE	−

Additional specific knowledge
See case material.

Analysis and synthesis

N.D.   *Dependence/independence struggle*. It appears that the client's choice in this dilemma is reliance, despite its negative components. The dependence stance is known and familiar but vulnerable to challenge.

N.D.   *Absent support system*. Increased supportive measures from the clinician, the only viable support system available, must be begun with increased presence, feedback, and affirmation.

N.D.   *Unrealistic expectations in relationships*. In all relationships the client expects to be "taken care of," but according to her rules. She seems to need to protect her vulnerability even at the expense of increased physical pain.

N.D.   *Interpersonal relationship disturbance*. Fantasy relationships, such as the one the client maintains with her brother, provides a false sense of security and none of the demands of real-life relationships.

N.D.   *Low stress tolerance*. The fear of the unknown or of what might happen causes the client to retreat to physical illness symptoms rather than cope with the reality of a visit to her brother.

N.D.   *Psychophysiological reaction to stress*. The protective illness stance is resorted to whenever stress is perceived. Since her physical discomfort is real, it is notable that the desired visit to Edward must be perceived as an extremely unpleasant and uncertain occasion.

N.D.   *Self-centered life focus*. Uncomfortable in all life encounters, the client clings to her painful and falsely secure life stance rather than risk uncertain new encounters. Tremendous energy is used in maintaining her position at all cost, since sameness seems to equal safety.

4B—Design of action

N.D.   Dependence/independence struggle, absent support system, unrealistic expectations in relationships, interpersonal relationship disturbance, low stress tolerance, psychophysiological reaction to stress, self-centered life focus.

1. Plan
    a. Institute a spontaneous visit for client and brother to facilitate client's verbal wish.
2. Strategy
    a. Maintain a nonnegotiable stance for established limits.
    b. Maintain a firm, matter-of-fact but supportive stance for client's positive action.
    c. Assess brother-sister relationship.
3. Expected outcomes
    a. Completion of visit with client's brother.
    b. Positive interaction between siblings.
    c. Plans for regular visits and telephone contacts in the future.
4. Criteria
    a. Observation of the visit and relationship dynamics.
    b. Therapy interaction concerning telephone conversations and future visits.

Betty talked about her brother and how she missed him. Verbally, she posed the question: "Maybe I should be moved into his nursing home." Then, she reasoned, her life would be wonderful. Plans were made to visit Edward, but many well-designed visit schedules were aborted. Volunteer drivers and taxicabs drew up to the door to find Betty "just too ill to go." Repeated lack of adherence to any plan that Betty proposed resulted in a nurse-instituted spontaneous visit to Edward by Betty accompanied by the nurse-clinician. Energy directed to action-oriented behaviors was the only intervention to impede Betty's tremendous energy used in plans to visit Edward that were never intended to succeed.

After several empty threats of "I'll throw up," "I'll fall," "I can't," the duo arrived at Edward's nursing home to find he was confined to bed with multiple contractures. He appeared pale, gaunt, and physically compromised. He demonstrated emotional withdrawal by giving little verbal or nonverbal response to Betty's reticent conversation. He groaned and grunted responses, initiating very limited amounts of interaction. After 10 minutes he told Betty and the clinician to leave.

Nursing staff at the facility validated Edward's compromised physical and emotional state, his tremendous physical pain, disability, and dependence, which appeared obvious to the clinician. Furthermore, he had several decubitus ulcerations and a breathing impairment related to his immobility. Betty's emotions were difficult to assess. She did not cry. Furthermore, she refused to discuss her feelings, and she emphatically stated that she wanted to go home. She spent the next 3 days bedridden with a migraine headache, nausea, and vomiting. Thereafter, Betty spoke her brother's name in a passing manner, as if he did not actually exist anymore, when she finally allowed his name to reenter the therapy conversation. She relentlessly and somatically refused to talk about the visit to Edward. Now her brother would never take care of her. There would be no one to meet the expectation of Betty's bottomless need to be saved from the daily living stress and her need to be cared for in a totally infantile manner. Therapy attempts to work through her grief reaction to her separation from family were only met by increased, painful somatic behavior.

One could hypothesize at some length about Betty's attitude toward males, her own sexuality, and the corresponding events in her growth and development years. She was definitely not flirtatious or seductive with men. In the presence of men she was blatantly hostile, offering cutting remarks under her breath. Her own bodily stance was extremely tense in male company.

In like manner her own sexuality was painstakingly denied. Her menstrual period had a carefully maintained aura of mystery. It was always accompanied by many and diverse somatic sufferings and was referred to as "her visitor." She often made contrary and quarrelsome remarks at any outward appearance of the therapist that denoted femininity, especially anything that enhanced her womanly attributes. All possible measures to detract from her own femininity were part of Betty's self-camouflage.

She had taken careful steps to insulate herself from having to cope with her own femaleness. The cocoon this woman had spun around herself for protection and security succeeded in limiting her life with impenetrable walls. Surprisingly, no hallucinatory material surfaced, nor was there any indication of such dormant pathology. No psychological testing had ever been completed. Maintenance of illness and eluding suitable help became tightly entwined inner goals for this client.

PROCESS IMPLEMENTATION

1—Evaluation

N.D. *Dependence/independence struggle*
  S "I'll throw up." "I'll fall." "I can't." "I want to go home." "Take me home." "I'm too sick to talk."
  O Reticent conversation during visit. Spent 3 days after visit bedridden with a migraine headache, nausea, and vomiting. Refused to talk about visit with Edward.

N.D. *Absent support system*
  S "I'll throw up." "I'll fall." "I can't." "I want to go home." "Take me home." "I'm too sick to talk."
  O Reticent conversation during visit. Spent 3 days after visit bedridden with a migraine headache, nausea, and vomiting. Refused to talk about visit with Edward.

N.D. *Unrealistic expectations in relationships*
  S "I'll throw up." "I'll fall." "I can't." "I want to go home." "Take me home." "I'm too sick to talk."
  O Reticent conversation during visit. Spent 3 days after visit bedridden with a migraine headache, nausea, and vomiting. Refused to talk about visit with Edward.

N.D. *Interpersonal relationship disturbance*
  S "I'll throw up." "I'll fall." "I can't." "I want to go home." "Take me home." "I'm too sick to talk."
  O Reticent conversation during visit. Spent 3 days after visit bedridden with a migraine headache, nausea, and vomiting. Refused to talk about visit with Edward.

N.D. *Low stress tolerance*
  S "I'll throw up." "I'll fall." "I can't." "I want to go home." "Take me home." "I'm too sick to talk."
  O Reticent conversation during visit. Spent 3 days

after visit bedridden with a migraine headache, nausea, and vomiting. Refused to talk about visit with Edward.

N.D. *Psychophysiological reaction to stress*
  S "I'll throw up." "I'll fall." "I can't." "I'm too sick to talk."
  O Spent 3 days after visit bedridden with a migraine headache, nausea, and vomiting.

N.D. *Self-centered life focus*
  S "I'll throw up." "I'll fall." "I can't." "I want to go home." "Take me home." "Im too sick to talk."
  O Reticent conversation during visit. Spent 3 days after visit bedridden with a migraine headache, nausea, and vomiting. Refused to talk about visit with Edward.

Actual outcome
  Visit completed. Client's refusal to discuss visit and its ramifications. For 3 days following visit, client bedridden with migraine headache, nausea, and vomiting. Brother-sister relationship does not appear positive or show potential for future development.

2A—Assessment

N.D. *Dependence/independence struggle*
  S "They can't throw me out if I'm this sick." "I'm glad to be gone from there."
  O Revealed that client had verbal outbursts, door slamming, object throwing, and blatant verbal harassment of other residents. Screaming at therapist. Covered head with bedclothes. Took to her bed with a migraine headache.

N.D. *Psychophysiological reaction to stress*
  S "They can't throw me out if I'm this sick."
  O Took to her bed with a migraine headache. Covered head with bedclothes.

N.D. *Acceptance of the illness role*
  S "They can't throw me out if I'm this sick."
  O Took to her bed with a migraine headache. Covered head with bedclothes.

N.D. *Passive resistance*
  S "They can't throw me out if I'm this sick." "I'm glad to be gone from there."
  O Took to her bed with a migraine headache. Covered head with bedclothes. No words of farewell to former living companions.

N.D. *Interpersonal relationship disturbance*
  S "They can't throw me out if I'm this sick." "I'm glad to be gone from there."
  O Revealed that client had verbal outbursts, door slamming, object throwing, and blatant verbal harassment of other residents. Screaming at therapist. Covered head with bedclothes. Took

to her bed with a migraine headache. No words of farewell to former living companions.

N.D. *Absent support system*

    S   *

    O Social Services personnel secured a room. Therapist and social worker packed Betty's possessions. No words of farewell to former living companions.

N.D. *Inability to perform required tasks of daily living*

    S "My headache is getting worse." "I'm too sick to move."

    O Social Services personnel secured a room. Therapist and social worker packed Betty's possessions. No words of farewell to former living companions.

N.D. *Lack of insight*

    S "They can't throw me out if I'm this sick." "I'm glad to be gone from there." "My headache is getting worse." "I'm too sick to move."

    O Social Services personnel secured a room. Therapist and social worker packed Betty's possessions. No words of farewell to former living companions.

N.D. *Financial stress*

    S *

    O Extremely limited resources. No knowledge of cost of living.

3—Additional nursing diagnosis
None

4A—Variables

Reality timing	−3
Relationships	−5
Stressors and/or crisis	−5
Coping resources	−5
Significant emotional strength	−3
Significant emotional limitations	−5
Therapy relationship	0
Physical health status	−3
Physical and emotional readiness dimension	−5
Available support system	−5
Meaning significance	−5
Values and belief impact	−5
Other	
BALANCE	−

Additional specific knowledge
See case material.

Analysis and synthesis
N.D. *Dependence/independence struggle.* The residence change will renew the struggle and force

the client to initiate autonomous behaviors. Support for such measures is mandatory.

N.D. *Psychophysiological reaction to stress.* Illness will not prevent the residence change, precipitated by this client's unacceptable behavior. This will be a prime time to replace illness behavior with new, healthy behavior.

N.D. *Acceptance of the illness role.* Retreat to bed and complete withdrawal from the living activity around her suggests inner fear and uncertainty. The necessity of an actual residence move will precipitate clinging to old behaviors and an opportunity to experience new behaviors and coping methods.

N.D. *Passive resistance.* The new living situation will negate the effectiveness of previous passive behaviors. Survival will demand an increase of direct confrontational approaches to living.

N.D. *Interpersonal relationship disturbance.* The absence of other than caregiver relationships indicates the person void and emotional deprivation in this client's life.

N.D. *Absent support system.* Rejections of most attempts to build a support system make the client alone and dependent. Renewed therapy effort in this area is mandatory.

N.D. *Inability to perform required tasks of daily living.* The learning of several new tasks will be necessary to maintain client's existence. The potential for adjustment is available, but past performance suggests that the client may not adjust.

N.D. *Lack of insight.* Self discernment and understanding are not acknowledged or are quickly denied.

N.D. *Financial stress.* Limited finances restrict comfort and create task boundaries.

4B—Design of action
N.D. Dependence/independence struggle, psychophysiological reaction to stress, acceptance of the illness role, passive resistance, interpersonal relationship disturbance, absent support system, inability to perform required tasks of daily living, lack of insight, financial stress.

1. Plan
   a. Facilitate move and adjustment to new living arrangement.
2. Strategy
   a. Assist with exploration of environment.
   b. Assist with settling-in process.
   c. Support and encourage autonomous action.
   d. Encourage feeling expression.

---

*Absence of verbal comment indicates intensity of problem.

3. Expected outcomes
   a. Gradual, limited adjustment to new living arrangement.
4. Criteria
   a. Participation in settling-in process.
   b. Participation in environmental exploration.
   c. Beginning autonomous life action.
   d. Beginning feeling disclosure in therapy.

Like floods and tornadoes, some life crises cannot be avoided. Unfortunately for Betty, all the signs of her impending crisis were clear but remained masked to her. The therapist unsuccessfully attempted to have Betty confront the facts as they emerged. Betty could or would not be helped, forced, or coerced into coping with this large, looming problem. She had received an eviction notice from her residence, which was based on her disruptive, uncooperative, and trouble-producing behaviors. The eviction order was definitely nonnegotiable. The management of the residence had reached the limits of their tolerance for Betty's unacceptable behaviors. At this point her previously hidden loud verbal outbursts, door slamming, object throwing, and blatant verbal harassment of the other residents were revealed by the management. Predictably, Betty took to her bed with a migraine headache. Her only verbal interaction was to scream at the therapist, "They can't throw me out if I'm this sick," and then cover her head with the bedclothes. This threat to her security was real and unavoidable.

Social Services personnel secured a room with a bath in a transient hotel, but no food service was available. The therapist and a social worker packed Betty's meager possessions into cardboard boxes. She was up and dressed, watching the work and complaining about how poorly she felt while she slowly and hesitantly followed the group to the car with no words of farewell to her former living companions. A brighter mood descended after a short time lapse in the car, and she strongly announced, "I'm glad to be gone from there." Reality could not longer be avoided.

Reality was not pleasant. A small, dark, eighth-floor room in need of cleaning and paint, smelling stale and mouldy, greeted Betty. Its one window was 3 feet from the brick wall of the next building. One could see the street at a distance. The bed was soft and lumpy. The bathroom had only a shower, stool, and sink. Betty loudly lamented, "I need a tub. I need a tub." A small closet, a two drawer dresser, a dim ceiling light, and an even dimmer reading light did little to enhance this room. One wooden chair and threadbare matching beige spread and draperies along with a dark, worn rug completed Betty's new home. She seemed unable to move, and she could not verbally respond. Her affect was flat. This was not the hoped-for milieu improvement.

Betty received her meager financial allotment for the week. The nurse-therapist attempted some planning in this matter, with no demonstrated enthusiasm from Betty. She responded in a compliant, robot fashion to the nursing supervision of the settling-in of her personal possessions. She seemed stunned but cooperative. Finally, she was directed to go with the nurse to locate the nearest eating establishment. Docilely, Betty obeyed. After ordering her meal, she was given the therapist's home telephone number and told she would return at 9:00 A.M. the following day. Ultimately, she was reminded of the location of her magazines, and she was asked to repeat the directions back to her room as the therapist left Betty to have her sandwich and tea alone.

At 9:00 A.M. the next day, Betty appeared in a more conforming mood than she had been in for the past several weeks. This woman had tremendous strength if it could be channeled for health and positive achievement. Direct feeling expression was more prominent than in past nurse-client sessions. She did not like the hotel, and she did not withhold her anger. After some data clarification, she understood clearly that there was no turning back. There were no other available living places, and she would have to cope with this situation, such as it was. This arrangement was acknowledged as a considerably less desirable state of existence by both parties.

The therapist offered to make daily visits for 1 week and then, gradually, over a month, tapered nursing home visits back to 1 or 2 hours a week. Furthermore, the therapist stated that they would explore the adjacent physical environment. Formulation of a program of activities for Betty was begun, and she showed increased positive initiative and involvment in the plan.

The level of resistance from Betty was fluctuating and unpredictable. Some days she was ready to leave her room and even had suggestions for the therapy hour activity. On one occasion she wished to find a beauty shop to make an appointment for a haircut. The task was accomplished with Betty agreeing to return alone to the shop later that week. Betty's hair was cut, and she reported some satisfaction on both a task and interpersonal level. Task completion and achievement was a rare experience for this client. Pleasure from interpersonal encounters was also new and an experience helping to fill an identified void.

The earlier suggestion of a trip to explore the library was begun several times and finally completed. The three-block walking caused Betty's legs to ache, and the library procedure for obtaining a book and learning policies for using the library were confusing to her. Retention of verbal and written orientation material was short lived. She did not return to the library or did she initiate or become involved in a discussion of a return visit. Betty continued to say that she wanted reading material, and she pouted when the therapist would not provide materials for her reading pleasure.

Betty began to speak of ''the good old days at the home,'' and of the many friends she had there. At times she wondered out loud if she could return. Isolation and loneliness were self-precipitated and self-enforced but highly problematical.

Her meager allowance permitted little funding to help enhance her desolate room. Betty did purchase a small radio. All other milieu measures suggested by the therapist were rejected. Unless the therapist chose to complete the task with her, Betty would only assume the role of a passive observer, despite her seeming enjoyment of any noticeable enhancement. The therapist refused to be pressured into assuming responsibility for Betty's task completion. Occasional, pointed hostile comments were made by the client to the nurse about this therapy stance. Validation of reality was an ongoing nursing intervention.

Betty's nutritional status was becoming compromised as she began to skip meals. Her excuses for failure to eat were not plausible, but they were firmly adhered to. Her therapy and medical team refused to supply her with home-delivered meals. She had to leave her room for restaurant meals and be responsible for her nutrition. Betty's complaintive and psychosomatic behavior became increasingly prominent as the stress of her life increased.

The decrease of nurse psychotherapy and the coming vacation of the nurse-clinician were a threat to the dependence of this client. Substitute supportive people were introduced before the therapist's planned departure. On the therapist's return, Betty was a nursing-home patient out of the nurse's usual jursidiction. Factual data supplied to the therapist validated another poor adjustment for Betty, despite the quality and amount of professional care provided to her. In her infantile psychological state, Betty chose illness over health. Her stance and energy were directed to negative rather than to positive ends. The need satisfaction achieved through her life role was perceived as secure once more. The threat and uncertainty of life modification had been too enormous and overpowering for her.

Evaluation through the technique of nursing process assists in professional and personal objectivity and lack of self-recrimination for the therapist. The almost impenetrable pathology of this client occurs in some therapy situations. Community-based care could no longer be considered the treatment of choice for this client. An objective evaluation and assessment of the client-therapist relationship will support and renew the therapists skills in situations where similar pathology must be encountered, with a positive end goal and a renewed self-energy and an affirmative care-concern attitude. Success is not always the most reliable measure of the value in therapy. Measurement that applies the sole criterion of goal accomplishment rather than the recognition of the helping nature of the therapy process is not a valid evaluation tool. Betty's victory was specious, but her perceived triumph was sad. One skilled person cannot perform a therapeutic miracle, but two persons, client and nurse, committed to similar goals, are an intricate part of the working mechanism of a successful therapy treatment program.

SUMMARY PERSONAL PROFILE*
Social adjustment

S ⎱ Confined in a skilled care facility. Ineffective coping style, impaired interacting manner, and negative behavior patterns unO ⎰ altered and retained as immutable.

---

*A revised plan of action could be initiated with an available nurse-clinician from within the system of the confined setting. The boundaries of the setting may allow for a new, more structured intervention restricting the client to fewer illness options. It is important to note that this is a crucial time for decision making regarding the initiation of an intense treatment regimen in a psychiatric setting. The option may be viewed as the last or only turning point for positive behavior change for this client. A diminished capacity to alter life-style and an atrophy of living skills becomes a variable influencing the client's behavior when chronicity is integrated into her life stance. The 3 years of nurse-client interaction provide accurate data to plan a new comprehensive inpatient treatment program. This terminated relationship can also provide the impetus for intial relationship dynamics that contain fewer impediments to bonding, growth, and healthy interpersonal encounters.

Emotional health status

S ⎱ Confined in a skilled care facility. Ineffective coping style, impaired interacting manner, and negative behavior patterns O ⎰ unaltered and retained as immutable.

Physical health status

S ⎱ Confined in a skilled care facility. Ineffective coping style, impaired interacting manner, and negative behavior patterns O ⎰ unaltered and retained as immutable.

Spiritual dimension

S ⎱ Confined in a skilled care facility. Ineffective coping style, impaired interacting manner, and negative behavior patterns O ⎰ unaltered and retained as immutable.

Daily living skill performance

S ⎱ Confined in a skilled care facility. Ineffective coping style, impaired interacting manner, and negative behavior patterns O ⎰ unaltered and retained as immutable.

Coping skill repertoire

S ⎱ Confined in a skilled care facility. Ineffective coping style, impaired interacting manner, and negative behavior patterns O ⎰ unaltered and retained as immutable.

Maturational struggle according to Erikson's developmental stages

S ⎱ Confined in a skilled care facility. Ineffective coping style, impaired interacting manner, and negative behavior patterns O ⎰ unaltered and retained as immutable.

Self-integration

S ⎱ Confined in a skilled care facility. Ineffective coping style, impaired interacting manner, and negative behavior patterns O ⎰ unaltered and retained as immutable.

Quality of life

S ⎫ Confined in a skilled care facility. In-
  ⎪ effective coping style, impaired interacting
  ⎬ manner, and negative behavior patterns
O ⎭ unaltered and retained as immutable.

SUGGESTED READINGS

American Nurses' Association: Standards of psychiatric mental-health nursing practice, Kansas City, 1973, The Association.

Becker, M. H.: The health belief model and sick role behavior, Nursing Digest **6:**35-40, Spring, 1978.

Beland, I.: Clinical nursing, ed. 2, New York, 1970, Macmillan Publishing Co., Inc.

Chavegny, K.: Psychosomatic illness and personality, Journal of Psychiatric Nursing **7:**261-266, Dec., 1967.

Kerr, N.: Anxiety: Theoretical considerations, Perspectives in Psychiatric Care **16:**36-40, Jan./Feb., 1978.

Kolb, L.: Modern clinical psychiatry, Philadelphia, 1977, W. B. Saunders Co.

Peplau, H.: Professional closeness, Nursing Forum **8**(4):342-360, 1969.

Price, K.: Treating psychosomatic disorders with behavior therapy, Nursing Digest **3:**12-17, Nov./Dec., 1975.

Ray, O.: Drugs, society, and human behavior, ed. 2, St. Louis, 1978, The C. V. Mosby Co.

Rodman, M., and Smith, D.: Pharmacology and drug therapy in nursing, Philadelphia, 1968, J. B. Lippincott Co.

Rouhani, G.: Understanding anxiety, Nursing Mirror **146:**25-27, March 9, 1978.

Rubin, T.: The angry book, New York, 1969, Collier Books.

Selye, H.: The physiology and pathology of exposure to stress, Montreal, 1950, Acta.

Selye, H.: The stress of life, New York, 1976, McGraw-Hill Book Co.

Shontz, F.: The psychological aspects of physical illness and disability, New York, 1957, Macmillan Publishing Co., Inc.

Sloboda, S.: Understanding patient behavior, Nursing '77 **7:**74-77, Sept., 1977.

Uhely, G.: What is realistic emotional support? American Journal of Nursing **68:**758-762, April, 1968.

Woolstone, A. S.: Stress—a call for a humane approach, Nursing Times **74:**599-600, April 6, 1978.

Yoder, J.: Alienation as a way of life, Perspectives in Psychiatric Care **15:**66-71, Jan./Feb., 1977.

CHAPTER 8

MARY M *manifests*

PROBLEMATIC LIFE CONDUCT

evidenced by

ANGER AND SELF-DESTRUCTIVE BEHAVIOR

INTRODUCTORY PERSONAL PROFILE
Social adjustment

S "Hello! You must be my nurse." "I've been waiting for you. Come on up. I have hot coffee and fresh cake ready." "I know it's early to eat, but I made this just for you. You can't disappoint me with a no to my cake. I'll have just a little piece. You know I'm on a diet."

O Receives adequate alimony support. Has no marketable employment skill. Talked at length and uninterruptedly about her divorce, her hospitalization, her child-rearing years, and how much better her life was now. Noticeably absent from her conversation is mention of friends or significant other people in her life.

Emotional health status

S "Hello! You must be my nurse." "I've been waiting for you. Come on up. I have hot coffee and fresh cake ready." "I know it's early to eat, but I made this just for you. You can't disappoint me with a no to my cake. I'll have just a little piece. You know I'm on a diet."

O Order or lack of order in home evidences stress level. Constant fatigue. Talkcd at length and uninterruptedly about her divorce, her hospitalization, her child-rearing years, and how much better her life was now. Noticeably absent from her conversation is mention of friends or significant other people in her life.

Physical health status

S "I feel OK. I'm not sick, so why should I take pills?"

O Height 5 feet, 2 inches. Weight 350 pounds. Hypertension. Breathing difficulty on exertion. Constant fatigue. Limited exercise. Repeated refusal to follow prescribed medical regimen.

Spiritual dimension

S "I wasn't brought up to go to church." "Never seemed to want to join a church; thought about it when the kids were little."

129

O   Does not subscribe to a defined religious denomination or belief.

Daily living skill performance

S   "I've been waiting for you. Come on up. I have hot coffee and fresh cake ready." "I know it's early to eat, but I made this just for you. You can't disappoint me with a no to my cake. I'll have just a little piece. You know I'm on a diet." "I'm too tired to go out much." "I'm all right here." "Some of my friends don't like me anymore." "I feel OK. I'm not sick, so why should I take pills?"

O   Usually clean, bright, tasteful home environment. Food and kitchen are center of life activity. Frequent rest periods. Frequent T.V. viewing. Neat, clean appearance. Clothing pulled and torn at seams.

Coping skill repertoire

S   "I've been waiting for you. Come on up. I have hot coffee and fresh cake ready." "I know it's early to eat, but I made this just for you. You can't disappoint me with a no to my cake. I'll have just a little piece. You know I'm on a diet."

O   Talked at length and uninterruptedly about her divorce, her hospitalization, her child-rearing years, and how much better her life was now. Noticeably absent from her conversation is mention of friends or significant other people in her life.

Maturational struggle according to Erikson's developmental stages

S   "I like it here, I have no need to go out." "You can't disappoint me with a no to my cake." "Some of my friends don't like me anymore."

O   Basic trust vs. basic mistrust.
Dependence vs. independence.
Intimacy vs. isolation.

Self-integration

S   "I like it here, I have no need to go out." "I'm too tired to go out much." "Some of my friends don't like me anymore." "I feel OK. I'm not sick, so why should I take pills?" "I know it's early to eat, but I made this for you. You can't disappoint me with a no to my cake. I'll have just a little piece. You know I'm on a diet."

O   Order or lack of order in home environment evidences stress. Talked at length and uninterruptedly about her divorce, her hospitalization, her child-rearing years, and how much better her life was now. Noticeably absent from her conversation is mention of friends or significant other people in her life.

Quality of life

S   "I like it here, I have no need to go out." "I'm too tired to go out much." "Some of my friends don't like me anymore." "I feel OK. I'm not sick, so why should I take pills?"

O   Usually clean, bright, tasteful home environment. Talked at length and uninterruptedly about her divorce, her hospitalization, her child-rearing years, and how much better her life was now. Noticeably absent from her conversation is mention of friends or significant other people in her life.

Time span: 3 years

Mary M is a 45-year-old divorced woman who lives alone in a small one-bedroom, centrally located apartment. Alimony payments, received on the fifteenth day of each month, are adequate support to provide for her needs. Mary has not had steady, gainful employment since she married at 20 years of age. She also has not completed high school and has no marketable employment skill. On occasion, she babysits for friends of her grown children.

Mary was divorced at 38 years of age. She

has three married children, two daughters and a son, but none of her children lives within a hundred miles of her home. They telephone and write to their mother regularly. They verbally express an affectionate relationship with her, although none of them expresses a desire or willingness to spend any lengthy time with her. They accept their mother as she is but tend to view her as an eccentric person.

Mary is 5 feet, 2 inches tall and weighs 350 pounds. Her enormous size seems to overshadow her round, pretty face. Her features are especially attractive when she applies makeup tastefully, styles her hair, and smiles. On first impression, despite her size, this woman portrays a meek and defenseless stance. Her initially soft-spoken manner does not betray an inner hostility or her erratic but covert negative acting-out behaviors.

Mary's apartment is tastefully decorated with contemporary-style furnishings. The rooms are usually clean, bright, warm, and comfortable. The personal mood of this client is reflected either in the orderliness or in the lack of order in her home. The usual harmony and tidiness become quickly disheveled when Mary is experiencing fragmented thinking and stress beyond her low level of tolerance for anxiety. At these times she becomes unkempt in appearance, speaks loudly with pressured speech, and often resorts to foul language. The dichotomy between Mary's behavior under stress and her behavior at less anxious times is striking and announced by her living environment.

Mary received treatment in a state psychiatric facility for two months immediately following her divorce. An available record review provides little history or treatment data about this episode or the consequent follow-up care. Apparently her psychiatric therapy depended on her erratic and uncooperative behavior rather than on a restoration or maintenance program. She was referred for nurse psychotherapy for both assessment and treatment of her obesity and stress-related problematical behaviors. It

was expected from the onset that a consistent treatment program would provide a more homogeneous state for this client. At the point of referral, Mary did not take any psychotropic medication. She did, however, have a prescription for an antihypertensive medication and potassium supplements. Mary openly admitted she took this medicine only when she felt like it rather than according to the twice-daily regimen prescribed by her physician. "I feel O.K. I'm not sick, so why should I take pills," was Mary's protective rationale, a faulty cover for her low self-concept.

Unpredictably, according to past caregivers' records, Mary was open to and even sounded eager for a home visit when the clinician telephoned to arrange for the first appointment. Mary gave the nurse adequate directions and was observed watching the nurse's arrival from her apartment window. Her door was open and she was smiling. "Hello! You must be my nurse," she called from the top of a narrow, steep flight of stairs that led from the outside entrance to her apartment. "I've been waiting for you. Come on up. I have hot coffee and fresh cake ready," was Mary's loud welcome as the nurse cautiously climbed the treacherous stairs.

Mary's hostessing efforts were an attempt to please, but they were overpowering. Her speech was pressured as she tried to make the clinician welcome and comfortable. Name introductions and other comments about the environment were exchanged as Mary ushered the nurse to the table saying, "I know it's early to eat, but I made this just for you. You can't disappoint me with a no to my cake. I'll have just a little piece. You know I'm on a diet."

All comments to redirect the conversation were futile. The client and therapist ate as Mary talked at length and uninterruptedly about her divorce, her hospitalization, her child-rearing years, and how much better her life was now. A hint of loneliness crept through her monologue. Noticeably absent from this speech was any mention of friends or significant other people

Mary's self-protective maneuver was revealing in itself.

After 2 hours and a second piece of cake for the therapist, Mary seemed less anxious. Her speech was less rapid, her body less rigid, and her smile more relaxed and visible. The clinician's nursing judgment concluded that the establishment of trust and the formation of bonds in this professional relationship would take time. Initial rapport had been established, but a climate of trust and an atmosphere promoting growth would stabilize with exposure and experiential realizations for the client.

In an attempt to summarize and close the initial interview, the therapist made several statements in a warm, caring manner but with authority. Mary was complimented on her cake but asked to reserve her culinary delights for future, special occasion visits that the client and nurse would plan together. The nurse stated distinctly that the therapy purpose was to help Mary cope with present stress and problems and not to focus on past events. Mary was requested to reflect on this message and be ready to help plan her therapy goals with the nurse on the next visit. In a less verbal stance but without hesitation Mary agreed to a time for a second visit during the following week.

Initial visits would have to be strictly structured by the therapist to assist the client's fragile psyche and faulty self-esteem and to maintain a focus on the defined therapy problems and resultant goals.

Nursing assessment and a review of available medical and psychiatric records assisted the clinician in formulating the following nursing diagnosis:

Anxiety
Dependence/independence struggle
Low self-concept
Suicide potential
Thought disorder
Trust/mistrust struggle
Suspicious behavior
Interpersonal relationship disturbance

Emotional deprivation
Faulty support system
Loneliness
Faulty self-image
Low stress tolerance
Unstructured life-style
Lack of insight
Antisocial and abusive behavior
Obesity
High blood pressure

The second nurse-client session was important to the overall therapy and the professional relationship itself. In such a case the clinician must present the problematical areas in an open and honest manner while decreasing the perceived threat of therapy. Interpersonal relationships of any kind were a risk for this client. Previous hurtful relationship experiences had left Mary frightened and vulnerable. She did not know how to begin or to proceed, and she had an insatiable need to be liked by others. The thin facade she wore for this end achievement also prevented her from reaching the desired and reasonable goal. Mary needed to feel liked through self-achieved positive encounters.

PROCESS IMPLEMENTATION

1—Evaluation

N.D.   *Anxiety*

   S   "I've been waiting for you. Come on up. I have hot coffee and fresh cake ready."

   O   Watching nurse's arrival from apartment window. Speech loud and pressured. Conversation focus on things and events; noticeably absent is mention of friends or significant others. After 2 hours' time, speech less rapid, body less rigid, smile more relaxed and apparent.

N.D.   *Low self-concept*

   S   "I know it's early to eat, but I made this just for you. You can't disappoint me with a no to my cake. I'll have just a little piece. You know I'm on a diet."

   O   Conversation focus on things and events; noticeably absent is mention of friends or significant others.

N.D.   *Loneliness*

   S   "Oh, yes, come anytime to visit." "You can come today if you wish."

O Conversation focus on things and events, noticeably absent is mention of friends or significant others.

N.D. *Obesity*

S "I've been waiting for you. Come on up. I have hot coffee and fresh cake ready." "I know it's early to eat, but I made this just for you. You can't disappoint me with a no to my cake. I'll have just a little piece. You know I'm on a diet."

O Height 5 feet, 2 inches. Weight 350 pounds.

N.D. *Hypertension*

S "I feel OK. I'm not sick, so why should I take pills?"

O Medical history validates hypertension.

Actual outcome

Initial rapport established.

2A — Assessment

N.D. *Anxiety*

S "My 'nerves' are bad." "You won't tell anyone about me?"

O Speech loud and pressured. Some pacing.

N.D. *Obesity*

S "I'll think about what to do, but I like food and I don't eat much."

O Height 5 feet, 2 inches. Weight 350 pounds.

N.D. *High blood pressure*

S "No, you can't take my blood pressure." "I don't want you snooping in my pills."

O Medical history validates hypertension.

N.D. *Low self-concept*

S "There is no help for me. There is nothing that will work." "My 'nerves' are bad." "You won't tell anyone about me?"

O Inability to accept physical health problems.

N.D. *Trust/mistrust struggle*

S "My 'nerves' are bad." "You won't tell anyone about me?" "There is no help for me. There is nothing that will work." "No, I don't want you snooping in my pills."

O Many questions testing nurse's motivation and action.

N.D. *Dependence/independence struggle*

S "You won't tell anyone about me?" "I'll think about what to do, but I like food and I don't eat much." "No, you can't take my blood pressure." "I don't want you snooping in my pills." "There is no help for me. There is nothing that will work." "My 'nerves' are bad." "You won't tell anyone about me?"

O Faulty decision-making mechanisms.

3 — Additional nursing diagnosis

None

4A — Variables

Reality timing	−2
Relationships	−3
Stressors and/or crisis	−2
Coping resources	−3
Significant emotional strength	−3
Significant emotional limitations	−3
Therapy relationship	−1
Physical health status	−2
Physical and emotional readiness dimension	−4
Available support system	−3
Meaning significance	−3
Values and belief impact	−3
Other	
BALANCE	−

Additional specific knowledge

See case material.

Analysis and synthesis

N.D. *Anxiety.* Chronic, intense anxiety and loneliness motivate the client to reach out, but her harsh manner and stress-related behaviors seem to have an unwanted effect on interaction with others.

N.D. *Obesity.* Food provides satisfaction and comfort, needs that are not currently met from limited available person resources. Lifestyle must be broadened to find new sources of need gratification.

N.D. *High blood pressure.* Unable to cope effectively with the existence of an actual health problem and its resultant increase of uncertainty in her life. Client denies the problem, since she "feels good."

N.D. *Low self-concept.* Withdrawal, obesity, and pressured interaction style seem to elicit negative feedback and reinforce negative self-esteem.

N.D. *Trust/mistrust struggle.* A life stance of mistrust multiplied by negative interactions, dwelling on the past, and holding grudges block present trust relationships. Open questioning, inner pain, and the actual dependence of the client may decrease some of the restrictions to trust within the therapy relationship.

N.D. *Dependence/independence struggle.* Unmet dependency needs, chronic stress, and inaccurate perception of a caregiver as strong, nurturing, supportive, and all-giving provide the client with a false sense of autonomy.

4B — Design of action

N.D. Anxiety, obesity, high blood pressure, low self-concept, trust/mistrust struggle, dependence/independence struggle.

1. Plan
   a. Focus on acknowledged problems of stress, obesity, and high blood pressure.
   b. Involve Mary in plan to alleviate problems.
2. Strategy
   a. Structure interview.
   b. Demonstrate warm, care-concern manner and interest.
   c. Expect client to participate in plan but allow for limitations and negotiation.
   d. Actively listen to actual client message.
3. Expected outcomes
   a. Involvement in diet plan and execution.
   b. Weekly monitoring of blood pressure and antihypertensive drugs.
   c. Limited, here-and-now disclosure of stress-related problems.
4. Criteria
   a. Initial weight loss.
   b. Weekly monitoring of blood pressure and antihypertensive drugs.
   c. Self-disclosure in therapy.

The clinician approached the second interview with a structured format and a warm care-concern manner. First, she honestly complimented Mary on extending herself to the nurse. "You made me feel very comfortable last week, Mary. I know you went to a lot of work preparing for my coming. You don't have to do anything out of the usual for my visits. I prefer that you save your energy for our work." The sessions were defined as health work. The therapist acknowledged that Mary had problems with stress, obesity, and hypertension.

Mary agreed with the therapist's broad assessment of her problematic areas but offered no other comments. On questioning, Mary stated that she had contemplated her concerns but that "There is no help for me. There is nothing that will work." As the hour progressed, the therapist proposed a plan for the identified areas. Mary objected to routine blood pressure monitoring and refused to allow the clinician to evaluate her medication regimen. Mary could not deny that she was obese, and she reluctantly agreed to spent the next visits developing an acceptable weight-reduction program. "I'll think about what to do, but I like food and I don't eat much." Surprisingly, Mary seemed eager to

have someone help her with her "nerves." An expansion of the confidential nature of the relationship reassured Mary that the nurse "wouldn't tell anyone about her." The second session drew to an end with the nurse refusing a piece of fresh banana cream pie. Intellectually, the therapy plan was outlined and agreed on. The planned intervention would not be easy to begin or achieve, since Mary was not emotionally committed to the stated goals.

Negotiation of a compromised physical health status is not usually a sound principle of beginning therapy, especially when these considerations can be detrimental to life. Weight and stress reduction would assist with containing Mary's hypertension. She needed personal space to allow for a feeling of self-control in the face of her extremely fragile and faltering person and overall low self-concept. Extensive, confining limits would negatively affect the therapy climate and the bonding of the professional relationship. Mary was free to reject the acknowledgement of one problem, but the other two problems had to be encountered to a degree of resolution. Reasonable limits for therapy would further establish trust and confidence and would promote self-growth within a sturdy framework built around a care concern, durable interpersonal encounter.

The third visit began with a reaffirmation of the agreed-on goals and supportive measures to enhance Mary's inner feelings that she was, indeed, a good, likeable, and acceptable person. She rambled on about being unhappy and expounded on many past hurts. All intervention measures to focus on the present were thwarted or greeted with a vague, inconclusive response.

The therapist redirected the topic to the broad focus of obesity. Mary had no plan, commenting, "I'm just fat. Nothing works." She was asked to share past weight-reduction efforts. It was revealed that she had begun many diets, including medically supervised plans, group efforts, and fad reduction programs. Most of these struggles were only temporarily effective and resulted ultimately in an increased weight gain. Mary had tears in her eyes as she told of the thousands of pounds she had lost in her lifetime. "It's just no good," she said. Assuringly, she was informed that she must begin again.

The therapist asked Mary to reconstruct her average day, week, and month as the therapy visits stretched over several months. This dialogue provided the therapist with information about Mary's life-style. She had little exercise each week, resting for the greater amount of each day to ease her fatigue. The passivity of T.V. viewing consumed many hours. Outside excursions were food centered for a meal or to grocery shop. Mary had no meal plan or time schedule. She ate when she was hungry, often whatever was available. It was true that Mary ate in small quantities, but she also ate very frequently. Pleasurable, high-calorie foods were always available in her home. Her limited energy was used to pursue her highly developed culinary talents. There is no doubt that she was an accomplished and talented cook. Mary acknowledged the existence of few friends or acquaintances, and actual encounters with these people were even fewer in number.

An initial effort for her to begin walking outside her apartment was met with strong verbal resistance and the lament, "I can't go. I have no clothes," and "The stairs are too hard for me to walk. My legs hurt, and I can't breathe so good." Mary continued to have little if any emotional investment in weight reduction. Her lament of, "I want to but I can't, I've tried, too many times before, it won't work anyway," continued in a whiny, helpless little girl's voice and posture.

PROCESS IMPLEMENTATION

1—Evaluation

N.D. *Anxiety*

S "I'm so unhappy" (Repeated four times.) "My feelings were hurt when . . ." (Repeated six times.)

O Whiny voice. Helpless posture. Verbally resistive to helping measures.

N.D. *Obesity*

S "I'm just fat. Nothing works." "It's just no good."

O Had little exercise, resting for the greater part of each day to ease fatigue. T.V. viewing consumed many hours. Activity food centered for a meal or to grocery shop. Ate *often* in small quantities. Talented cook.

N.D. *High blood pressure*

S "I'm just fat. Nothing works." "It's just no good."

O Had little exercise, resting for the greater part of each day to ease fatigue. T.V. viewing consumed many hours. Activity food centered for a meal or to grocery shop. Ate *often* in small quantities. Talented cook.

N.D. *Low self-concept*

S "I'm so unhappy." (Repeated four times.) "My feelings were hurt when . . ." (Repeated six times.) "I want to but I can't. I've tried, too many times before. It won't work anyway."

O Talented cook. Few friends or acquaintances. Tears. Whiny voice. Helpless posture.

N.D. *Trust/mistrust struggle*

S "I'm so unhappy." (Repeated four times.) "My feelings were hurt when . . ." (Repeated six times.) "I want to but I can't. I've tried, too many times before. It won't work anyway."

O Whiny voice. Helpless posture. Tears.

N.D. *Dependence/independence struggle*

S "I'm so unhappy." (Repeated four times.) "My feelings were hurt when . . ." (Repeated six times.) "The stairs are too hard for me to walk. My legs hurt, and I can't breathe so good." "I want to but I can't. I've tried, too many times before. It won't work anyway."

O Whiny voice. Helpless posture. Tears.

Actual outcome

Resistant to dietary management. Refusal to allow monitoring of blood pressure and medication. Conversation oriented to past, unable to focus on present. Increased assessment data gathered.

2A—Assessment

N.D. *Low self-concept*

S "I want to but I can't. I've tried, too many times before. It won't work anyway." "I have nothing to wear." "I'm just fat."

O Had little exercise, resting for the greater part of each day to ease fatigue. T.V. viewing consumed many hours. Activity food centered for a meal or to grocery shop. Ate *often* in small quantities. Talented cook.

N.D. *Faulty self-image*

S "I want to but I can't. I've tried, too many

times before. It won't work anyway.'' ''I have nothing to wear.'' ''I'm just fat.''

O   Had little exercise, resting for the greater part of each day to ease fatigue. T.V. viewing consumed many hours. Activity food centered for a meal or to grocery shop. Ate *often* in small quantities. Talented cook.

N.D.   *Trust/mistrust struggle*

S   ''I want to but I can't. I've tried, too many times before. It won't work anyway.''

O   Whiny voice. Helpless posture. Verbally resistive to helping measures.

N.D.   *Dependence/independence struggle*

S   ''I want to but I can't. I've tried, too many times before. It won't work anyway.'' ''I have nothing to wear.'' ''I'm just fat.''

O   Had little exercise, resting the greater part of each day to ease fatigue. T.V. viewing consumed many hours. Activity food centered for a meal or to grocery shop. Ate *often* in small quantities. Talented cook.

N.D.   *Low stress tolerance*

S   ''I want to but I can't. I've tried, too many times before. It won't work anyway.'' ''I have nothing to wear.'' ''I'm just fat.''

O   Had little exercise, resting the greater part of each day to ease fatigue. T.V. viewing consumed many hours. Activity food centered for a meal or to grocery shop. Ate *often* in small quantities. Talented cook.

N.D.   *Obesity*

S   ''I'm just fat. Nothing works.'' ''It's just no good.''

O   Had little exercise, resting for the greater part of each day to ease fatigue. T.V. viewing consumed many hours. Activity food centered for a meal or to grocery shop. Ate *often* in small quantities. Talented cook.

N.D.   *Unstructured life-style*

S   ''I'm just fat. Nothing works.'' ''It's just no good.''

O   Had little exercise, resting for the greater part of each day to ease fatigue. T.V. viewing consumed many hours. Activity food centered for a meal or to grocery shop. Ate *often* in small quantities. Talented cook.

3 — Additional nursing diagnosis

None

4A — Variables

Reality timing	-1
Relationships	-2
Stressors and/or crisis	-3

Coping resources	-1
Significant emotional strength	-1
Significant emotional limitations	-3
Therapy relationship	0
Physical health status	-2
Physical and emotional readiness dimension	$+1$
Available support system	-1
Meaning significance	$+1$
Values and belief impact	$+1$
Other	
BALANCE	$-$

Additional specific knowledge

See case material.

Analysis and synthesis

N.D.   *Low self-concept.* Client's self-perception as a person unable to begin or complete a desired task must be altered. Simple tasks that can be begun and completed will encourage self-esteem and provide corrective feedback on actual abilities.

N.D.   *Faulty self-image.* Obesity, an ''I can't'' life stance, and mistrust combine to reinforce a negative self-image. Simple task completion will help reinforce an expanding and positive view of the self.

N.D.   *Trust/mistrust struggle.* Self-trust is absent. Simple task completion will provide a medium for positive feedback and affirmation. Slower therapy movement allowing space and time for trust development in a free-floating, nondemanding climate may help.

N.D.   *Dependence/independence struggle.* The ''I can't'' life stance has reinforced her dependency and has received limited but desired response from caregivers in the past. Important to note, client really believes she is incapable.

N.D.   *Low stress tolerance.* Therapy expectations seem to have precipitated stress beyond the norm. Client interaction seems to be a method of escaping the expectations as impossible to meet.

N.D.   *Obesity.* Being overweight is an objective health problem that is critical to both her physical and psychological health status.

N.D.   *Unstructured life-style.* Client seems to have no purpose or direction in life other than self-protection and comfort.

4B — Design of action

N.D.   Low self-concept, faulty self-image, trust/mistrust struggle, dependence/independence struggle, low stress tolerance, obesity, unstructured life-style.

   1. Plan

a. Reduce stress perceived by client.
b. Develop bonds of nurse-client relationship.
c. Further assess client strengths and limitations.
2. Strategy
a. Decrease focus on problems.
b. Allow therapy relationship to evolve in a less structured setting.
c. Select an appropriate task-centered activity.
d. Assess and intervene as therapy relationship evolves and client readiness is apparent.
3. Expected outcomes
a. Decreased tension-related behaviors.
b. Increased pertinent dialogue.
c. Increased willingness to begin defined therapy tasks.
4. Criteria
a. Involvement in a task-centered activity.
b. Increased self-disclosure in therapy.
c. Present focus in therapy.
d. Beginning limited exercise program.

The therapist decided to decrease the strain anticipated by the client in the coming interviews by allowing time for increased self-expression and a relatively free-floating environment. This would help to provide a better footing for the interpersonal relationship and for future goal orientation. A new focus on Mary's clothing problems encouraged her to produce attractive material, a pattern, a sewing machine, and more know-how than she apparently wished to reveal. Decreased urgency to attack the problems eased her distress and created a renewed feeling of openness.

During several task-centered sessions, Mary and the nurse adjusted a pattern and sewed a new dress. Often Mary pleaded ignorance to have the therapist complete the task. In reality, Mary was a much more accomplished seamstress than the nurse. When the task was completed, Mary was pleased with her new dress, surprised to be better at something than the nurse was, and also was increasingly free with her existing stress-related concerns. Her self-concept had received a needed boost. Mary agreed to walk a stated distance outside her apartment at the next scheduled home visit.

Affirmative experiences increased her readiness, availability, and understanding of the urgency to proceed with the agreed-on plan.

Reluctantly, but without verbal protest, Mary walked downstairs and around one square block, accompanied by the nurse. There was no doubt that she had trouble carrying her body weight this distance. She stopped to rest twice on her return ascent to the apartment. Breathless and weary, she reclined in a comfortable chair. Now 4 months into therapy, Mary was informed she must join a prescribed weight-reduction group, but it was another 4 months before Mary complied.

In the meantime she sprained her left ankle in an accident never clearly described. The obviously bruised, edematous, painful leg had been examined by a physician. Mary took to her bed, unable to cope with the discomfort. Physical nursing care along with an honest care-concern element were consumed by this emotionally starved client. The duration of this episode lasted long beyond the curing of her injured ankle. Mary's emotional scars could not be so easily healed. Years of emotional unfulfillment, isolation, and high anxiety levels led to a conflicting resistance and a desire for restorative measures to ease her emotionally impoverished state.

Again and in a more forceful manner, the therapist outlined the necessity for adequate exercise and proper diet. Not in an attempt to frighten but as a tactic to force reality, the consequences of recurrent negative and resistive behavior in this matter were outlined clearly, graphically, and strongly. Weepingly, Mary said she would begin daily walks and think about a weight-reduction program. She did walk daily, increasing her distance very slowly. Sometimes she walked to a nearby café for a piece of pie or cake, but she did increase her exercise and she did not always treat herself to tasty food. Some weeks later, Mary, in her new dress and delivered to the door by her therapist, joined a structured weight-control group. Over the next 2 years she remained on the prescribed diet in a fluctuating pattern and with vacillating changes. Extremely slowly she lost 100 pounds and maintained a weight loss of 75 pounds. Mary most assuredly needed to lose more weight, but this was a new beginning for her, the most success she had experienced in a lifetime of effort to establish a healthy and proper diet and weight reduction.

PROCESS IMPLEMENTATION

1—Evaluation

N.D. *Low self-concept*
   S   "Nothing fits me anymore." "You don't know how? I can do it." "The dress looks nice." "You do it for me."
   O   Dress-making task completion. Affirmation received.

N.D. *Faulty self-image*
   S   "Nothing fits me anymore." "You don't know how? I can do it." "The dress looks nice." "You do it for me." "I'm just fat." "Yes, but I just can't."
   O   Dressmaking task completion. Affirmation received. Unable to cope with discomfort of her sprained ankle. Withdrew to bed long after physical healing process.

N.D. *Trust/mistrust struggle*
   S   "You don't know how? I can do it." "You do it for me."
   O   Dressmaking task completion. Affirmation received.

N.D. *Dependence/independence struggle*
   S   "It hurts!" "I can't take care of myself." "No one really cares about me." "Yes, but I just can't." "You do it for me."
   O   Unable to cope with discomfort of her sprained ankle. Withdrew to bed long after physical healing process. Reluctantly, but without verbal protest, began walk of one block, accompanied by nurse. Weepingly, began daily walks. Sometimes treated self to cake or pie. Eight months after first walk joined weight-reduction group at therapist's insistence.

N.D. *Low stress tolerance*
   S   "It hurts!" "I can't take care of myself." "No one really cares about me." "Yes, but I just can't." "You do it for me."
   O   Unable to cope with discomfort of her sprained ankle. Withdrew to bed long after physical healing process.

N.D. *Obesity*

   S   "I'm just fat." "The dress looks nice." "Yes, but I just can't." "You do it for me."
   O   Reluctantly, but without verbal protest, began walk of one block, accompanied by nurse. Weepingly, began daily walks. Sometimes treated self to cake or pie. Eight months after first walk joined weight-reduction group at therapist's insistence.

N.D. *Unstructured life-style*
   S   "No one really cares about me." "Yes, but I just can't." "You do it for me." "I don't know how." "Things just happen." "I don't know how to plan."
   O   Reluctantly, but without verbal protest, began walk of one block, accompanied by nurse. Weepingly, began daily walks. Sometimes treated self to cake or pie. Eight months after first walk joined weight-reduction group at therapist's insistence.

Actual outcome
   Completed task of making new dress with therapist's assistance. Therapy dialogue has a present focus. Physical health problem precipitates withdrawal and decreased coping abilities. Gradually begins exercise and structured weight-reduction activities.

2A—Assessment

N.D. *Thought disorder*
   S   "The man in the next apartment is talking about me. I hear him through the walls. I'm afraid of him. He'll hurt me."
   O   Person and environment disheveled and untidy. Speech loud and pressured. Trembling. Hesitant.

N.D. *Suspicious behavior*
   S   "The man in the next apartment is talking about me. I hear him through the walls. I'm afraid of him. He'll hurt me."
   O   Trembling. Hesitant. Frightened. Hostile and angry.

N.D. *Suicide potential*
   S   "The man in the next apartment is talking about me. I hear him through the walls. I'm afraid of him. He'll hurt me."
   O   Trembling. Hesitant. Frightened. Hostile and angry.

N.D. *Lack of insight*
   S   "The man in the next apartment is talking about me. I hear him through the walls. I'm afraid of him. He'll hurt me."
   O   Reassurance with actual facts only angered client.

2B—Validation by assessment

N.D. *Thought disorder*

   S "The man in the next apartment is talking about me. I hear him through the walls. I'm afraid of him. He'll hurt me."

   O Person and environment disheveled and untidy. Speech loud and pressured. Trembling. Hesitant. Reassurance with actual facts only angered client.

N.D. *Suspicious behavior*

   S "The man in the next apartment is talking about me. I hear him through the walls. I'm afraid of him. He'll hurt me."

   O Trembling. Hesitant. Frightened. Hostile and angry. Reassurance with actual facts only angered client.

3—Additional nursing diagnosis

None

4A—Variables

Reality timing	−5
Relationships	−5
Stressors and/or crisis	−5
Coping resources	−5
Significant emotional strength	−5
Significant emotional limitations	−3
Therapy relationship	−3
Physical health status	−5
Physical and emotional readiness dimension	−5
Available support system	−5
Meaning significance	−5
Values and belief impact	−5
Other	
BALANCE	−

Additional specific knowledge

See case material.

Analysis and synthesis

N.D. *Thought disorder.* Reality validates the hallucinatory episode. Therapy efforts must be directed to assist the client to a more intact and stable state or renewed equilibrium.

N.D. *Suspicious behavior.* A basic nontrusting, self-protective life stance erupts into a decompensation episode with marked paranoid ideation.

N.D. *Suicide potential.* The decompensation episode is accompanied by ineffective reality coping, lack of an adequate support system, and perceptual disturbance. Alertness to self-destructive measures is a priority.

N.D. *Lack of insight.* Faulty perception and self-discernment block the development of healthy self-knowledge. Insight development through positive task and interaction experiences in therapy can prevent further decompensation episodes.

4B—Design of action

N.D. Thought disorder, suspicious behavior, suicide potential, lack of insight.

  1. Plan

    a. *Assess* and evaluate reality.

    b. Intervene with supportive measures to alleviate crisis.

    c. Secure medication; monitor medication intake.

    d. Initiate frequent, short home visits.

    e. Provide concise, reality messages and support. Be alert to suicidal clues.

  2. Strategy

    a. Validate reality.

    b. Give clear, distinct verbal messages.

    c. Make frequent, short home visits until crisis period is alleviated.

    d. Assess client perception.

  3. Expected outcomes

    a. Decompensation episode will resolve.

  4. Criteria

    a. Client will take medication.

    b. Hostility and anger will decrease.

    c. Personal appearance and environmental surroundings will return to norm.

    d. Therapy dialogue will return to previous interaction level.

    e. Medication can be decreased.

Gradually, dormant sides of Mary's personality exposed themselves. At one visit she was in a personal and environmental turmoil. Her speech was loud and pressured, and her self-composure was noticeably shaky and faltering. Aided by proved trust in the therapist, a durable relationship, and helpfulness, Mary confided her pressing problem. "The man in the next apartment is talking about me. I hear him through the walls. I'm afraid of him. He'll hurt me." Investigation proved that the one apartment next door was rented to a frail, elderly widow. Nothing could be heard through the walls by the clinician. Reassurance with these facts only angered Mary. The auditory hallucinations were very real to her.

A prescription for trifluoperazine, 5 mg t.i.d., was secured from her physician. This had been an effective treatment for previous transitory hallucinatory episodes. Mary's suspicious psyche was apparently recontained within 2 weeks. In 1 month the medication dosage was reduced to 2 mg b.i.d. In 3 months the medication was discontinued with no return of the episodic behavior until 6 months had elapsed and at a point of increased intrinsic and extrinsic stress.

The strained therapy climate and rapport weakened by Mary's decompensation demanded a renewed effort by the therapist. During the initial 2 weeks of medication treatment, home visits were made every other day but for only 20 to 30 minutes. At each encounter, medication for the next 48 hours was apportioned. Mary was directed to take the blue pills from a medication container on the kitchen counter, Written, understandable directions concerning time and amount of medication were attached to the compartmentalized dispenser. The information and special medication container helped prevent error for the distraught client. Mary was simply and distinctly informed that "the blue pills will help your nerves." She was reminded that they had decreased her stress when she previously experienced such episodes.

Some suspicious psychotic clients undergoing a fragmented thinking process will not take prescription drugs as directed. There are no guarantees that the medications are not disposed of when the therapist leaves, especially when paranoid ideation is prominent. Time to evaluate the effect of the drug treatment will define the actual ingestion.

The second purpose of frequent short home visits was the assessment of Mary's mental status. The therapist carefully noted any positive or negative changes from the defined deviations and observed the emergence of behavior that indicated a return to the norm. Gradual improvement in her thought process showed that medication was being taken as prescribed. No other intervention had been attempted except for the presence of the therapist and short, un-

clouded, honest messages about Mary's overall improved mental status accompanied by honest affirmation messages. Therapy was limited to these measures until a renewed but relative equilibrium was restored. Hostility waned, and Mary had weathered the stress and decompensation again. A concentrated therapy effort was started to aid her to begin more successful coping measures and to keep her psyche intact.

Mary's self-enforced social isolation, dependency, obesity with resultant traumatized body image, autistic thinking, and low stress tolerance were behaviors which indicated prevalence of an overall self-destructiveness. The ineffectiveness of her coping behaviors in relation to her obesity and her blatant defiance and resistance to measures aimed at reducing her elevated blood pressure further validated this nursing judgment. Failure in her passive measures to destroy her person and inability to cope effectively with the realities of living had precipitated Mary's transient psychotic state. It was this condition that her family members usually referred to as eccentricity.

High self-gratification needs and a low insight level were elements that often deterred positive therapy progress. Mary expressed a desire to change, but she wanted the therapist to do the needed work for her. The transition was supposedly to happen in a miraculous manner. The task of adaptation loomed as monumental. Mary's perception of the energy involved in the transformation made, in her mind, the living of the change experience insurmountable. At times she did try, but for a relatively short time. No matter how much support she was given, when the crucial periods arrived, she could or would not act. Almost all turning points in Mary's therapy were marked by a return to previously defective coping patterns and a rejection of new coping devices. In such a situation it is therefore more important to note the degree of progress and the degree of adaptation or change than the overall achievement of early defined therapy goals. Small inroads of different or new positive behavior did increase Mary's quality of life and her day-to-day life comfort and need satisfaction. There is no easy antidote or cure for life.

PROCESS IMPLEMENTATION

1—Evaluation

N.D. *Thought disorder*

S No verbal messages indicative of thought disorder or fragmented thinking.

O Personal grooming returned to norm. Environment returned to norm. Therapy interaction returned to previous level.

N.D. *Suspicious behavior*

S No verbal messages indicative of suspicious behavior.

O Personal grooming returned to norm. Environment returned to norm. Therapy interaction returned to previous level.

N.D. *Suicide potential*

S No verbal messages indicative of self-destructive behavior.

O Personal grooming returned to norm. Environment returned to norm. Therapy interaction returned to previous level.

N.D. *Lack of insight*

S "I can't remember." "I didn't do that." "Is the weather nice today?"

O Unable or unwilling to explore the episodic behavior. Agitation apparent when discussion attempted or pursued.

Actual outcome

Client took medication as prescribed for 6 months. Personal grooming and environment returned to norm. Decreased anger and hosility. Therapy interaction returned to previous level.

2A—Assessment

N.D. *Dependence/independence struggle*

S "When he's sober, he is a nice guy; then he stays here. We go dancing. I cook for him. He makes me happy." "I don't like it when he's mean to me and then I throw him out, but he always comes back."

O Low voice. Restless. Smiley. Noticeable weight gain. Agitation increased with nurse's normal voice tone.

N.D. *Interpersonal relationship disturbance*

S "Don't talk so loud." "Hush!" "He's in the bedroom, sleeping. He works at night."

O Low voice. Restless. Smiley. Noticeable weight gain. Agitation increased with nurse's normal voice tone.

N.D. *Emotional deprivation*

S "When he's sober, he is a nice guy; then he stays here. We go dancing. I cook for him. He makes me happy." "I don't like it when he's

mean to me and then I throw him out, but he always comes back." ". . . so it don't go to waste."

O Low voice. Restless. Smiley. Noticeable weight gain. Agitation increased with nurse's normal voice tone.

N.D. *Low self-concept*

S "When he's sober, he is a nice guy; then he stays here. We go dancing. I cook for him. He makes me happy."

O Low voice. Restless. Smiley. Noticeable weight gain. Agitation increased with nurse's normal voice tone.

N.D. *Antisocial and abusive behavior*

S "I don't like it when he's mean to me and then I throw him out, but he always comes back."

O Low voice. Restless. Smiley.

N.D. *Obesity*

S "When he's sober, he is a nice guy; then he stays here. We go dancing. I cook for him. He makes me happy." ". . . so it don't go to waste."

O Noticeable weight gain.

N.D. *Loneliness*

S "When he's sober, he is a nice guy; then he stays here. We go dancing. I cook for him. He makes me happy."

O Low voice. Restless. Smiley. Noticeable weight gain. Agitation increased with nurse's normal voice tone.

3—Additional nursing diagnosis

None

4A—Variables

Reality timing	−2
Relationships	−2
Stressors and/or crisis	0
Coping resources	−2
Significant emotional strength	−2
Significant emotional limitations	−2
Therapy relationship	+4
Physical health status	−1
Physical and emotional readiness dimension	0
Available support system	−3
Meaning significance	−1
Values and belief impact	−1
Other	
BALANCE	−

Additional specific knowledge

See case material.

Analysis and synthesis

N.D. *Dependence/independence struggle.* Autonomy is perceived by client as outside her grasp. Both client and boyfriend are dependent on one another in an unhealthy manner.

Interdependent experiences may help client validate healthy life choices.

N.D. *Interpersonal relationship disturbance.* Providing medium to experience positive encounters and emotions will help client to expand self-concept and decision-making skills.

N.D. *Emotional deprivation.* A life deprived of positive feeling experiences makes the client cling to perceived security, no matter how transient.

N.D. *Low self-concept.* Client's negative self-worth encourages her to accept relationship with Howard, since she feels that she can do no better and is fortunate to have him.

N.D. *Antisocial and abusive behavior.* When pressed and vulnerable, client resorts to physical force to protect herself. Needs to adapt a new stance somewhere between force and helplessness.

N.D. *Obesity.* Weight gain was a result of increased inner conflict and transient need satisfactions related to the tenuous relationship with Howard. Ambivalence must be resolved and sound decision-making skills begun.

N.D. *Loneliness.* In the client's perception the relationship with Howard, despite its negative and erratic nature, was better than a life void of relationships. Client needs to experience new, healthy relationships to realize that she does indeed have a reality choice.

4B—Design of action

N.D. Dependence/independence struggle, interpersonal relationship disturbance, emotional deprivation, low self-concept, antisocial and abusive behavior, obesity, loneliness.

1. Plan
    a. Expand client's social activity and contacts.
    b. Encourage problem solving, decision making, and autonomy.
2. Strategy
    a. Maintain a nonjudgmental stance.
    b. Introduce and encourage other-centered activities to encourage positive self-esteem.
    c. Increase positive feedback and person affirmation.
3. Expected outcomes
    a. Participation in an activity-centered social group.
    b. Return to weight-control group and renewed weight loss.
    c. Increased commitment to therapy.
    d. Increased autonomous stance in client's relationship with Howard.

4. Criteria
    a. Participation in an activity-centered social group on a regular basis.
    b. Return to weight-control group and weight reduction.
    c. Therapy participation and self-growth.
    d. Decreased emotional dependence on Howard.

One afternoon at the midpoint of Mary's therapy, the nurse arrived to be greeted by Mary in a low voice. In the course of the interview, she often asked the nurse to speak in a more hushed tone. Mary's nonverbal behavior was restless and smiley. It was noticeable that Mary had stopped losing weight again and had regained some of her laboriously lost pounds.

The nurse commented on the observations concerning Mary's weight. Defensively, the client stated that the nurse was wrong. She admitted, however, that she had not been to her weight-control group for a few weeks. The nurse's normal voice tones increased Mary's agitation. After half an hour of verbal gymnastics, the therapist directly asked, ''Mary, is something troubling you today? You seem restless and nervous and the tone of my voice appears to upset you. Let me help you with the unsettled feelings you seem to have.''

Embarrassed, Mary uncomfortably admitted, ''He's in the bedroom, sleeping. He works at night.'' ''He'' was Mary's boyfriend, Howard. They had a fluctuating relationship during the previous several years. Howard was an admitted alcoholic, and he would disappear for weeks and months. His employment record was sporadic. Mary commented, ''I don't like it when he's mean to me and then I throw him out, but he always comes back.'' She smiled when she stated that he always returned. She continued, ''When he's sober, he is a nice guy; then he stays here. We go dancing. I cook for him. He makes me happy.''

The therapist took a nonjudgmental stance regarding Mary's obvious embarrassment over the sexual relationship she had with Howard.

Part of her discomfort was the anticipation of the nurse's disfavor. Client and nurse need not share the same values and beliefs to execute a helping relationship. Respect for the other person allows one to accept differing significant emphasis in basic beliefs while honoring the other's worth. Nurse and client agreed to meet when Howard was not sleeping. In the next weeks the therapist met Howard. He was obviously fond of Mary and also openly negative, even jealous, toward the nurse-client relationship. "She is OK. She don't need a nurse," he repeated at each encounter.

The conflict between two significant relationships caused an unneeded, increased stress for Mary. In a staunch manner, Mary informed Howard in the therapist's presence that she did need the nurse and that the two would continue to meet. Furthermore, Howard was expected to leave Mary's apartment during the interviews. Not pleased by this ultimatum but unwilling to offend Mary, he complied. The therapist affirmed Mary's assertive stance and her self-assured posture toward therapy. The Mary-Howard relationship did not appear positive to the therapist. Coming events would validate this nursing judgment.

Intense persuasion was needed to convince Mary to return to her weight-control group. Several weeks later and after an increase of 20 pounds, Mary finally succumbed to the therapist's adamant pressure and returned to the dietary program. In the interval, Mary had made homemade bread, pies, cakes, and other high-calorie delicacies for thin Howard. He ate one or two pieces, commented profusely on his enjoyment of these delights, and Mary ate the remaining food "so it don't go to waste." Mary would have been comfortable to drift along in this less stressed state and the false security of this tenuous relationship if it had not been for her budding appetite for health acquired through nurse psychotherapy.

Ambivalently, Mary began to complain about Howard in the therapy sessions. He was drinking heavily, and she didn't like him when he was intoxicated. Mary did not experience such intense loneliness when Howard was present. He gave her money for the rent, and he also bought her groceries. She was fearful whenever he arrived in a drunken state. Mary asked the therapist to tell her what to do, despite the previously learned knowledge that the nurse would not supply the answers. Mary had to decide for herself, but assistance with her own problem-solving method could be given in the therapy hours.

An activity-centered social group was introduced into Mary's life by the therapist during her state of indecision, and Mary was open to this maneuver. Readily and with relative ease, Mary made several new friends and began to join regularly in weekly activities as well as in monthly outings with this group. Mary no longer relied on Howard as her sole source of socialization. She expressed happy feelings related to these new activities and acquaintances. Some of them were as alone in the world as Mary was. Sharing lonely feeling is one method of dissolving loneliness. Finding other individuals in the same living status does not stop the experiencing, but it does broaden one's own perspective.

The current episode of the Howard-Mary relationship came to an abrupt end when Howard arrived at the apartment one evening in a very intoxicated state. The therapist hypothesized that Mary, too, may have been drinking, although she firmly and repeatedly denied it. She did, however, state that at other times she did imbibe with Howard, "but never as much as he does." On the evening in question the client and her boyfriend had a heated quarrel. Mary could not recall the issue over which they disagreed. "I got mad and threw him out. He'll be back. I have his glasses, but he can't stay here anymore," she declared.

Further discussion revealed that Howard had struck Mary during the disagreement. At that point, Mary, who usually maintained a helpless stance, removed Howard's glasses, struck him in return and then bodily threw him out of the apartment and down the stairs. Several days later, Howard meekly returned to the apartment to request his glasses. Mary returned them, but remained adamant about ending their relationship. Although the therapist could not condone the method of termination of this faulty relationship, Mary was supported in her decision to end it and its consequent conflicts. Howard did reenter Mary's life again but not until many months later. Mary was vulnerable to Howard when her own life pivot was loneliness and absence of human warmth and contacts. This relation would always be unsound for both parties, marked by destructiveness, abusiveness, mutual enabling, and disruptive antisocial behaviors. The clinician was not accepting of Mary's dependent helpless stance during subsequent therapy encounters. Rather, her energy was directed toward positive outlets for self-protection, self-satisfaction, and decided self-concept development.

PROCESS IMPLEMENTATION

1—Evaluation
N.D. *Dependence/independence struggle*
S "I had a good time." "She seems to like me." "I got mad and threw him out. He'll be back. I have his glasses, but he can't stay here anymore." "I do need my nurse." "What should I do about Howard?"
O Removed Howard's glasses, struck him in return, and then bodily threw him out of the apartment and down the stairs.
N.D. *Intepersonal relationship disturbance*
S "I had a good time." "She seems to like me." "I got mad and threw him out. He'll be back. I have his glasses, but he can't stay here anymore."
O Made several new friends. Began to join regularly in weekly activities and monthly group outings. Removed Howard's glasses, struck him in return, and then bodily threw him out of the apartment and down the stairs.
N.D. *Emotional deprivation*
S "I had a good time." "She seems to like me."
O Made several new friends. Began to join regu-

larly in weekly activities and monthly group outings.
N.D. *Low self-concept*
S "He likes me fat." "I got mad and threw him out. He'll be back. I have his glasses, but he can't stay here anymore." "I do need my nurse."
O Made several new friends. Began to join regularly in weekly activities and monthly group outings.
N.D. *Antisocial and abusive behavior*
S "I got mad and threw him out. He'll be back. I have his glasses, but he can't stay here anymore."
O Removed Howard's glasses, struck him in return, and then bodily threw him out of the apartment and down the stairs.
N.D. *Obesity*
S "I eat just what's left over." "He likes me fat."
O Twenty-pound weight gain. Returned to weight-control group as mandated by therapist.
Actual outcome
Increased commitment, disclosure, and activity in therapy. New involvement in an activity-centered social group. Return to weight-control group. Partial resolution of her emotional dependence on Howard.

2A—Assessment
N.D. *Interpersonal relationship disturbance*
S "I'll just be in the way." "Maybe they (grandchildren) won't like me."
O Usually did not accept children's invitation to visit. Familial connections were maintained through regular letters and telephone calls.
N.D. *Emotional deprivation*
S "I'll just be in the way." "Maybe they (grandchildren) won't like me."
O Usually did not accept children's invitation to visit. Familial connections were maintained through regular letters and telephone calls.
N.D. *Faulty support system*
S "I'll just be in the way." "Yes, I want to go." "Can you help me?"
O Her children and their spouses were open to Mary's visit. The only qualification was that Mary learn to control her abusive language while in her children's home. Grown children agreed to establish the stated boundary during Mary's visit.
N.D. *Lack of insight*
S "I'll just be in the way." "Maybe they (grandchildren) won't like me."

O Usually did not accept children's invitation to visit.

N.D. *Low self-concept*
S "I'll just be in the way." "Maybe they (grandchildren) won't like me." "Yes, I want to go." "Can you help me?"
O Usually did not accept children's invitation to visit.

N.D. *Low stress tolerance*
S "I can't control myself." "I've always cussed like this." "Can you help me?"
O The only qualification was that Mary learn to control her abusive language while in her children's home. Grown children agreed to establish the stated boundary during Mary's visit.

N.D. *Antisocial and abusive behavior*
S "I've always cussed like this." "Can you help me?"
O The only qualification was that Mary learn to control her abusive language while in her children's home. Grown children agreed to establish the stated boundary during Mary's visit.

N.D. *Unstructured life-style*
S "I've always cussed like this." "Can you help me?"
O The only qualification was that Mary learn to control her abusive language while in her children's home. Grown children agreed to establish the stated boundary during Mary's visit.

3—Additional nursing diagnosis
None

4A—Variables

Reality timing	+3
Relationships	+3
Stressors and/or crisis	+3
Coping resources	+3
Significant emotional strength	+2
Significant emotional limitations	0
Therapy relationship	+4
Physical health status	−1
Physical and emotional readiness dimension	+3
Available support system	+3
Meaning significance	+4
Values and belief impact	+4
Other	
BALANCE	+

Additional specific knowledge
See case material.

Analysis and synthesis
N.D. *Interpersonal relationship disturbance*. Renewed family relationships encouraged inner strength, feelings of self-worth, and other life relationships. An increased autonomous life stance is now possible.

N.D. *Emotional deprivation*. Withdrawal from the mainstream of life increased the client's feelings of emptiness. Openness, trust, and growth were possible once the client could experience "good" feelings.

N.D. *Faulty support system*. Renewing family ties will strengthen a viable support system. Renewed availability of family members will foster self-development.

N.D. *Lack of insight*. "Trying on" or experiencing new behaviors provided beginning self-realization, which in turn encouraged further self-development and behavior experimentation.

N.D. *Low self-concept*. Insights, new and renewed relationships, positive life experiences, especially positive emotional experiences, expanded the client's overall self-concept, encouraging initiative, interaction, and other-centered activity.

N.D. *Low stress tolerance*. Modification of unacceptable language provides motivation to try to cope with anxiety and a medium to experience increased stress with new and positive coping devices.

N.D. *Antisocial and abusive behavior*. Control of unacceptable behavior to significant others will strengthen self-concept and provide objective corrective feedback and needed person affirmation.

N.D. *Unstructured life-style*. Family ties and planning life events with significant persons creates a thread throughout one's life-span to add order and meaning to life and life events.

4B—Design of action
N.D. Interpersonal relationship disturbance, emotional deprivation, faulty support system, lack of insight, low self-concept, low stress tolerance, antisocial and abusive behavior, unstructured life-style.

1. Plan
   a. Plan and prepare for visit to grown children.
2. Strategy
   a. Frequent feedback of positive actions during therapy.
   b. Structured learning experience in therapy hour to assist with unacceptable language control.
   c. Verbal preparation in therapy for each visit.
3. Expected outcomes
   a. Acknowledgment of self-growth.

    b. Beginning acceptable control of abusive language.
    c. Beginning insight concerning her behavioral effect on others.
    d. Preparation for family visits.
    e. Actual visits to family with positive outcome.
4. Criteria
    a. Self-initiated verbal self-disclosure regarding insight.
    b. Modification of behavior regarding abusive language.
    c. Sharing preparations for family visits in therapy.
    d. Actual visits to family without incident and renewed family bonds developing.

Mary's association with her children was usually positive in nature. They were all in their early years of marriage with small children and vast responsibilities. Familial connections were maintained through regular letters and telephone calls. Visits by necessity were short and infrequent. Mary was repeatedly invited to their homes for limited visits, but she never accepted these invitations. "I'll just be in the way," she said.

At the end of 2 years of therapy, the therapist encouraged Mary to make a brief visit to each child's home as a summer project. Mary needed familial ties. Her children and their spouses were open to this plan. Mary could become acquainted with her grandchildren and proudly demonstrate her weight loss efforts to genuinely concerned family members. Willing but frightened, Mary embarked on the planned visits, each of which would last for 5 to 7 days.

Mary had told her children about "her nurse." With her consent the therapist had a telephone conversation with each daughter and son. They agreed to the plan, even expressing some enthusiasm for the proposal. The only qualification they all wished to put on their mother was that she "learn to control her abusive language" while she was in their homes. Mary's frequent swearing, cursing, and loud insulting language were not a social asset. This rough-hewed part of Mary's person would conflict with the child-rearing patterns her chil-

dren had established for her grandchildren. The therapist agreed to confront this perplexing behavior. Mary's grown children also agreed to be responsible for establishing this boundary as the only expressed condition regulating Mary's behavior while in their homes.

Self-control was a deviation from Mary's usual norm, calling for modification of old life patterns. The client introduced the issue into the therapy hour shortly after her family extended their invitations. Mary was reminded of the number of inescapably positive actions she had completed in the past 2 years. Most of these accomplishments she had previously considered impossible. Her weight loss was pointed to as a hallmark of self-control, along with her healthy choice concerning the termination of her relationship with Howard and her new life-style choices regarding activities.

Unacceptable language was defined by Mary as she understood the issue. Accordingly, the inner control of her expression began in the therapy hour. A tally of her deviations from the established acceptable norm was kept by both parties during encounters. Improvement was measured by decreased negative expression and increased positive expression from week to week. Mary was directed to attempt more verbal restraint in her activity and weight-control groups. Her ebbing insight expressed itself as she reported to the therapist that "people seem to like me better when I don't cuss and swear."

At times, Mary felt she could not control her language, especially when frustration and stress loomed immovably and threateningly. Personal space to allow her usual expression was defined. She was encouraged to vent her feelings in her accustomed style but in a controlled setting—only in her apartment when she was alone. Mary was directed to remove herself to the bathroom or her bedroom while visiting her family if she felt she could not control her language. She was to use this space for expression and return to the group when her inner controls returned. If this was not effective, she was directed to leave the home and go for a long walk as another more acceptable energy outlet.

Mary expressed satisfaction while achieving this self-control. She heard an honest and warm, ''Thank you, mother'' from her family. The therapist also expressed a true joy for Mary's growth. Some of Mary's rough-edged personality would not change or did it need to be changed. Positive perception from honest life experiences decreased her pent-up frustration, reducing the need for expressive, emphatic, verbal hostility.

Prior therapy encounters also assisted with her involvement in this new and satisfying adventure. Mary bought gifts for her grandchildren and several new dresses for herself. She found old and favorite cookie recipies she had used during her children's early years and reintroduced them to her grandchildren as a thread between family generations. The happy excitement and anticipation effected a less self-centered concern and also provided Mary with topics of conversation to share with the members of her activity group and weight-control group. A renewed family tie linked Mary to a past and a future existence.

Significantly, Mary commented that she was too busy for nurse psychotherapy. Frequency of sessions was decreased from once a week to twice a month. Summer therapy would occur once a month between visits to her grown children. Mary was given support through the option of calling the therapist if she felt the need for additional time. Many verbal comments were given reaffirming her growth during therapy hours. She continued to have difficult days, even difficult weeks, of stress, but they were becoming fewer in number and shorter in duration. Gradually, there were as many positive days as negative days in Mary's life. A new sense of balance and homeostasis created an increased even tenor and cohesion in her present existence.

Mary's trips were uneventful but pleasant. She proudly returned with photographs of herself with her children and with her grandchildren. Stories abounded of pleasant family dinners, picnics, and outings. Future trips were planned, to the delight of all family members. Mary had definite plans for Thanksgiving, Christmas, and Easter and was even formulating arrangements for the following summer. Lonely feelings would be less traumatizing to her with these plans and a new sense of meaning in her life.

Therapy hours would help her solve problems effectively and complete some anticipatory activities for each visit. The therapist coached her in organization and execution of ideas. Mary had not previously indulged her grandchildren with gifts, but now Christmas and birthday presents were bought on sale so that Mary could remain within a reasonable budget. Needed exercise resulted from the shopping trips. Money saved for bus tickets could not be spent on high-calorie foods and tasty treats. Mary's cakes and cookies could be exploited as gifts on the next family visit.

Her daughters and daughter-in-law were in agreement and felt fortunate to be able to turn their kitchen over to Grandma when she visited. In her turn she provided these young women with a needed change of pace and relaxation in their busy child rearing and family life. Freely given comments by these young mothers helped to reinforce and bolster Mary's self-image, self-confidence, and overall self-concept.

Before Mary left for her third and last summer visit to see her son and his family, she agreed to telephone the therapist on her return to establish an appointment time. However, 3 weeks passed with no message from Mary. The therapist attempted to telephone her, but a dozen calls produced no answer. One more call would be made, and if no answer was received the therapist, motivated by concern, would make an unscheduled home visit.

Mary answered the telephone the next afternoon loudly and expressively, asking the nurse where she had been and why she hadn't called

Mary as agreed. All verbal attempts to clarify the misunderstanding only increased the client's anger and hostility. Mary was allowed to talk in a nonstop manner for 20 minutes. As her energy and anger waned, the therapist asked if Mary wanted an appointment. Her answer was, "Of course I do," and a home visit was arranged for later that same week.

During the session, the therapist took the initiative to rectify the misunderstanding. Mary was surprised to find neither party had to be identified as the wrong one but that the blame could be shared without either person having to concede defeat. Communication errors are a part of life. Mary expressed astonishment at the therapist's statement that she could have misunderstood the nurse-client agreement. In all communication breakdowns it is not the winning or losing that is of primary importance but the resolution of conflict or misunderstanding. This new concept was foreign to Mary's life stance, but because of her trusting relationship with the therapist, the notion was intriguing. Later in the hour, she revealed an inner fear following her demonstrative telephone conversation with the therapist. Mary would probably always expect her negative behaviors to produce rejection by significant other people. Experiencing new behaviors and new coping styles in a therapy situation can be the beginning of a transference of these mechanisms to other life situations.

Mary's life-style alterations precipitated new insightful comments that she shared in therapy. She eagerly and excitedly told the clinician, "Sometimes I feel good now. I have reason to live." A meaning for living had been reestablished, and Mary agreed to return to her physician for an evaluation of her hypertension. She completed the evaluation and began taking daily medication. She also allowed the nurse to monitor her blood pressure during home visits. Mary had a renewed zest, spirit, and reason for taking part in life. No hallucinatory episodes were noted. Howard reentered the scene on oc-

casion, but he did not live in Mary's apartment or was he the total focus of her life. They had an occasional evening out dancing, transient sexual encounters, and more subdued arguments. Mary was no longer dependent on Howard to fill an empty life. This void was partially filled with new and renewed relationships and activities.

On occasion, grown friends of her children called Mary to babysit for them. Now a more reliable person and able to emit warmth, she found these child-caring services a frequent request. The additional revenue was welcome to further her other expanding areas of interest. Now Mary had choices to make. In therapy, she laughingly complained of having too many decisions to make and too much to do.

Mary continued to have distress episodes related to intrinsic and extrinsic stress, and these would continue despite modification and transformations related to therapy. Decompensation was the outgrowth of unresolved pathology. Fatigue and depressed initiative often multiplied in her constant battle with obesity and were deterrents to a healthy, active life-style. A life of self-centered protectiveness and high immediate need gratification led to recurrent feelings of depression and sadness. Withdrawal from other-centered activities and relationships would add to the negative effect of unsettled episodes. Like most human beings, Mary coped more effectively with the good, the positive, the sanguine feeling. She certainly had her share of the bad, the negative, the low experiences of life and their resultant cumbersome antagonistic feelings. Mary rarely found effectual methods of coping with critical situations. It seemed impossible to her to confront the crux of a troublesome issue or the recurrent stumbling blocks in her life without some guidance.

The introduction of positive activities and healthy relationships decreased the tenuousness and imbalance of her existence. Involvement in real-life experiences provided a positive anticipatory outlook, decreasing self-destructive thoughts and the nebulous sadness she felt. Some early need gratification could be achieved through expectation, preparation, and anticipation of definitely planned coming events. Loneliness was quashed by this maneuver. An aloneness is contained or negated by the effective coping devices deployed to fill the empty time spaces. Isolation only expands aloneness.

Termination of therapy was a gradual process, allowing the client the actual decision of when to conclude the association. The relationship was to remain on an open-ended basis for many months. This maneuver in itself offered a supportive presence to Mary. She did negotiate for services during crisis and before actual crisis periods peaked. Reentry to therapy was accompanied by a relative level of insight from the past encounters. Reestablished contacts were for short durations.

The readiness and availability factors of the helping relationship were primary variables, allowing Mary's growth toward a more fulfilling, comfortable, and enjoyable life. Nursing process was the tool advancing the clinician's objectivity and realistic goal-oriented direction. Interpersonal dynamics of any nurse-client relationship are clarified and developed by the applied nursing process framework. This procedure allows the intervention base a strong grounding in both objective and subjective data as well as in proved theoretical knowledge. The acquired information concludes in measures, tasks, or health work that employ the available client's energy and therapist's skill toward possible positive outcomes. For Mary and the clinician this process brought about limited agreed-on goals and intensified the professional interpersonal relationship.

SUMMARY PERSONAL PROFILE
Social adjustment

S   ". . . people seem to like me better when I don't cuss and swear." "Look what I bought for . . ." "I'm going to my son's for Christmas."

O   Increasing self-disclosure. Developing insight. Active participation in both activity and weight-reduction groups. Increased and stronger affiliation with adult children and grandchildren.

Emotional health status

S   ". . . people seem to like me better when I don't cuss and swear." "My grandchildren like my sugar cookies." "I thought you might be mad at me for . . ." "Howard took me out to dinner Saturday, but I came home early. He began to drink too much."

O   Increasing self-disclosure. Developing insight. New problem-solving skills. Increasing self-control. No new hallucinatory episodes noted. Limited relationship with Howard. Limited emotional dependence on Howard. Sufficient initiative to negotiate for mental health services when needed. Ability to plan and make choices.

Physical health status

S   "I lost 3 pounds this month." "I take those pills every day now." "Yes, you can take my blood pressure. Is it better?"

O   Weight 275 pounds. Taking daily hypertensive drugs as prescribed. Allowed nurse to monitor blood pressure. Active involvement in weight-reduction group. Increased exercise.

Spiritual dimension

S
O } No acknowledged or observable change.

Daily living skill performance

S   "I lost 3 pounds this month." "I take those pills every day now."

O   Active participation in both activity and weight-reduction group. Increased exercise. Taking daily hypertensive drugs as prescribed. New problem-solving skills.

Coping skill repertoire

S   "I lost 3 pounds this month." "I take those pills every day now." "Yes, you can take my blood pressure. Is it better?" "I thought you might be mad at me for . . ." "Howard took me out to dinner Saturday, but I came home early. He began to drink too much."

O   Increasing self-disclosure. Developing insight. New problem-solving skills. Increasing self-control. No new hallucinatory episodes noted. Limited relationship with Howard. Limited emotional dependence on Howard. Sufficient initiative to negotiate for mental health services when needed. Ability to plan and make choices.

Maturational struggle according to Erikson's developmental stages

S   ". . . people seem to like me better when I don't cuss and swear." "I thought you might get mad at me for . . ." "I'm going to my son's for Christmas."

O   Basic trust vs. basic mistrust—increasing drive and hope.
Dependence vs. independence—increasing autonomy.
Intimacy vs. isolation—beginning affiliation.

Self-integration

S   ". . . people seem to like me better when I don't cuss and swear." "My grandchildren like my sugar cookies." "I thought you might be mad at me for . . ." "Howard took me out to dinner Saturday, but I came home early. He began to drink too much." "I'm busy now but I feel better." "I used to feel lonely."

O   Increasing self-disclosure. Developing insight. New problem-solving skills. Increasing self-control. No new hallucinatory episodes noted. Limited relationship with Howard. Limited emotional dependence on Howard. Sufficient initiative to negotiate for mental health services when needed. Ability to plan and make choices.

Quality of life

S   "I'm busy now but I feel better." "I used to feel lonely."

O   Active participation in both activity and weight-reduction groups. Increased and stronger affiliation with adult children and grandchildren. Limited emotional dependence on Howard.

SUGGESTED READINGS

Aiken, L.: Patient problems are problems in learning, American Journal of Nursing 70:1916-1918, Sept., 1970.

American Nurses' Association: Standards of psychiatric mental-health nursing practice, Kansas City, 1973, The Association.

Collins, M.: Communication in health care, St. Louis, 1977, The C. V. Mosby Co.

Colten, S., et al.: Social concerns for psychiatric rehabilitation, Psychosocial Rehabilitation Journal 2:16-23, 1978.

Curtin, L.: Human values in nursing—toward a philosophy of human kind, Supervisor Nurse 9:21-23, March, 1978.

delCampo, E.: Psychiatric nursing therapy, philosophy and methods, Journal of Psychiatric Nursing 16:34-37, Aug., 1978.

Dixon, B.: Interviewing when the patient is delusional, Journal of Psychiatric Nursing 69:25-34, Jan./Feb., 1969.

Fidler, G. S. et al.: Doing and becoming: purposeful action and self-actualization, American Journal of Occupational Therapy 32:305-310, May/June, 1978.

Kline, N., and Davis, J.: Psychotropic drugs, American Journal of Nursing 73:54-62, Jan., 1973.

Koehne-Kaplan, N. S., and Levy, K. E.: An approach for facilitating the passage through termination, Journal of Psychiatric Nursing 16:11-14, June, 1978.

Kolb, L.: Modern clinical psychiatry, Philadelphia, 1977, W. B. Saunders Co.

Lewis, C. W.: Body image and obesity, Journal of Psychiatric Nursing 16:22-24, Jan., 1978.

Mitchell, H., et al.: Nutrition in health and disease, Philadelphia, 1976, J. B. Lippincott Co.

O'Brien, M.: Communications and relationships in nursing, ed., 2, St. Louis, 1978, The C. V. Mosby Co.

Ray, O.: Drugs, society, and human behavior, ed. 2, St. Louis, 1978, The C. V. Mosby Co.

Robinson, C.: Basic nutrition and diet therapy, New York, 1970, Macmillan Publishing Co., Inc.

Rubin, T.: The angry book, New York, 1969, Collier Books.

Selye, H.: Stress in health and disease, Woburn, Mass. 1976, Butterworths Publishing, Inc.

Shapiro, D. H., Jr., et al.: Medications and psychotherapeutic effects, Archives of General Psychiatry **35**:294-302, March, 1978.

Shontz, F.: The psychological aspects of physical illness and disability, New York, 1975, Macmillan Publishing Co., Inc.

Sumner, F. C., et al.: A nurse for suicidal patients, American Journal of Nursing **76**:1792-1793, Nov., 1976.

Wallston, K., et al.: Increasing nurse's person centeredness, Nursing Research **27**:156-159, May/June, 1978.

Yoder, J.: Alienation as a way of life, Perspectives in Psychiatric Care **15**(2):66-71, 1977.

Yura, H., and Walsh, M.: The nursing process, ed. 2, New York, 1973, Appleton-Century-Crofts.

CHAPTER 9

MABEL E *manifests*

PROBLEMATIC LIFE CONDUCT

evidenced by

WITHDRAWAL AND FEAR

INTRODUCTORY PERSONAL PROFILE
Social adjustment

S "It's useless anyway. I'm hospitalized every fall. Nothing can be done about it." "I really don't want you to come." "It won't do any good anyway." "I can't."

O Long blocks of time when marketing is only venture outside of home. Sleeps much of day. Usual daytime attire is worn black pants, faded cotton blouse, and soiled grey sweater. Often appears in old blue robe and worn flannel pajamas. Often goes for more than a week without combing or shampooing hair.

Emotional health status

S "It's useless anyway. I'm hospitalized every fall. Nothing can be done about it." "I really don't want you to come." "It won't do any good anyway." "I can't."

O Medication regimen: chlorpromazine, 200 mg q.i.d., and benztropine mesylate, 2 mg b.i.d. Usual daytime attire is worn black pants, faded cotton blouse, and soiled grey worn flannel pajamas. Often goes for more

than a week without combing or shampooing hair. Harry does all family meal preparation, most of the cleaning, and other family household maintenance duties. Harry insists she help with marketing. Sleeps much of day. Competent family financial management.

Physical health status

S *

O Height 5 feet, 4 inches. Weight 145 pounds. Medication regimen: chlorpromazine, 200 mg q.i.d., and benztropine mesylate, 2 mg b.i.d.

Spiritual dimension

S *

O Abandoned religious practice of weekly church attendance and active participation in her faith.

---

*Absence of subjective data indicates limited verbal exchange, extended periods of silence in therapy, or lack of comment to clinician's queries.

Daily living skill performance

S   "It's useless anway. I'm hospitalized every fall. Nothing can be done about it." "I really don't want you to come." "It won't do any good anyway." "I can't."

O   Usual daytime attire is worn black pants, faded cotton blouse, and a soiled grey sweater. Often appears in old blue robe and worn flannel pajamas. Often goes for more than a week without combing or shampooing hair. Harry does all family meal preparation, most of the cleaning, and other family household maintenance duties. Harry insists she help with marketing. Sleeps much of day. Competent family financial management.

Coping skill repertoire

S   "It's useless anyway. I'm hospitalized every fall. Nothing can be done about it." "I really don't want you to come." "It won't do any good anyway." "I can't."

O   No effort made to bridge the communication gap with children. To avoid conflict, Mable and Harry do not acknowledge the chemically dependent behavior or the implicit sexual behaviors of their son. Usual daytime attire is worn black pants, faded cotton blouse, and soiled grey sweater. Often appears in old blue robe and worn flannel pajamas. Often goes for more than a week without combing or shampooing hair. Harry does all family meal preparation, most of the cleaning, and other family household maintenance duties. Harry insists she help with the marketing. Sleeps much of day. Competent family financial management.

Maturational struggle according to Erikson's developmental stages

S   "It's useless anyway. I'm hospitalized every fall. Nothing can be done about it." "I really don't want you to come." "It

won't do any good anyway." "I can't."

O   Basic trust vs. basic mistrust.
Dependence vs. independence.
Intimacy vs. isolation

Self-integration

S   "It's useless anyway. I'm hospitalized every fall. Nothing can be done about it." "I really don't want you to come." "It won't do any good anyway." "I can't."

O   Usual daytime attire is worn black pants, faded cotton blouse, and soiled grey sweater. Often appears in old blue robe and worn flannel pajamas. Often goes for more than a week without combing or shampooing hair. Harry does all family meal preparation, most of the cleaning, and other family household maintenance duties. Harry insists she help with marketing. Sleeps much of day. Competent family financial management. Medication regimen, chlorpromazine, 200 mg q.i.d., and benztropine mesylate, 2 mg b.i.d.

Quality of life

S   "It's useless anyway. I'm hospitalized every fall. Nothing can be done about it." "I really don't want you to come." "It won't do any good anyway." "I can't."

O   Usual daytime attire is worn black pants, faded cotton blouse, and soiled grey sweater. Often appears in old blue robe and worn flannel pajamas. Often goes for more than a week without combing or shampooing hair. Harry does all family meal preparation, most of the cleaning, and other family household maintenance duties. Harry insists she help with marketing. Sleeps much of day. Competent family financial management.

Time span: 6 years

Mr. and Mrs. E, Harry and Mabel, have been married for 25 years and have four children. Harry is a skilled laborer who does seasonal work, and his earned income is supplemented by unemployment compensation. The E's own several pieces of commercial property. Mabel has not been employed outside the home since her marriage to Harry, although one of her covert strengths is competent bookkeeping and management of their joint income properties and family financial matters.

Harry is 62 years old, stands 6 feet tall, and weighs 200 pounds. He is broad shouldered and muscular, and his dark brown hair is thinning. His ruddy cheeks and calloused hands are the results of years of strenuous manual labor. Harry's marriage to Mabel is his third marriage. He has a history of alcoholism. Periodically, Harry drinks heavily for several days and then returns to a state of sobriety for many months, at times for more than a year. He is not involved in Alcoholics Anonymous, although he has sporadically been an active member, seemingly committed to the A.A. philosophy. Harry states that he is comfortable with his life-style and acknowledges no reason for any change for himself.

Both of the E's two older sons, ages 25 and 24 years, are high school dropouts and are serving in the military service. They contact their parents rarely, and often Harry and Mabel do not know where they are stationed. Both sons were arrested on felony charges in their early teen years. Neither parent evidences concern for their sons as persons or family members. When they are mentioned by name, neither parent reflects facial expression or voice inflection. Their attitude appears to be one of relief at their sons' physical and emotional distance as well as a welcome deliverance from any parental responsibilities, care, or concern. One quickly reached a gut-level reaction that Harry and Mabel had disassociated these grown children from their conscious minds.

One daughter, 22 years of age, also a high school dropout, is married, has four small children, and lives in a nearby farming community. She was 7 months' pregnant and 17 years of age when she married her husband. At 15 years of age she had been charged with shoplifting for the third time. She visits her mother several times a month, usually accompanied by her young, undisciplined children. The mother-daughter interaction during these visits is superficial and centered on the daughter's complaints and on her recurrent family and marital problems. Concerns of both mother and daughter seem to be self-centered with a nongiving attitude pervading both sides of this stressful, thorny relationship. One concludes that the relationship was never viewed as satisfactory by either party but that its unhealthy pattern contributes to the pathology of both individuals. Neither mother nor daughter has the strength to sever these unhealthy emotional ties.

The E's youngest son, Henry, 16 years of age, has recently dropped out of high school after a third and final suspension for blatant misconduct and is on legal probation as a juvenile offender. Under duress from both parents and an assigned probation officer, he is employed as a dishwasher at a local restaurant 6 days a week, often working split shifts and irregular hours and earning a minimum wage. He is required by his father to pay board and room. He also makes regular monthly payments on his second-hand motorcycle, which he uses for transportation to and from work.

Henry does not plan to return to school. He is relatively uncommunicative with his parents, and they make no effort to bridge the communication gap with him. He is a regular user of marijuana, occasionally experimenting with other illegal drugs, and is a heavy drinker of hard liquor. Henry's girl friend frequently spends the night with him. To avoid conflict, Mabel and Harry do not acknowledge the chemically dependent behavior or the implicit sexual behaviors of their son. Avoidance of conflict, discomfort, and stress has become a life-style coping pattern within this family.

Harry and Mabel own their family dwelling, an older, small, two-story, three-bedroom building in great need of paint, both on the inside and on the outside. Their furniture is sparse and worn, although a comfortable new, blue floral living room couch with a matching chair is pointed to with pride by Mabel when she shows her home. She maintains a savings account earmarked for new carpeting for the living room. Harry has painted the kitchen and papered its adjacent eating area and has painted their bedroom a soft green. He promises to paint the living room, and they both hope to save sufficient money for him to paint the exterior of the house.

Finances have always been a stressor for Harry and Mabel. They had no savings when they married. Harry's employment record shows a sporadic pattern of work. Their income property was inherited from Mabel's relatives and is expensive and time consuming to maintain adequately. Often they are fortunate to balance actual real estate income and the actual expenses at the end of each year. Their own home was mortgaged until a 20-year mortgage contract was completed. Harry's erratic work pattern and drinking habits have been costly, as has Mabel's psychiatric care. Child-rearing financial stressors were often viewed as prohibitive, and they were multiplied by Mabel's inability to cope with required daily living tasks and by her frequent absences from home because of psychiatric hospitalization. The instability of this family system is a prominent factor at almost every stage in this marriage relationship, family development, and the frequent and recurrent crisis states.

Mabel is the identified psychiatric client in this family. She has experienced multiple hospitalizations over the past 30 years. At the onset of therapy, Mabel is 56 years of age. Her overt thought process appears to be in control, but her outward life-style is one of withdrawal and passivity and is structured by pervading inner fears. She is maintained on a medication regimen of chlorpromazine, 200 mg q.i.d., and benztropine mesylate, 2 mg b.i.d.

Mabel is 5 feet, 4 inches tall and weighs 145 pounds. Her hair is an attractive salt and pepper color when it is regularly washed and styled, but often more than a week passes without her shampooing or even combing her hair. Her daytime attire is black pants, a faded cotton blouse, and soiled, grey sweater. Significantly, Mabel often appears in an old blue robe and worn blue flannel pajamas when the therapist calls.

Mabel shows little expression, often staring into space for long lapses of time. When she does speak, her voice tone is deep and sounds harsh. She replies in as few words as possible and initiates no conversation. Eye-to-eye contact is avoided. Nonverbally, Mabel quickly lets one know that she is not interested in a relationship or a person-to-person encounter of any kind for any reason. Her challenge is, "It's useless anyway. I'm hospitalized every fall. Nothing can be done about it." Mabel's loss of hope, apathy, and acceptance of *being* mentally ill is devastating to her, to her family, and to anyone allowed into her territorial space. An air of helplessness and hopelessness pervades her life.

Harry does all the family meal preparation, most of the cleaning, and many of the other family household maintenance tasks and duties. He does insist that Mabel accompany him when he does the grocery shopping. She frequently expresses a wish not to partake in this task, but Harry insists that he needs her help with the marketing. There are blocks of time when this is her only venture outside the safety of her home. Years before, Mabel abandoned her religious practice of weekly church attendance and active participation in her faith.

Once each month Mabel visits her psychiatrist, her progress being defined as unremarkable but stable. She was referred for nurse psychotherapy specifically with the goal of helping her avoid further hospitalization. Weekly home nursing visits were prescribed by her psychiatrist. Mabel was extremely reluctant, apprehensive, and fearful, but apathetically she agreed after a 2-hour encounter to begin supportive nurse psychotherapy, forewarning the therapist that she really "doesn't want it" and that "it won't do any good anyway." From the start her resistance and lack of investment were defined clearly and openly. Her declaration against the relationship was explicit. Mabel had untapped inner strength. The force of her resistance needed to be harnessed to a positive outcome rather than to the maintenance of illness.

Collaboration with her psychiatrist, a record review of limited available data, and four weekly home visits led to the following nursing diagnosis:

Anxiety

Dependence/independence struggle

Low self-concept

Perceptual disturbance

Fear

Acceptance of the mental illness role

Apathy

Affect disturbance

Short concentration span

Interpersonal relationship disturbance

Family disruption

Inability to solve problems effectively

Inability to perform required tasks of daily living

Initial therapy encounters were taxing for both client and therapist. It was evident that Mabel's goal was to abort this health effort as quickly as possible. Positive health and change were extremely threatening to her. In the first months during home visits, Mabel wore her pajamas and robe, and her appearance remained unkempt. She appeared to have gotten out of bed only after the therapist persistently rang the doorbell. Twice in 2 months she did not answer the door, despite the therapist's perseverance. In a later telephone conversation with the therapist, she insisted that she had forgotten the visit, and, furthermore, she had "gone out with Harry."

During the first encounters, Mabel would lie on the living room couch, often focusing on the ceiling and always turning her body at least partially away from the therapist to avoid eye contact. Despite physical distance of only 4 to 6 feet, Mabel created an invisible shield to counteract any maneuver of the therapist to create rapport, a climate of security and trust, and a relationship bond. Social-emotional distance protectively sheltered Mabel from investment in the relationship and perceived hurt, whether real or unreal.

Consistency, sameness, thereness, care, concern, and skill in both verbal and nonverbal communication became nursing intervention tools of choice to ground this relationship. One must diligently apply proficient and knowledgeable, deliberate communication when strong resistance to help, such as a total energy commitment to illness, is encountered. Self-imposed imprisonment and the perpetuation of distress are always perplexing to encounter. In itself, this energy for remaining ill is the focus for the reversal of the illness process. Mabel not only believed she was ill, but she also believed that the forces of disease controlled her very being. She appeared to work at perpetuating this belief system for herself and for all significant others within her sphere of possible control.

The many limitations of these encounters made strength assessment a questionable exercise but critical to any goal achievement. The harnessing of this resistance and rechanneling of Mabel's energy in a positive direction would be the pivot to change and adaptation, but one needs sufficient data to begin a process. For several visits Mabel was accepted as she was and where she was, but this intervention alone was not sufficient to initiate any therapeutic measures. It was a bleak state, and progress was at an absolute standstill. With Mabel's apathetic, reluctant consent, the therapist invited Harry to join one of the sessions in an assessment endeavor to expand the substance and dimensions of the data base.

PROCESS IMPLEMENTATION*

1—Evaluation

N.D. *Anxiety*

S †

O Wore pajamas and robe. Appearance unkempt. Did not answer door when therapist arrived for appointment. During initial encounters would lie on couch, focusing on ceiling and turning body away from therapist. Direct eye contact avoided.

N.D. *Affect disturbance*

S †

O Affect flat without noticeable change during initial interviews.

N.D. *Short concentration span*

S "What did you say?" (Repeated four times.) "I can't remember."

O Unwilling or unable to become involved in therapy interaction.

N.D. *Acceptance of the mental illness role*

S †

O Wore pajamas and robe. Appearance unkempt. Did not answer door when therapist arrived for appointment. During initial encounters would lie on couch, focusing on ceiling and turning body away from therapist. Direct eye contact avoided.

N.D. *Apathy*

S †

O Wore pajamas and robe. Appearance unkempt. Did not answer door when therapist arrived for appointment. During initial encounters would lie on couch, focusing on ceiling and turning body away from therapist. Direct eye contact avoided.

Actual outcome

Rejection of the therapy relationship.

---

*It is important to note the limited data in this case. Adaptation, change, and/or progress was extremely slow. The relative lack of both initial and new data signifies extent of distress when chronicity is well established. *Assessment* therefore becomes a *critical factor* in nursing process. Ongoing assessment is vital to unfold new data and to validate the establishment of patterns of behavior and growth and the meaning of these recurring patterns. This information is essential in examining overall client profiles when planning nursing intervention.

†Absence of subjective data indicates limited verbal exchange, extended periods of silence in therapy, or lack of comment to the clinician's queries.

2A—Assessment

N.D. *Anxiety*

S "Yes." "Harry doesn't want me to go back to the hospital." "I don't know." "I don't know. I always go every year. I can't help it."

O Harry did all the household tasks. Harry explained a vague fear his wife had relating to the family laundry task. Looked away and left the room. Did not become involved in conversation.

N.D. *Dependence/independence struggle*

S "Yes." "Harry doesn't want me to go back to the hospital." "I don't know." "I don't know. I always go every year. I can't help it."

O Harry did all the household tasks. Did not become involved in conversation.

N.D. *Low self-concept*

S "Yes." "Harry doesn't want me to go back to the hospital." "I don't know." "I don't know. I always go every year. I can't help it."

O Harry did all the household tasks. Harry offered that his wife was a good cook and managed household and business finances. Did not become involved in conversation.

N.D. *Acceptance of the mental illness role*

S "Yes." "Harry doesn't want me to go back to the hospital." "I don't know." "I don't know. I always go every year. I can't help it."

O Harry did all the household tasks. Looked away and left the room. Did not become involved in conversation.

N.D. *Apathy*

S "Yes." "Harry doesn't want me to go back to the hospital." "I don't know." "I don't know. I always go every year. I can't help it."

O Harry did all the household tasks. Looked away and left the room. Did not become involved in conversation.

3—Additional nursing diagnosis

None

4A—Variables

Reality timing	0
Relationships	−3
Stressors and/or crisis	−5
Coping resources	−5
Significant emotional strength	0
Significant emotional limitations	−3
Therapy relationship	−4
Physical health status	0
Physical and emotional readiness dimension	−3
Available support system	−1

Meaning significance   −3
Values and belief impact   −3
Other   BALANCE   −

Additional specific knowledge
See case material.

Analysis and synthesis

N.D.   *Anxiety.* Alteration of an accepted pattern causes stress with which the client cannot cope. The protectiveness of an "I can't" stance and withdrawal are resorted to for safety.

N.D.   *Dependence/independence struggle.* Dependency has become a comfortable life-style. Reinitiation of the struggle for autonomy is not perceived as desirable by the client.

N.D.   *Low self-concept.* Self-perception is vividly displayed in personal grooming, absence of social interaction, and the "I can't" stance.

N.D.   *Acceptance of the mental illness role.* Chronicity with a pattern of hospitalization once a year, during the fall season, has become an accepted life-style.

N.D.   *Apathy.* A diminished capacity to experience life is accepted as a positive, protective quality by the client. Withdrawal to a position where emotional experiences seem reduced in size or intensity is equated with a position of personal safety.

4B — Design of action

N.D.   Anxiety, dependence/independence struggle, low self-concept, acceptance of the mental illness role, apathy.

   1. Plan
     a. Expect client to prepare one evening meal each week.
   2. Strategy
     a. Express expected task performance clearly and explicitly.
     b. Involve Harry in supporting client's task involvement.
     c. Express positive, supportive, and corrective feedback for task performance and completion.
   3. Expected outcomes
     a. Preparation of one evening meal each week.
     b. Discussion of meal preparation tasks in therapy hour.
   4. Criteria
     a. Completion of meal preparation task.
     b. Discussion of meal preparation in therapy hour.

In later evaluation of the situation, a continuous strength for Mabel was the fact that

Harry seemed to truly love and care for her. He also desired and was willing to work for a more functional state for his wife, offering, "I want her to be able to enjoy life."

Harry provided information that was helpful. He related that Mabel would not go to the basement to do the family laundry because she was afraid. He added that he himself did not like to wash clothes. He had purchased a new washer-dryer combination for his wife on her last birthday, but this had not helped ease her fears or facilitated the task. Mabel was silent. Harry's explanation of Mabel's perceived fear was vague in nature.

Harry did all the meal preparation and stated that he didn't mind this job. He also added that Mabel was an excellent cook and he wished she would prepare some of the meals that he really enjoyed. He even listed specific foods he was hungry for, meals she prepared especially well.

It also came to light that Mabel spent several hours each week managing both the family and the business finances. She was accurate and astute in the financial management of their lives. When the therapist finally saw some demonstration of this skill, the observations helped validate assessment of Mabel's potential for wellness.

Harry expressed a desire to extend beyond home more often in the company of his wife. He said that they both enjoyed going out for a lunch or dinner when finances permitted. "Mabel is real pretty when she gets dressed up," he remarked.

Harry was emphatic about not wanting his wife to return to the hospital. Furthermore he stated, "If she takes her pills, she's all right. I'll see to that. The kids are mostly gone, so there's no commotion. Henry has to be good and keep his job or he goes to reform school."

During all of Harry's talking, Mabel offered few comments, looked away, and left the room several times. At one point Harry had to find her and bring her back to the meeting. When Mabel was asked if she had heard what Harry said, she would say, "Yes." She could repeat that

"Harry doesn't want me to go back to the hospital." When asked how she felt about Harry's desire for her to remain at home, she would only say, "I don't know." When she was asked how she felt about returning to the hospital, she said, "I don't know. I always go every year. *I can't help it.*" Her response was a posture of acceptance and predestination to cope with a comfortable, accepted pattern of behavior.

Shortly after this visit, the therapist had a collaborative planning session with Mabel's psychiatrist, who thought that telling Mabel she was "not sick enough" to be hospitalized could be risked. Therapy then proceeded with a total push program of focusing on change of significant negative behaviors and a reprogramming with messages of "I am *not* sick" and "I can." The old coping pattern of "I am too sick" had to be abandoned.

To intervene effectively with individuals whose condition is labeled as chronic, one must possess a strong sense of one's own personhood. The words "I can't" must be foreign to the tongue of the nurse-therapist. The negative "I can't" attitude is a destructive factor to growth and is often prominent in the ideation of the person who is emotionally distressed over a long period of time. It produces a negative circular phenomenon in one's thinking. This defeatist syndrome must be stopped or broken to begin a new and healthful behavior pattern. If one says and acts as if "I can't," this sets up one's own negative reinforcement, pushing down growth and health and multiplying the destructive variables that counter positive self-concept development. The most effective barrier to "I can't" is an assured "I can" attitude of the nurse-therapist. One must believe that the client can. This may be the first encountered positive belief imposed by another individual, and it must pervade the relationship.

Reality must be accepted. For example, if one says, "I can't spend money on a new car if I don't have the cash," or "I can't paint a picture because I am not very artistic," these are realistic coping methods. Everyone has authentic limitations to be accepted. Change is necessary when the unrealistic theme of "I can't" becomes a coping style that prevents trying a new behavior, despite the discomfort of the old behavior habits. It is when the "I can't" phrase protects illness as security that it must be countered with new coping to promote healthy feelings of safety. Chronically emotionally disabled individuals need concentrated guidance and convincing support to reach the assurance of initiating thinking with an "I can" attitude that comes with an increased self-esteem and self-integration. False security is replaced with the actual security of a functioning person.

Therapy plans called for Mabel to begin preparing one evening meal a week, the menu to be chosen by Harry. As the expectation was being laid out, Mabel's affect was flat and she avoided eye contact. Her verbal responses were "I don't know" and "I can't." With generous encouragement dispersed at regular intervals and with enormous verbal support, Mabel grudgingly said she would try to prepare a baked chicken the following week, adding "but I won't make the dressing and gravy." Bargaining may not always be helpful and it is manipulative in nature, but in this case it was forward movement and growth from the "I can't" stance. Shortly, Mabel baked a small chicken. Once she was in the kitchen, she helped Harry with the dressing so "he would get it right," but she went to rest when it was time to fix the gravy. Harry enjoyed the meal despite all his assistance and involvement. He seemed not only to enjoy Mabel's chicken but also to gain pleasure from working cooperatively with her. Mabel received immense positive feedback from her husband. Harry enjoyed doing a task with his wife, companionship being relatively absent from their marriage.

On the therapist's next visit, Mabel's achievement was reinforced with additional positive verbal feedback. She did not show a sense of satisfaction, but she could relay that she knew that Harry did enjoy the meal. She was less distant with the therapist during the interview, indicating that her shielded self could be penetrated. Nonverbally, she quietly accepted the expectation as fact that she would be preparing a main meal each week. Growth was measured several months after the initiation of this task when Mabel began to prepare the menu of her choice. Now she was also preparing the total meal unassisted. Harry often sat in the kitchen and visited with his wife while she worked in the kitchen. Over several years Mabel grew to preparing four, five, and even six meals a week. She smiled when she was complimented on this achievement, and her growth and sense of satisfaction were indicated by an occasional appropriate smile and increased verbalization.

Henry did not eat with his parents. Mabel was asked to invite her son to join his parents for one of her meals. She strongly refused with, "He doesn't want to. He's never home. He doesn't like my cooking." She was noticeably agitated and uncomfortable with the topic of her son. It was noted that she avoided his presence and withdrew emotionally if the therapist chose to talk about him. If the topic was pursued, she also withdrew physically by leaving the room. Harry was quiet and noncommittal about his son, and he would not force this issue with his wife. One sensed an attitude of parental denial regarding Henry. It was as if he did not exist, except perhaps as a roomer in the back upstairs bedroom. Child-rearing experiences had been painful and nonrewarding for this couple.

PROCESS IMPLEMENTATION*

1—Evaluation

N.D.   *Anxiety*
       S   "I don't know." "I can't."

---

*It is important to note the limited data in this case. Adaptation, change, and progress was extremely slow. The relative lack of both initial and new data signifies extent of distress when chronicity is well established. *Assessment* therefore becomes a *critical factor* in nursing process. Ongoing assessment is vital to unfold new data and to validate the establishment of patterns of behavior and growth and the meaning of these recurring patterns. This information is essential in examining overall client profiles when planning nursing intervention.

O   Affect flat. Avoided eye contact.

N.D.   *Dependence/independence struggle*
       S   "I don't know." "I can't." " . . . so he'll get it right." "But I won't make the dressing and gravy." "Harry liked the chicken."
       O   Prepared meal. Became less distant with therapist. Quietly accepted expectation that she prepare one main meal each week.

N.D.   *Low self-concept*
       S   "I don't know." "I can't." " . . . so he'll get it right." "But I won't make the dressing and gravy." "Harry liked the chicken."
       O   Prepared meal. Became less distant with therapist. Quietly accepted expectation that she prepare one main meal each week.

N.D.   *Acceptance of the mental illness role*
       S   "I don't know." "I can't." " . . . so he'll get it right." "But I won't make the dressing and gravy." "Harry liked the chicken."
       O   Prepared meal. Became less distant with therapist. Quietly accepted expectation that she prepare one main meal each week.

N.D.   *Apathy*
       S   "I don't know." "I can't." " . . . so he'll get it right." "But I won't make the dressing and gravy." "Harry liked the chicken."
       O   Prepared meal. Became less distant with therapist. Quietly accepted expectation that she prepare one main meal each week.

Actual outcome
       Client completed the task of preparing one evening meal assisted by her husband.

2A—Assessment

N.D.   *Dependence/independence struggle*
       S   "I can't."*
       O   Average day reconstructed as rising at noon, napping much of the afternoon, and retiring for the day at 7 P.M. Preferred therapist's visit at 2 P.M.

N.D.   *Acceptance of the mental illness role*
       S   "I can't."*
       O   Average day reconstructed as rising at noon, napping much of the afternoon, and retiring for the day at 7 P.M. Preferred therapist's visit at 2 P.M. Wore pajamas and robe for interview. Personal appearance unkempt.

N.D.   *Low self-concept*
       S   "I can't."*

---

*Absence of subjective data indicates limited verbal exchange, extended periods of silence in therapy, or lack of comment to the clinician's queries.

O Average day reconstructed as rising at noon, napping much of the afternoon, and retiring for the day at 7 P.M. Preferred therapist's visit at 2 P.M. Wore pajamas and robe for interview. Personal appearance unkempt.

N.D. *Inability to perform required tasks of daily living*

S "I can't."*

O Average day reconstructed as rising at noon, napping much of the afternoon, and retiring for the day at 7 P.M. Preferred therapist's visit at 2 P.M. Wore pajamas and robe for interview. Personal appearance unkempt.

N.D. *Apathy*

S "I can't."*

O Average day reconstructed as rising at noon, napping much of the afternoon, and retiring for the day at 7 P.M. Preferred therapist's visit at 2 P.M. Wore pajamas and robe for interview. Personal appearance unkempt.

3 — Additional nursing diagnosis

None

4A — Variables

Reality timing	0
Relationships	+1
Stressors and/or crisis	0
Coping resources	+1
Significant emotional strength	+1
Significant emotional limitations	−3
Therapy relationship	+1
Physical health status	0
Physical and emotional readiness dimension	−2
Available support system	+1
Meaning significance	−2
Values and belief impact	−2
Other	
BALANCE	−

Additional specific knowledge

See case material.

Analysis and synthesis

N.D. *Dependence/independence struggle.* Acceptance of the illness role is a method of reinforcing dependency. Autonomy is perceived as an unwanted, negative commodity.

N.D. *Acceptance of the mental illness role.* Since this is the way things have always been, there is no motivation to seek a new or better existence. The client and family belief system views the client's position of illness as immutable.

---

*Absence of subjective data indicates limited verbal exchange, extended periods of silence in therapy, or lack of comment to the clinician's queries.

N.D. *Low self-concept.* The escapism of extended hours in sleep suggests the client's dissatisfaction and discomfort with life. Initiating structured expectation can provide a medium for the client to learn positive self-perception.

N.D. *Inability to perform required tasks of daily living.* Withdrawal by sleeping for 20 out of 24 hours reinforces the unworthy life stance. This pattern prevents the establishment of a medium for positive, corrective feedback and reinforces valueless feelings.

N.D. *Apathy.* This seeming insensibility to others and emotional coldness or unconcern is difficult to encounter. Flat affect further veils the client from disclosing the emotional self.

4B — Design of action

N.D. Dependence/independence struggle, acceptance of the mental illness role, low self-concept, inability to perform required tasks of daily living, apathy.

1. Plan
   a. Promote necessary daily living skills through structured daily routine.
2. Strategy
   a. Expect client to spend less time in bed.
   b. Expect client to be well groomed for interview.
   c. Gradually establish interview hour in morning.
   d. Enlist Harry's supportive assistance.
   e. Accompany client on outdoor walks.
3. Expected outcomes
   a. Increasing amounts of daytime hours spent out of bed.
   b. Improved personal grooming.
   c. Increased participation in activities of daily living.
4. Criteria
   a. Reported increasing hours up and about.
   b. Improved grooming for therapy interview.
   c. Weekly outdoor walks by client accompanied by therapist.
   d. Established therapy hour of 10 A.M.

Mabel slept for the greater part of each day. After interview data collecting, her average day was reconstructed as rising at noon, napping much of the afternoon, and retiring for the day at 7:00 P.M. Mabel was up more hours on the days when she prepared dinner, on grocery shopping days, and on her bookkeeping days.

She preferred that the therapist visit her around 2:00 P.M. Over a 1-year time span, the visit was gradually moved back to 10:00 A.M. Once she was up and given carefully defined tasks, Mabel would remain up and about for an increasingly longer time. Imposed expectations were necessary to achieve any therapy goals with this client who could or would not participate in the real world. Mabel's self-perception as an emotionally crippled person precluded her growth.

It also became evident that Mabel's medication was being taken in the amount prescribed but consumed during her waking hours. In effect, Mabel had 800 mg of chlorpromazine between noon and 7 P.M., resulting in restlessness, drowsiness, and occasional postural hypotension by early evening. As her day was lengthened and she was directed to take the medication over a minimum of 12 hours rather than in a 7-hour time span, the intended effect was more apparent. Evening restlessness and drowsiness resulting from medication were greatly reduced. Postural hypotension was minimal and rare. Mabel seemed more amenable to therapy, and periods of agitation were decreased.

As the interviews were moved to the morning hours, Mabel continued to greet the therapist in robe and pajamas and with a very unkempt personal appearance. Not to be deterred, the therapist insisted that Mabel be dressed for the visits. One must view personal grooming as a necessity to promote and accompany person-social-emotional growth. Harry again assisted by frequently complimenting his wife when she was clean, dressed, and groomed.

Mabel and the therapist began to walk outside during the visits. The fresh air and exercise were healthful and invigorating. Often Mabel would say, ''I can't walk today,'' as nurse and client left the home. Her resistance came in the form of words and slowness of action but rarely as direct refusal. Direct refusals came only with the thorny issue of her adolescent son. Some of her resistance was habit and some was actual wariness and fear of new experiences, but some of it was also due to her perceptual distortion. Progress was oiled with large dosages of corrective feedback and affirmation. Personal grooming would never be a chosen priority with Mabel, but by the second year of her nurse psychotherapy, she was usually dressed in clean attire and conservatively well groomed for the day by 10 A.M.

Mabel did not return to the hospital in the fall after the initiation of home-based nurse psychotherapy or in any of the following fall seasons. Her attitude seemed to remain that eventually she would return for an episode of confined psychiatric care. Her relationship with the clinician was never easy to define. There was a prominent insensitivity in Mabel's stance. She remained passive-resistant to therapy measures and goals. She was noncommittal to the relationship and its involvements. In the first year she often stated that the therapist did not have to come back. Occasionally, she even said, ''Do not come next week.'' With the therapist's firm approach about the need for encounters, Mabel would agree to an alternate appointment the following week. Verbal resistance stopped as time proved the durability and helpfulness of the relationship. One does not have to be liked by the client to be effective. The therapy and/or the therapist can be the target for direct healthy-angry expression.

Mabel began to converse more easily and at greater length. Conversations with the therapist were sometimes on a superficial level, but Mabel had an emerging initiative to be encouraged. Her apathy and withdrawal were less prominent, except when stressors were at high or peak level. As a person, she had a lack of refinement in behavior and language. These coarse edges of her personality remained constant. Despite these qualities, she could project a pleasant manner when she was relaxed.

PROCESS IMPLEMENTATION*

1—Evaluation

N.D. *Dependence/independence struggle*
- S "Sooner or later I'll go back to the hospital." "I took a walk alone yesterday." "Harry likes this outfit." "I can't."
- O Usually dressed and conservatively well groomed for the day by 10 A.M. Less resistance to therapy expectation.

N.D. *Acceptance of the mental illness role*
- S "Do not come next week." "Sooner or later I'll go back to the hospital." "I can't."
- O Usually dressed and conservatively well groomed for the day by 10 A.M. Less resistance to therapy expectation.

N.D. *Low self-concept*
- S "Sooner or later I'll go back to the hospital." "I took a walk alone yesterday." "Harry likes this outfit." "I can't."
- O Usually dressed and conservatively well groomed for the day by 10 A.M. Less resistance to therapy expectation.

N.D. *Inability to perform required tasks of daily living*
- S "I can't."
- O Usually dressed and conservatively well groomed for the day by 10 A.M. Less resistance to therapy expectation.

N.D. *Apathy*
- S "Sooner or later I'll go back to the hospital." "I can't."
- O Usually dressed and conservatively well groomed for the day by 10 A.M. Less resistance to therapy expectation.

Actual outcome

Client's grooming improved. Increasing participation in daily living tasks such as meal preparation and household routines. Therapy hour established as 10 A.M. Client dressed and groomed for therapy hour.

---

*It is important to note the limited data in this case. Adaptation, change, and progress was extremely slow. The relative lack of both initial and new data signifies extent of distress when chronicity is well established. *Assessment* therefore becomes a *critical factor* in nursing process. Ongoing assessment is vital to unfold new data and to validate the establishment of patterns of behavior and growth and the meaning of these recurring patterns. This information is essential in examining overall client profiles when planning nursing intervention.

2A—Assessment

N.D. *Anxiety*
- S "I can't." "I won't." "I don't like the basement." "I can't stay down there." "It's like bad dreams."
- O Rigid body posture when in laundry room. Difficulty expressing self. Pressure of speech. Hyperventilation. Flushed face. Perspiration. Tremors.

N.D. *Fear*
- S "I can't." "I won't." "I don't like the basement." "I can't stay down there." "It's like bad dreams."
- O Rigid body posture when in laundry room. Difficulty expressing self. Pressure of speech. Hyperventilation. Flushed face. Perspiration. Tremors.

N.D. *Inability to solve problems effectively*
- S "I don't know why." "I just don't like it." "I can't stay down there."
- O Avoidance of laundry facility. Refusal to examine remodeled room.

N.D. *Inability to perform required tasks of daily living*
- S "I don't know why." "I just don't like it." "I can't stay down there."
- O Avoidance of laundry facility. Refusal to examine remodeled room.

N.D. *Perceptual disturbance*
- S "I can't." "I won't." "I don't like the basement." "I can't stay down there." "It's like bad dreams." "I can't."
- O Rigid body posture when in laundry room. Difficulty expressing self. Pressure of speech. Hyperventilation. Flushed face. Perspiration. Tremors.

N.D. *Dependence/independence struggle*
- S "I can't." "I won't." "I don't like the basement." "I can't stay down there." "It's like bad dreams."
- O Rigid body posture when in laundry room. Difficulty expressing self. Pressure of speech. Hyperventilation. Flushed face. Perspiration. Tremors.

N.D. *Low self-concept*
- S "I can't." "I won't." "I don't like the basement." "I can't stay down there." "It's like bad dreams."
- O Rigid body posture when in laundry room. Difficulty expressing self. Pressure of speech. Hyperventilation. Flushed face. Perspiration. Tremors.

3 — Additional nursing diagnosis
None

4A — Variables

Reality timing	0
Relationships	−3
Stressors and/or crisis	−3
Coping resources	−3
Significant emotional strength	0
Significant emotional limitations	−3
Therapy relationship	+2
Physical health status	0
Physical and emotional readiness dimension	+1
Available support system	+1
Meaning significance	−5
Values and belief impact	−5
Other	
BALANCE	−

Additional specific knowledge
See case material.

Analysis and synthesis

N.D.   *Anxiety.* Stress builds to an almost explosive state. The unknown and associative quality of the task and the environment cause mounting distress.

N.D.   *Fear.* This most unpleasant state of turbulent feelings must be examined and placed in perspective. Fear has a reality base. Exposing the fear for what it is can decrease the discomfort of the feeling.

N.D.   *Inability to solve problems effectively.* A lifetime of ineffective problem-solving approaches and unreliable coping does not prepare the client with the necessary decision-making skills. Anxiety and fear further complicate the thought process.

N.D.   *Inability to perform required tasks of daily living.* The task in this instance is not as important as the meaning and association of the environment. Alternatives to this task performance are possible, but task completion is essential to desensitization of the fear response.

N.D.   *Perceptual disturbance.* Perceiving shock therapy as an inevitable but unpleasant experience and unable to repress negative emotions, causes perceptual distortion and associative disturbance.

N.D.   *Dependence/independence struggle.* Dependency as a life stance becomes a reliable coping device. Stress is increased when the clinician refused to accept the "I can't." syndrome.

N.D.   *Low self-concept.* A deterrent to significant therapy interaction was the client's low self-concept. Client has repressed fears rather than cope with the reality of having had shock treatments and their meaning to her.

4B — Design of action

N.D.   Anxiety, fear, inability to solve problems effectively, inability to perform required tasks of daily living, perceptual disturbance, dependence/independence struggle, low self-concept.

1. Plan
   a. Structure laundry task.
   b. Begin desensitization process.
2. Strategy
   a. Divide task to simplest forms.
   b. Time structure the task.
   c. Initially provide support through nurse's presence.
   d. Gradually withdraw presence but continue verbal support.
   e. Involve Harry in supporting client's task.
3. Expected outcomes
   a. Gradual desensitization to environment.
   b. Assumption of family laundry task as structured.
4. Criteria
   a. Observation of less anxious behavior while in laundry room.
   b. Task completion.
   c. Task completion without noticeable distress.

The time came to deal directly with the problem of the family laundry. Mabel did not want to talk about it. She emphatically did not want to do the laundry. As the topic was pursued, she swore at the therapist loudly and vigorously. Her strength of resistance indicated the depth and possible pathological ramification of this issue. Both client and therapist were adamant in opposing directions. The therapist had set the stage, so to speak, in encountering previous problem areas. Mabel grudgingly agreed that she must cope with this task too.

To further assess the situation and its relevant stressor and in an attempt to decrease the blatant hostility, the therapist asked to see the laundry facilities. Willingly, but with obvious anxiety-related behaviors, Mabel did show her basement laundry facility. It was dark and dreary and had a damp and depressing air.

Mabel's body seemed to relax somewhat as she quickly left the basement room. After the therapist secured Mabel's reluctant agreement, Harry's assistance to clean and paint the laundry room was enlisted. Mabel remained uninvolved in the project. After 6 weeks, Harry completed his remodeling by installing adequate lighting fixtures and a dehumidifier. Mabel did not even want to look at the refurbished room.

Mabel's defensive resistance to doing the laundry was like bucking against a solid wall. Penetration of this wall seemed impossible, even with Harry's urging and with his firm refusal to do the laundry himself until forced to do so by lack of clean clothes. Before exploring alternatives to doing the laundry, the therapist attempted to elicit the meaning of the task to Mabel.

After several more weeks of emotional conflict and a therapist-client power and control struggle, Mabel spontaneously volunteered helpful information. She didn't like the basement. It made her anxious, and she felt she couldn't stay in the basement for any amount of time. As the therapy hour progressed, it became clear that the physical environment of her basement conjured up memories of her surroundings after receiving electroshock treatment. It created a fear feeling for her that amounted to a phobia. In addition, her entrapment in the "I can't" syndrome perpetuated the task as being totally impossible. The positive element was that she took the risk within the confines of her relationship with the therapist to disclose her inner conflict.

Reluctantly, Mabel agreed to try a plan to embark on the laundry task. The desensitization process began with daily limited trips to the laundry room. Next the dirty clothes were sorted within a controlled time space. Another step was taken when Mabel started one load of clothes for washing. Nurse and client would return to the living room until this wash cycle was completed. Then they returned to the room to put these laundered clothes into the dryer.

Again both parties waited in the living room until the drying cycle was completed. Finally, the clothes were gathered up and brought upstairs for folding.

This was a very slow and tedious, step-by-step project. Task initiation and task completion were months apart. At first, Mabel hyperventilated while sorting laundry. Verbal support and short durations of exposure to the room helped control her anxiety. Matter-of-fact verbal comments on her health, her emotional growth, the length of time since her last hospitalization, and a professional opinion about her not presently needing electroshock therapy were helpful interventions during the desensitization project. These comments were given in short, explicit statements, often couched in just one theme. Sometimes a reassuring hand on Mabel's shoulder and verbal comment, such as "I'm here with you" were helpful. Harry's expressed satisfaction with Mabel's accomplishing the laundry task reinforced and replenished her. Both husband and therapist stated that they knew how difficult this process was for Mabel.

After several weeks, Mabel did not hyperventilate while she was in the laundry room. She could complete a load of clothes alone if she had some support to begin the task. She was being visited by the therapist only twice a week, and she washed one load of clothes on each of those days. To make this a more routine procedure and to complete the necessary weekly amount of family laundry, Mabel agreed to follow a schedule set up for her if she "didn't have to" remain in the basement alone for long.

The working schedule was as follows:

9:30	Get up and put coffee pot on.
9:45	Go to basement, sort clothes, and begin *one* load of washing.
10:00	Eat breakfast.
10:30	Put clothes in dryer.
10:45	Bathe, dress, make beds.
11:30	Remove clothes from dryer and fold clothes upstairs.
	WASHING DONE FOR TODAY

This schedule was posted on the bathroom mirror, bedroom mirror, and refrigerator door.

Mabel followed this schedule on most days. With time and increased self-confidence, Mabel would choose to do a second load of laundry only if it were necessary. The schedule did not give Mabel time to worry or procrastinate. In addition, it provided a set time for personal hygiene, forced her to be up and about for additional hours each day, and provided a medium for Harry to give needed positive feedback. Mabel followed this routine relatively well over a long period. The time came, as reported by Mabel, when she did not experience a gripping fear at entering her basement. She never enjoyed doing the laundry, but she completed it and eventually had little need to talk about her subsiding feelings of fear. Wellness decreased the likelihood of further electroshock therapy. With the actual imminent threat removed, the fear was reduced. Acclimation to the environment of her laundry room removed the perceived threat and stress of any impending danger. Completing the task without harm provided space to experience reality and to facilitate change by reinforcement of effective problem-solving devices.

PROCESS IMPLEMENTATION*

1—Evaluation

N.D. *Anxiety*

    S   "I'll try if I don't have to stay down there." "I don't feel so tight when I go down there."

    O   Decreased hyperventilation. Completed task alone. Initiated second load of laundry when necessary.

---

*It is important to note the limited data in this case. Adaptation, change, and/or progress was extremely slow. The relative lack of both initial and new data signifies extent of distress when chronicity is well established. *Assessment* therefore becomes a *critical factor* in nursing process. On-going assessment is vital to unfold new data and to validate the establishment of patterns of behavior and growth and the meaning of these recurring patterns. This information is essential in examining overall client profiles when planning nursing intervention.

N.D. *Fear*

    S   "I'll try if I don't have to stay down there." "I don't feel so tight when I go down there." "I'm not so afraid anymore."

    O   Decreased hyperventilation. Completed task alone. Initiated second load of laundry when necessary.

N.D. *Inability to solve problems effectively*

    S   "I'll try if I don't have to stay down there." "I don't feel so tight when I go down there." "I did two loads of laundry yesterday."

    O   Decreased hyperventilation. Completed task alone. Initiated second load of laundry when necessary.

N.D. *Inability to perform required task of daily living*

    S   "I'll try if I don't have to stay down there." "I don't feel so tight when I go down there." "I did two loads of laundry yesterday."

    O   Decreased hyperventilation. Completed task alone. Initiated second load of laundry when necessary.

N.D. *Perceptual disturbance*

    S   "I'll try if I don't have to stay down there." "I don't feel so tight when I go down there." "I'm not so afraid anymore." "I can manage OK."

    O   Decreased hyperventilation. Completed task alone. Initiated second load of laundry when necessary.

N.D. *Dependence/independence struggle*

    S   "I'll try if I don't have to stay down there." "I don't feel so tight when I go down there." "The schedule helps." "I did two loads of laundry yesterday."

    O   Decreased hyperventilation. Completed task alone. Initiated second load of laundry when necessary.

N.D. *Low self-concept*

    S   "I'll try if I don't have to stay down there." "I don't feel so tight when I go down there." "I can manage OK now."

    O   Decreased hyperventilation. Completed task alone. Initiated second load of laundry when necessary.

Actual Outcome

    Desensitization to laundry room and assumption of family laundry task without distress.

2A—Assessment

N.D. *Dependence/independence struggle*

    S   "Oh, I can't go without Harry." "No, I don't go to church anymore."

    O   Household daily living tasks completed. Improved personal appearance maintained. Extreme dependence on husband. Would not risk other relationships.

N.D. *Acceptance of the mental illness role*

S "I feel bad sometimes when he says . . ." "I don't like feeling . . ." "But I am sick."

O Beginning self-disclosure of feelings and concerns. Extreme dependence on husband. Would not risk other relationships.

N.D. *Interpersonal relationship disturbance*

S "Oh, I can't go without Harry." "I wouldn't know what to say in a group."

O Began to share some of her life concerns about Harry's drinking, about Harry himself, about unstable family finances, and about her children. Extreme dependence on husband. Would not risk other relationships.

N.D. *Family disruption*

S "Henry did have dinner with us." "I can't take the hassle when he's home."

O Henry remained on periphery of family. Mabel maintained a position of control through her illness.

N.D. *Apathy*

S "Oh, I can't go without Harry." "I wouldn't know what to say in a group." "No, I can't." "I can't take the hassle when he's home."

O Began to share some of her life concerns about Harry's drinking, about Harry himself, about unstable family finances, and about her children. Extreme dependence on husband. Would not risk other relationships. Some therapy hours passed with dialogue of little depth.

N.D. *Low self-concept*

S "Oh, I can't go without Harry." "I wouldn't know what to say in a group." "I feel bad sometimes when he says . . ." "I don't like feeling . . ." "But I am sick." "No, I can't." "I can't take the hassle when he's home."

O Began to share some of her life concerns about Harry's drinking, about Harry himself, about unstable family finances, and about her children. Extreme dependence on husband. Would not risk other relationships. Beginning self-disclosure of feelings and concerns.

3—Additional nursing diagnosis

None

4A—Variables

Reality timing	0
Relationships	−2
Stressors and/or crisis	0
Coping resources	+1
Significant emotional strength	+1
Significant emotional limitations	−1
Therapy relationship	+3
Physical health status	0
Physical and emotional readiness dimension	+1
Available support system	0
Meaning significance	0
Values and belief impact	0
Other	
BALANCE	+

Additional specific knowledge

See case material.

Analysis and synthesis

N.D. *Dependence/independence struggle.* The reinitiation of this struggle is evidence of progress.

N.D. *Acceptance of the mental illness role.* Periods of self-disclosure, concern, and emotional expression indicate that client may reach the point of examining this negative life stance.

N.D. *Interpersonal relationship disturbance.* Extension of relationships beyond husband is essential to growth. Interaction skills learned in therapy can be helpful to gain self-assurance in relationships.

N.D. *Family disruption.* Limited but positive acknowledgment of and interaction with son decreases client's boundaries. At some point family therapy may be helpful.

N.D. *Apathy.* Less prominent but problematic, this behavior must become reduced in relation to other positive behavior patterns and new coping styles.

N.D. *Low self-concept.* Self-disclosure risks in therapy help expand self-esteem. The feeling of personal dignity is new to this client.

4B—Design of action

N.D. Dependence/independence struggle, acceptance of the illness role, interpersonal relationship disturbance, family disruption, apathy, low self-concept.

1. Plan
   a. Continue assessment, intervening in defined areas as readiness develops.
2. Strategy
   a. Encourage beginning self-disclosure.
   b. Continue to expect defined task performance.
   c. Actively listen and encourage increasing verbalization in therapy.
   d. Allow client space for growth.
   e. Encourage socialization skills.
3. Expected outcomes
   a. Initial self-disclosure.
   b. Adequate task performance.
   c. Increased verbal content of therapy hour.
   d. Limited openness to new ideas.

4. Criteria
   a. Initiative in task performance.
   b. Self-identification of areas of concern.
   c. Expression of concern in therapy.

Henry remained a distressed youth on the periphery of this family. His probation officer demonstrated a combined consistent firmness and genuine interest in him. In late adolescence Henry came under the umbrella of mental health care, precipitated by his drug dependency and related behaviors. His instability remained prominent. Collaboration among caregivers commenced with several family therapy hours. All family members presented anxiety, resistance, conflict, and hostility. Their energy was directed toward the aborting of this therapy effort. The fact that they sat in the same room and were unified in their covert efforts to disrupt and obstruct these sessions was evident and held potential for future growth and positive family cohesion.

One might question the focus of therapy on Mabel rather than on the family itself. Mabel was the identified client and the entry of the therapist into the family system. It was apparent that Mabel's distress was not only spilling over on the other family members but also that her pathological behavior was having a controlling effect on the family. No progress would be achieved without targeting assistance at the source of the family distress. Health changes for Mabel did affect the family as well. Her position of control through her illness had to be relinquished.

Often many months of encounters with Mabel were unremarkable as to change or progress, and evaluation showed little growth. Often a conclusion of no change was viewed as a plateau period when new healthy behaviors, such as household task completion and improved personal appearance, were maintained. Continued time structuring impeded the client's involvement in thought disorder and negativism during these time spans. Plateau periods were times to seed new health concepts and nurture these concepts through an embryonic stage with a goal of producing budding new healthy behaviors.

Verbal exchange took place with ease after the first 2 years of therapy, but conversation often remained on a superficial level. Mental checklists of task achievement, medication maintenance, and body language assessment were constant evaluative measures by the nurse-therapist in all weekly encounters. New expectations had to be planted with care and a casual manner. Time to nurture the idea was a primary requirement to accomplish the expectation. Often new behaviors appeared to be spontaneous when they were, in reality, the germination of a long-cultivated idea. For example, Henry began to be invited to share a meal with his parents. This family meal became a twice-a-month occasion, apparently enjoyed by all parties.

In a seemingly spontaneous manner but fostered by a realistic security in the professional relationship, Mabel began to share some of her life concerns about Harry's drinking, about Harry himself, about unstable family finances, and about her children. Expressions of concern and caring for others were new for her and perceived as an uncertain undertaking. Self-absorption had not prevented or protected her from being hurt in relationships. There were many fallacies in Mabel's thinking—concepts that were a part of her life-style. There were few answers to some of Mabel's self-blame and guilt. Ventilation of feelings produced a needed catharsis effect. Some of the past could not be changed, but the present could be coped with in new and more effective ways on a day-to-day basis. Mabel's positive coping with family financial affairs could be reinforced as potential for other healthful coping measures and would also affirm her positive self.

During the course of her relationship with the therapist, Mabel remained extremely dependent on her husband. She did not choose to risk other friendships outside her marriage. This was not a healthy stance, but the idea of activities outside her family sphere was presented with the expectation that at some point Mabel would feel strong enough to venture into the outside world. No group therapy experience was available.

Spontaneous changes occurred several times each year. Mabel began leaving the house more frequently with Harry. At times, she would recount encounters and dialogue with Henry, both positive and negative. These mother-son interactions indicated an attempt to cope more effectively within the family system. Some weeks, nurse therapy dialogue grappled with the core of her life dilemmas. Other weeks passed with dialogue of little depth. The therapist was constantly planting seeds of expectation and nurturing Mabel with verbal support and personal affirmation.

Termination was based on circumstances outside either person's control. Mabel had untapped potential for growth, adaptation, change, and health. Furthermore, based on the chronicity and duration of her mental health problems, she was a candidate for supportive nurse-psychotherapy over an extended rehabilitation period.

Mabel expressed no emotion over the termination experience itself. She withdrew from the process, unwilling to allow grief feelings and shielding herself from the turmoil that can be felt at the end of a significant relationship. The steps of reviewing growth, goal achievement, and expression of personal feelings about Mabel herself and about the relationship were verbalized by the therapist. Mabel was in the early infancy of her emotional development and could not cope positively with the termination experience. Role modeling honest expression of feelings would leave a mark for her future reference. As a technique of intervention, role modeling for a client can provide a passive emotional experience that does not necessitate the entrance to an area of perceived risk. Passage of time and repeated exposure to positive passive emotional experiences may provide the incentive to initiate the actual experiencing of such threatening feelings and encounters.

Restoration and maintenance measures applied through nursing process may mean that end evaluation is difficult to measure when healing has only begun. Chronicity, diminished emotional capacity, atrophy of living skills, apathy, and a reluctance to dissipate pathological behavior often counteract corrective nursing measures. Decompensation becomes a constant variable, even a life-style. Mabel would not be described as mentally healthy. In fact, behavioral assessment would place her within the limits of mental illness. Therefore it is important to note that her behavioral deviations were less severe and fluctuated less often. Mabel was increasingly functional. The quality of her life had changed, as had the quality of family life. Overall, therapy can frequently be judged by a positive change in the quality of life within the boundaries of each client's values.

SUMMARY PERSONAL PROFILE
Social adjustment

S   "Harry liked my chicken; I think I'll fix it again next week." "Henry had dinner with us." "Harry took me out for fish on Friday." "I can't go with him. . ." "I like to watch daytime T.V." "I've started reading a book my daughter gave me."

O   Limited interaction with son. Increased interaction with husband. Limited extension beyond the boundaries of her home.

Emotional health status

S   "Harry liked my chicken; I think I'll fix it again next week." "Henry had dinner with us." "It's not so bad to get the laundry done." "I can't go with him. . ." "No, I don't need to sleep all the time now." "I like to watch daytime T.V." "I've started reading a book my daughter gave me."

O   Up and dressed by 10 A.M. daily. Appearance neat and clean. Prepared five to seven meals a week. Completed laundry without distress. Accurate management of family finances. Limited interaction with son. Increased interaction with husband. Limited extension beyond the boundaries of her home.

Physical health status

S ⎱ No acknowledged or observable
O ⎰ change.

Spiritual dimension

S ⎱
O ⎰ No acknowledged or observable change.

Daily living skill performance

S   ''Harry liked my chicken; I think I'll fix it again next week.'' ''It's not so bad to get the laundry done.''

O   Up and dressed by 10 A.M. daily. Appearance neat and clean. Prepared five to seven meals a week. Completed laundry without distress. Accurate management of family finances.

Coping skill repertoire

S   ''Harry liked my chicken; I think I'll fix it again next week.'' ''Henry had dinner with us.'' ''It's not so bad to get the laundry done.'' ''I can't go with him . . .'' ''No, I don't need to sleep all the time now.'' ''I like to watch daytime T.V.'' ''I've started reading a book my daughter gave me.'' ''I can't take the hassle when he's home.'' ''Oh, I can't go without Harry.''

O   Up and dressed by 10 A.M. daily. Appearance neat and clean. Prepared five to seven meals a week. Completed laundry without distress. Accurate management of family finances. Limited interaction with son. Increased interaction with husband. Limited extension beyond the boundaries of her home.

Maturational struggle according to Erikson's developmental stages

S   ''It's not so bad to get the laundry done.'' ''I decided to try a new stew recipe.'' ''I can't go with him . . .''

O   Basic trust vs. basic mistrust—beginning limited drive and hope.
Autonomy vs. shame and doubt—beginning extremely limited autonomy.
Intimacy vs. isolation—isolation remains prominent.

Self-integration

S   ''Harry liked my chicken; I think I'll fix it again next week.'' ''Henry had dinner with us.'' ''It's not so bad to get the laundry done.'' ''I can't go with him . . .'' ''No, I don't need to sleep all the time now.'' ''I like to watch daytime T.V.'' ''I've started reading a book my daughter gave me.'' ''I can't take the hassle when he is home.'' ''Oh, I can't go without Harry.''

O   Up and dressed by 10 A.M. daily. Appearance neat and clean. Prepared five to seven meals a week. Completed laundry without distress. Accurate management of family finances. Limited interaction with son. Increased interaction with husband. Limited extension beyond the boundaries of her home.

Quality of life

S   ''No, I don't need to sleep all the time now.'' ''I like to watch daytime T.V.'' ''I've started reading a book my daughter gave me.'' ''Do you like my new sweater?'' ''I can't go with him . . .''

O   Up and dressed by 10 A.M. Appearance neat and clean. Prepared five to seven meals a week. Completed laundry without distress. Accurate management of family finances. Limited interaction with son. Increased interaction with husband. Limited extension beyond the boundaries of her home.

SUGGESTED READINGS

American Nurses' Association: Standards of psychiatric mental-health nursing practice, Kansas City, 1973, The Association.

Becker, M. H.: The health belief model and sick role behavior, Nursing Digest **6:**35-40, Spring, 1978.

Caplan, G., and LeGovia, S., editors: Adolescence: psychosocial perspectives, New York, 1969, Basic Books, Inc., Publishers.

Clement, J.: Family therapy: the transferability of theory to practice, Journal of Psychiatric Nursing **15:**33-37, Aug. 1977.

Craig, A., and Hyatt, B.: Chronicity in mental illness: a theory on the role of change, Perspectives in Psychiatric Care **16:**139-154, May/June, 1978.

Daniel, W.: Adolescents in health and disease, St. Louis, 1977, The C. V. Mosby Co.

Eichel, E.: Assessment with a family focus, Journal of Psychiatric Nursing **16:**11-14, Jan., 1978.

Gossop, M.: Drug dependence: the pattern of drug abuse, Nursing Times **74:**1060-1061, June 22, 1978.

Govani, L., and Hayes, J.: Drugs and nursing implications, New York, 1971, Appleton-Century-Crofts.

Huberty, D. H., et al.: Adolescent chemical dependency, Perspectives in Psychiatric Care **16:**21-27, Jan./Feb., 1978.

Kline, N., and Davis, J.: Psychotropic drugs, American Journal of Nursing **73:**54-63, 1973.

Knapp, M.: Non-verbal communication in human interaction, New York, 1972, Holt, Rinehart & Winston, Inc.

Kolb, L.: Modern clinical psychiatry, Philadelphia, 1977, W. B. Saunders Co.

Krieger, D.: Therapeutic touch: the imprimatur of nursing, American Journal of Nursing **75:**784-787, May, 1975.

Ray, O.: Drugs, society, and human behavior, ed. 2, St. Louis, 1978, The C. V. Mosby Co.

Rouhani, G.: Understanding anxiety, Nursing Mirror **146:**25-27, March 9, 1978.

CHAPTER 10

KIM P *manifests*

PROBLEMATIC LIFE CONDUCT

evidenced by

COMMUNICATION BARRIERS AND SELF-ABSORPTION

INTRODUCTORY PERSONAL PROFILE
Social adjustment

S   "Me Kim." "Why you come?"*
O   Employed as a factory assembly line work-
    er. Erratic work attendance due to high anx-
    iety level and psychotropic drug side ef-
    fects. Work production level high when
    present. Tolerated by other employees. Al-
    ternately praised and reprimanded by
    employer. On the surface mother and
    daughter appear to have an open, loving re-
    lationship. Available records characterize
    her as mute. Severe language barrier prom-
    inent.

Emotional health status

S   "Me Kim." "Why you come?"*
O   Withdrawn, passive posture. Flat affect.
    Frequent movements of hands and feet. Er-
    ratic work attendance due to high anxiety
    level and psychotropic drug side effects.
    On the surface mother and daughter appear

to have an open, loving relationship. Excessive reliance on husband. Available records characterize her as mute. Severe language barrier prominent.

Physical health status

S   *
O   Height 5 feet. Weight 105 pounds. Ques-
    tionable routine of drug maintenance. Fol-
    lows eating pattern of her family of
    origin.

Spiritual dimension

S   *
O   No present church affiliation.

Daily living skill performance

S   *
O   Neat, clean appearance. Home maintained
    in immaculate condition. Erratic work at-
    tendance due to high anxiety level and
    psychotropic drug side effects. Work pro-
    duction high when present. Daughter, neat,
    clean, well nourished. Available records
    characterize her as mute. Severe language
    barrier prominent.

---

*Absence of subjective data indicates limited verbal ex-
change, extended periods of silence in therapy, or lack of
comment to the clinician's queries.

Coping skill repertoire

S   "Me Kim." "Why you come?"*

O   Withdrawn, passive posture. Flat affect. Frequent movements of hands and feet. Erratic work attendance due to high anxiety level and psychotropic drug side effects. On the surface mother and daughter appear to have an open, loving relationship. Excessive reliance on husband. Available records characterize her as mute. Severe language barrier prominent.

Maturational struggle according to Erikson's developmental stages

S   "Me Kim." "Why you come?"*

O   Basic trust vs. basic mistrust.
     Autonomy vs. shame and doubt.
     Identity vs. role confusion.

Self-integration

S   "Me Kim." "Why you come?"*

O   Withdrawn, passive posture. Flat affect. Frequent movements of hands and feet. Erratic work attendance due to high anxiety level and psychotropic drug side effects. On the surface mother and daughter appear to have an open, loving relationship. Excessive reliance on husband. Available records characterize her as mute. Severe language barrier prominent.

Quality of life

S   *

O   Employed as a factory assembly line worker. Withdrawn, passive posture. Available records characterize her as mute. Severe language barrier prominent. On the surface mother and daughter appear to have an open, loving relationship. Excessive reliance on husband.

---

*Absence of subjective data indicates limited verbal exchange, extended periods of silence in therapy, or lack of comment to the clinician's queries.

Time span: 2 years

Kim is a 27-year-old woman of Asian descent. She is 5 feet tall, weighing 105 pounds, and dwells at length on the fact that she was a desirable and fragile 87 pounds before her marriage to Sam 9 years ago. Kim's Oriental features are highlighted by black, lustrous hair and a clear, clean complexion. Her eyes portray emotional distance, and during occasions of high stress they reveal a frightened inner feeling.

Kim at 16 years of age met her husband when he was on a tour of duty with the U.S. military service in the Far East. Sam spent his off-duty hours with Kim and her family. They were married when she was in the second trimester of her pregnancy with their daughter, Ann. For Kim this marriage was to consummate the expectation of a long-held fantasy: Sam would care for her, provide for her dependent person, and bring her to the United States.

Kim has a limited command of the English language and has not transferred her extreme dependence on her family of origin for emotional support and sustenance and for correct choices of successful life coping skills. Sam is 35 years of age and has no marketable employment skill. Since his discharge from the military service, he has been attending school under the G.I. Bill. He does not seem to have a defined educational objective, employment goal, or defined life direction. He completed a program of study for an associate degree in liberal arts and is presently commencing his third program in a vocational institute. He expresses little concern about his life-career ambition or family responsibilities and states that he is sure his present educational experience has great potential. One concludes that he expects to complete this 15-month course. He is quick to assure one that he likes this program better than the other courses of study he dropped after partial completion.

Kim is employed at a factory on an assembly line. Her employer views her as a good worker whose production level is high when she is present, but Kim is erratic in her work attendance. High anxiety and psychotropic drug side effects lead to absenteeism. Co-workers describe Kim as "unfriendly, different, and strange." Her language barrier, stress-related behaviors, and low self-concept do not create a medium for interpersonal contacts or friendly associations, even on a superficial level. In the work situation, Kim is tolerated by other employees and alternately praised and reprimanded by her supervisor, increasing her ambivalent emotions. The employer, aware of the problem, continues to employ Kim only because of her high productivity when she is present. Her asocial behavior adds to the employer's positive concept of Kim as not being associated with dissension and trouble making at the factory.

Ann, an 8-year-old only child, seems to be well adjusted but undisciplined. She has many material possessions and usually finds it easy to manipulate or control one or both parents. She attends public school, is accepted by her peers, and has a good command of the English language. On the surface, Ann and Kim appear to have an open, loving mother-daughter relationship. Further assessment, however, leads the therapist to question the structure of this relationship. Often Ann is observed by the therapist as the nurturing one, giving affection, guidance, and direction to Kim. To the observer, Kim seems like a lost child. Ann's cultural adjustment is stable, but her mother's adaptation to her present life is not rooted or durable.

Sam can be characterized as a drifter, often becoming verbally enthusiastic for a project or goal but rarely completing a task once the glow of newness evaporates. Responsible tasks of life confine him in a manner he cannot tolerate. Although extremely conversive, social, and pleasant during initial encounters with the therapist, he soon absented himself from the home during therapist's visits when perceived demands were placed on him and his role as husband.

The family rents a two-bedroom apartment that is part of an older home restructured as income property. Although this dwelling needs many repairs, Kim maintains it in an immaculate condition. No decorative items enhance the dark rooms, and one received an empty feeling in the clean but shabby and bare premises. Toys and games abound for Ann, and the color T.V. is constantly in use unless the therapist requests that this distraction be curtailed.

Kim has been hospitalized in three different psychiatric facilities in three different states since her arrival in the United States and after Ann's birth. The mobility of the family has not aided in Kim's adjustment. She presently takes no psychotropic medication, although she has a prescription for both chlorpromazine, 100 mg q.i.d., and trifluoperazine, 5 mg b.i.d. Available records indicate that medication management has always been a problem. Kim does take birth control pills as prescribed and with exactness. Later, she will confide in the therapist that she wants "no more babies." For Kim, newly arrived in this country with no family of origin, few English language skills, little understanding of the complex hospital procedures, a limited comprehension of the physiology of her body, and a husband who absented himself from the situation, the childbirth experience was a traumatic event. Kim's memory of it is intensely negative and personally devastating.

Kim's most recent year of outpatient therapy indicated that no progress had been achieved. She refused to take medication as prescribed. Although she arrived for scheduled outpatient appointments, she never verbally communicated with the therapist except in her native tongue. Presence in therapy does not indicate a commitment to becoming involved in the helping relationship. Kim was referred for nurse psychotherapy on a home visit basis for the expressed initial purpose of a mental status assessment and drug evaluation. It was hoped that a change of milieu from traditional office-centered therapy and the introduction of a female therapist might be helpful. Not encouraged by the comment, ''You won't get anywhere. She doesn't even speak English,'' the nurse began to form a plan to approach this client and therapy situation. Short-term therapy focusing on assessment and evaluation of the client would yield basic information for deciding on the choice of extended therapy involvement.

Available records presented meager data, underscoring the lack of understandable verbal exchange. An initial contact by telephone was not conducive to client rapport or to a climate of trust. Since Kim postured a complete language barrier stance, the first visit was arranged through her husband. This usual adaptation measure of reliance on Sam to speak for her and arrange her life was permeated with inner conflict and hostility.

At the appointed time the therapist arrived to meet the entire family. Kim nodded when introduced by Sam and retreated to the background of the room. Sam embarked on nonstop, highly emotive but pleasant conversation of stories about himself and his life. When he was not speaking, Ann verbally vied for time to tell her pressing tales. The child sat close to the therapist, taking her hand and commenting, ''I like you.'' Ann had unmet security needs vital to her development and emotional growth. Parental consistency, support, and guidance were missing elements to help her maintain her autonomy, initiative, emotional development, and self-growth. Kim viewed these interactions in a withdrawn, passive posture. Her affect was flat. Frequent movements of her hands and feet were clues to her inner restlessness and anxiety. She communicated a need for attention but less assertively than her husband and daughter. She would never be able to compete with the high English verbal skills and learned social pleasantries of Sam and Ann.

After 30 minutes of attentiveness to father and daughter and distant passive observation of the identified client, the therapist turned the focus of attention to Kim. ''I've enjoyed getting acquainted with you, Sam, and with you, Ann, but it is you, Kim, that I came to spend time with.''

''Oh, she doesn't talk,'' Sam answers.

The therapist responded by directly looking at Kim and asking if they could talk in the kitchen so as not to disturb Sam and Ann. Kim made no audible verbal or noticeable affective response but walked to the kitchen and sat at the table. The therapist followed suit. Affronted, Sam announced he was going out to the garage to work on his truck. Ann pouted and followed her mother and the therapist into the kitchen. Gently but firmly, the nurse directed Ann to use her crayons to complete a picture in her coloring book. She was further told that she could show her drawing to the nurse in half an hour. Unhappily expressing verbal resistance but finally compliant, Ann set about her assigned task.

The therapist began addressing Kim, facing her directly and talking slowly, simply, and distinctly. The nurse acknowledged Kim's existing language barrier and in addition disclosed an awareness that Kim did have a limited understanding of spoken English, as evidenced by her ability to follow directions and be productive on the job. The role of the nurse was defined for Kim as that of a helper and confidant. An initial schedule of weekly visits was established for a nondefined period. The setting of these visits would be at Kim's home. The therapist emphatically and repeatedly stated that these visits were for Kim herself. Client and therapist together would be expected to spend 1 hour a week away from the distraction of her family. Further acknowledgment was made of Kim's continual emotional turmoil and existing adjustment problems. The therapist expressed a desire, commitment, and belief that she could help Kim. In closing, the nurse asked Kim how she wished to be addressed. Her affect remaining flat, and staring at the therapist with the first observed eye-to-eye contact, she responded, ''Me Kim.'' A new appointment time was established by the therapist by pointing to the calendar and head nodding by the client. The time and date of this appointment were written on the kitchen calendar. Ann's drawing was praised as the child sat on the therapist's lap, and the first encounter drew to a close.

The content of the second interview was cast in the same mold, following a similar structured format. Sam was miffed at early termination of social conversation and left. Ann needed to be engaged in an activity with the promise of attention from the therapist later in the hour. Client and nurse sat in the kitchen facing one another. Again, slowly, simply, and distinctly the information from the first encounter was restated. Kim had increased, but fleeting, eye-to-eye contact. Her limbs moved restlessly, and she fidgeted, frequently changing sitting positions. When asked if she had any questions, Kim responded quietly, "Why you come?" Repetition of the already-given answers with emphasis on the care and concern helper role was elaborated in short, direct responses. Rudimentary rapport was commencing. A climate had been established for developing a trust relationship. Surprisingly, this interview ended with a statement of "You come back?" initiated by Kim. Ann received warm verbal and physical stroking for her task and for remaining in her defined limits.

Nursing judgment based on assessment of all available data led to the following nursing diagnosis:

Anxiety
Dependence/independence struggle
Low self-concept
Thought disorder
Perceptual disturbance
Autism
Interpersonal relationship disturbance
Emotional deprivation
Language barrier
Separation anxiety
Unresolved grief
Faulty support system
Short concentration span

Psychotropic medication side effects
Passive resistance
Communication disturbance within the marital relationship

It was vitally important to establish a communication pattern of interacting with Kim on an adult-to-adult level. In most previous adult relationships she was treated as a child. These communications held innuendos of incompetence, stupidity, and lack of personal worth, further decreasing her vulnerable self-concept and self-esteem. The need for precise clarity of speech and an extensive language barrier need not produce an impasse between two people. Understanding the reality and scope of the problem, patience, a carefully planned intervention, skilled ongoing assessment, and a true care and concern would help to define the limits of the total problem and provide data for further intervention. Nursing judgment concluded that consistent therapy for Kim over many months could achieve goals of resocialization, increased self-awareness, decreased anxiety, and overall cultural adjustment. The expected extended duration of therapy was now defined for Kim. She made no negative or positive response, and the therapist verbalized an understanding of passive agreement.

PROCESS IMPLEMENTATION

1—Evaluation
N.D. *Anxiety*
　　S "Why you come?"*
　　O Withdrawn, passive posture. Flat affect. Frequent movements of hands and feet. Fleeting eye-to-eye contact in the second interview.
N.D. *Dependence/independence struggle*
　　S *
　　O Withdrawn, passive posture. Flat affect. No audible verbal or noticeable affective response but walked to the kitchen as directed and sat at the table.
N.D. *Low self-concept*
　　S "Me Kim." "Why you come?"*

---

*Absence of subjective data indicates limited verbal exchange, extended periods of silence in therapy, or lack of comment to the clinician's queries.

O Withdrawn, passive posture. Flat affect. No audible verbal or noticeable affective response but walked to the kitchen as directed and sat at the table. Staring at the therapist with the first eye-to-eye contact at the end of the initial interview.

N.D. *Interpersonal relationship disturbance*
S "Me Kim." "Why you come?"*
O Withdrawn, passive posture. Flat affect. No audible verbal or noticeable affective response but walked to the kitchen as directed and sat at the table. Staring at the therapist with the first eye-to-eye contact at the end of the initial interview.

N.D. *Language barrier*
S "Me Kim." "Why you come?"*
O Withdrawn, passive posture. Flat affect. No audible verbal or noticeable affective response but walked to the kitchen as directed and sat at the table.

Actual Outcome
Initial rapport established.

2A — Assessment

N.D. *Anxiety*
S *
O Withdrawn, passive posture. Flat affect. Frequent movement of hands and feet. Silence.

N.D. *Dependence/independence struggle*
S *
O Withdrawn, passive posture. Flat affect. Frequent movement of hands and feet. Silence.

N.D. *Interpersonal relationship disturbance*
S *
O Withdrawn, passive posture. Flat affect. Frequent movement of hands and feet. Silence.

N.D. *Language barrier*
S *
O Withdrawn, passive posture. Flat affect. Frequent movement of hands and feet. Silence.

2B — Validation by assessment

N.D. *Anxiety*
S *
O Withdrawn, passive posture. Flat affect. Frequent movement of hands and feet. Silence. Over a duration of several months.

N.D. *Dependence/independence struggle*
S *

---

*Absence of subjective data in Kim's case indicates limited verbal exchange, extended periods of silence in therapy, or lack of comment to the clinician's queries *over a period of several months.*

O Withdrawn, passive posture. Flat affect. Frequent movement of hands and feet. Silence. Over a duration of several months.

N.D. *Interpersonal relationship disturbance*
S *
O Withdrawn, passive posture. Flat affect. Frequent movement of hands and feet. Silence. Over a duration of several months.

N.D. *Language barrier*
S *
O Withdrawn, passive posture. Flat affect. Frequent movement of hands and feet. Silence. Over a duration of several months.

3 — Additional nursing diagnosis
None

4A — Variables

Reality timing	0
Relationships	−3
Stressors and/or crisis	−3
Coping resources	−3
Significant emotional strength	−2
Significant emotional limitations	−3
Therapy relationship	0
Physical health status	0
Physical and emotional readiness dimension	0
Available support system	−2
Meaning significance	0
Values and belief impact	0
Other	
BALANCE	−

Additional specific knowledge
See case material.

Analysis and synthesis

N.D. *Anxiety*. Relationships present a fear of the unknown and fear of failure. A sense of apprehension may be due to the previously learned knowledge that a caregiver will have expectations of her. Sensitivity from the therapist is paramount to the state of rapport.

N.D. *Dependence/independence struggle*. Dependence seems to be accepted as an elementary position in client's communication. One has to wonder just how much this client really understands in her withdrawn state.

N.D. *Interpersonal relationship disturbance*. Usual stance of passivity, withdrawal, and reliance on husband does not encourage positive encounters or a sense of positive self-esteem for the client.

N.D. *Language barrier*. Bridging this obstacle will

establish the needed signals to facilitate evaluation of English language potential and a method of discernible communication between client and nurse.

4B — Design of action

N.D.   Anxiety, dependence/independence struggle, interpersonal relationship disturbance, language barrier.

1. Plan
   a. Clarify a method of comprehendible communication between client and nurse.
   b. Clarify verbal and nonverbal signals to indicate misunderstanding.
2. Strategy
   a. Demonstrate empathy and care-concern for client.
   b. Clarify and define structure, rules, and purpose of the relationship.
   c. Remain honest concerning comprehension of client's messages.
   d. Actively listen to client.
   e. Investigate language tutoring.
3. Expected outcomes
   a. Partial comprehension and understanding between client and nurse.
   b. Increased verbalization by client in the mutually understood language.
   c. Involvement in language tutoring.
4. Criteria
   a. Establishment of mutually acceptable nonverbal signals to understanding and misunderstanding.
   b. Establishment of acceptable verbal signals to understanding and misunderstanding.
   c. Expansion of English language skills.

The language barrier in this relationship demanded a careful assessment. Actual limits of the understanding of verbal communications, the boundaries of verbal expression, and methods and keys to clarification and comprehension of messages sent by each party must be identified by the therapist. Discernment of the variables affecting Kim's language barrier required hypotheses and validations. A mutual understanding between client and nurse had to be achieved regarding encoding and decoding of messages sent and received by each. Acceptable verbal and nonverbal signals for clarifying misunderstanding by client and nurse had to be established.

The initial months of contact, although laborious and tedious in nature, proved that Kim understood about 25% of the messages received, and careful repetition increased her comprehension by another 25%. Her verbal expression was extremely limited. Her cognitive process was in her native tongue, and she transcribed the subject matter with great effort into English. Her knowledge and command of the semantics of the English language were extremely limited. The communication problem was further magnified by the psychopathology of her faulty association and disassociation of ideas. This associative disorder magnified the problem of transcribing messages to an understandable form.

The care-concern manner and thoughtful approach of the therapist seemed to intrigue Kim. She would ask, "Why you see me?" She had no friends and was positioned both by choice and other member placement on the periphery of her nuclear family. She seemed to perceive the nurse with an aura of wonderment because therapy hours focused on Kim as a worthy adult person. Gradually, she could express to the therapist misunderstanding clues such as "no," and "don't know." Head shaking, hands waving, and rapid but uncomprehensive speech were signals of misinterpretation and lack of understanding. The bonds of this trusting professional relationship allowed Kim the freedom to risk verbal communication within a new and securely defined area with stated rules and consistency of structure. The therapist remained honest concerning her own level of comprehension from Kim's expression but always made several attempts to clarify expression when the frequent misunderstanding occurred. Kim seemed free to negate a statement when the therapist said, "Do you mean . . .?" As the relationship intensified, client and nurse could accept an inability to communicate clearly on a verbal level. They could even laugh at some misunderstandings. Nonverbal communication assumed increased importance in this interpersonal relationship. A calm stance and increased awareness by the therapist of the observable person and environment were of paramount importance for mutual understanding and meaning. Kim was able to take the initiative to uncloud several communication errors. It became significant to her for the nurse to actually hear what she had to say. This motivation assisted in Kim's effort and involvement in distinct and comprehendible message sending and reception.

Language tutoring was pursued. An available, knowledgeable professor had attempted to work with Kim the previous year. He was unwilling to begin the task again until Kim's attention span increased and until she had less distracting body gestures. During her previous tutoring session, Kim, motivated by an anxiety level close to panic, experiencing fear and agitation and a turbulent thought process, would quickly absent herself from the session without warning. Flight was her only available self-protection. Kim did not want to pursue tutoring now, nor did she have the inner control to meet the reasonable expectation of the only available teacher. The language tutoring program was tabled until both participants were open to negotiate the demands established for successful task completion.

PROCESS IMPLEMENTATION

1—Evaluation

N.D.   *Anxiety*
   S   "Why you see me?" "No." "Don't know." "Say again." "Me try." "What you say?"*
   O   Head shaking, hand waving, and rapid but uncomprehensive speech become signals of misinterpretation and lack of understanding. Unable to meet demands of language tutoring.

N.D.   *Dependence/independence struggle*
   S   "Why you see me?" "No." "Don't know." "Say again." "Me try." "What you say?"*

---

*Absence of subjective data indicates limited verbal exchange, extended periods of silence in therapy, or lack of comment to the clinician's queries. Less prominent factor of the interviews but continues to be significant.

   O   Head shaking, hand waving, and rapid but uncomprehensive speech become signals of misinterpretation and lack of understanding. Unable to meet demands of language tutoring.

N.D.   *Interpersonal relationship disturbance*
   S   "Why you see me?" "No." "Don't know." "Say again." "Me try." "What you say?"*
   O   Head shaking, hand waving, and rapid but uncomprehensive speech become signals of misinterpretation and lack of understanding. Unable to meet demands of language tutoring.

N.D.   *Language barrier*
   S   "Why you see me?" "No." "Don't know." "Say again." "Me try." "What you say?"*
   O   Head shaking, hand waving, and rapid but uncomprehensive speech become signals of misinterpretation and lack of understanding. Unable to meet demands of language tutoring.

Actual outcome

Increased comprehendible verbal exchange. Establishment of mutually acceptable verbal and nonverbal signals to understanding and misunderstanding. Language program tabled until readiness established.

2A—Assessment

N.D.   *Low self-concept*
   S   "He holler then." "Me feel bad." "Me no good." "Sometimes me get mad." "Me work hard." "He don't care." (Referring to husband).
   O   Demonstrated drowsiness, lethargy, and tardive dyskinesia in the form of involuntary movement of her limbs. Dryness of the mouth and constipation are other troublesome drug-related symptoms. Behaviors related to drug ingestion interfered with work productivity and relationships. Absence of durable relationships. Intensity and supportiveness of marriage relationship questionable.

N.D.   *Perceptual disturbance*
   S   "He holler then." "Me no good."
   O   Demonstrated drowsiness, lethargy, and tardive dyskinesia in the form of involuntary movement of her extremities. Dryness of the mouth and constipation are other troublesome drug-related symptoms. Behaviors related to drug ingestion interfered with work productivity and relationships. Absence of durable relationships. Intensity and supportiveness of marriage relationship questionable. Source of corrective feedback to validate perception absent.

N.D.   *Interpersonal relationship disturbance*
   S   "Me feel bad." "Me no good." "Sometime

me get mad.'' ''Me work hard.'' ''He don't care.'' (Referring to husband.)

    O Demonstrated drowsiness, lethargy, and tardive dyskinesia in the form of involuntary movement of her limbs. Dryness of the mouth and constipation are other troublesome drug-related symptoms. Behaviors related to drug ingestion interfered with work productivity and relationships. Absence of durable relationships. Intensity and supportiveness of marriage relationship questionable.

N.D. *Emotional deprivation*

    S ''Me feel bad.'' ''Me no good.'' ''Sometime me get mad.'' ''Me work hard.'' ''He don't care.'' (Referring to husband.)

    O Absence of durable relationships. Intensity and supportiveness of marriage relationship questionable.

N.D. *Psychotropic medication side effects*

    S ''He holler then.'' ''Me feel bad.'' ''It no good.'' ''It make me bad.''

    O Demonstrated drowsiness, lethargy, and tardive dyskinesia in the form of involuntary movement of her limbs. Dryness of the mouth and constipation are other troublesome drug-related symptoms. Behaviors related to drug ingestion interfered with work productivity and relationships.

3 — Additional nursing diagnosis
None

4A — Variables

Variable	Value
Reality timing	+2
Relationships	−4
Stressors and/or crisis	0
Coping resources	0
Significant emotional strength	0
Significant emotional limitations	−3
Therapy relationship	+3
Physical health status	0
Physical and emotional readiness dimension	+2
Available support system	−2
Meaning significance	+2
Values and belief impact	+2
Others	
BALANCE	+

Additional specific knowledge
See case material.

Analysis and synthesis

N.D. *Low self-concept.* Client integrates negative or perceived negative messages too readily. Can client hear positive messages? How much of her behavior is to protect her faulty self-concept?

N.D. *Perceptual disturbance.* Client withdrawn to a state of existence that only provides negative feedback, facilitating misperception and perceptual distortion. Positive and corrective feedback to validate reality perception is mandatory.

N.D. *Interpersonal relationship disturbance.* Client's different behaviors are partially because of her cultural adjustment and are viewed as ''strange.'' Unsure of how to respond, she continues her unacceptable behavior and low self-concept is reinforced.

N.D. *Emotional deprivation.* Unable or unwilling to make emotional contact with any significant person creates an empty helpless, alone feeling. One has to hypothesize that attempts at emotional closeness have been rejected or unsuccessful for the client.

N.D. *Psychotropic medication side effects.* Erratic patterns of drug ingestion prevent the intended effect. A controlled substance will permit ongoing assessment of both positive and negative effects. If thought disorder is a factor, psychotrophic medication should assist with language and interpersonal problems.

4B — Design of action
N.D. Low self-concept, perceptual disturbance, interpersonal relationship disturbance, emotional deprivation, psychotropic medication side effects.

  1. Plan
    a. Encourage self-disclosure.
    b. Evaluate drug regimen.
  2. Strategy
    a. Active listening.
    b. Validate reality.
    c. Initiate collaboration to evaluate and facilitate drug change.
    d. Educate concerning drug management.
  3. Expected outcomes
    a. Release of inner conflict and anxiety.
    b. Increased authentic self-perception.
    c. Increased comfort in relation to drug regimen.
    d. Understanding of need for drug maintenance.
  4. Criteria
    a. Relaxed posture.
    b. Increased verbalization in English.
    c. Expression of perceptions that are in alignment with reality.
    d. Expression of limited understanding concerning drug maintenance.

Kim gained strength as the duration and intensity of the nursing encounter grew. She could take the initiative to help structure the clinician-client time, removed from the demands of her husband and child. One must never underestimate the effect of a listening-hearing, other-centered concentration within a relationship. This type of focus can tap previously unsurfaced potential and provide a medium for freeing the client to risk personal growth. In this safe climate, Kim began to expose her hurt.

Prominent in therapy hours was the verbal release of Kim's inner feelings. Withheld anxieties and the expression of conflicts, anger, hostility, perceived hurt, and negative feelings were unburdened in a deliberate communication effort in therapy, yielding a catharsis effect for Kim. These expressive, emotive sessions, a renewed ability to trust another individual, and a feeling of less separation from human warmth encouraged Kim's ability to speak in the English language and a better literal application of the language while in therapy. New but passing positive emotions related to her self-concept and to a new therapy-related sensation of purification often created a short-lived euphoria for Kim. Feeling expression in therapy was a beginning of release from a negative emotional bondage. Kim was not ready or did she have the inner resources and needed healthy support system to allow a beginning adaptation in her daily living. Long hours of purgative listening-hearing interviews were needed to counteract negative, hurting emotions before an action-oriented relieving intervention could be initiated.

Kim was encouraged to express her feelings with a present, not past, orientation. A focus on today and the immediate was mandatory. Autistic thinking, frightening dreams, and obvious associative disturbances were present and did interfere with actual person availability to the therapist and energy for therapy goals. A tight, protective paranoid ideation produced reasons for not ingesting antipsychotic drugs as prescribed. Kim would not take her medication because of the color, or the size, or the shape of

the pills. Actual assessment seemed to verify that she did not like the feeling that the medication produced in her. She suffered from drowsiness, lethargy, and also tardive dyskinesia in the form of involuntary movement of her limbs. In addition, dryness of the mouth and constipation were prominent and troublesome drug-related problems. It seems that Kim's productivity at work suffered when she took high dosages of phenothiazine derivatives. "He holler then," she volunteered, referring to her supervisor. Any negative comment to Kim further lowered her already faulty, low self-concept and increased her negative feelings of self-degradation and self-debasement.

Intramuscular injections of fluphenazine hydrochloride elixir were begun at a low initial dosage and were also maintained at this low level on an every-3-week schedule. An antiparkinsonism drug was prescribed to control adverse reactions. Kim took the "white pill" daily as directed because it did help her feel better. Her discomfort was most prominent at the midway or peak point between injections, but this distress was minimal. Her overall attention span, availability to therapy, and functional living status were increased. Her thought process appeared to be more contained, as demonstrated by a significant decrease in flight of ideas and associative disturbance and an increased communication ability both as a sender and receiver of messages. Collaboration between nurse and psychiatrist yielded an agreement in judgment on the psychic desirability and soundness of an additional dosage level increase of fluphenazine hydrochloride, but overall consideration of the adverse effects on her daily living routine would negate any possible positive achievements from such an increment. The initial low dosage level of this drug became the maintenance level for the duration of nurse psychotherapy.

Kim's only valid complaint concerning her drug ingestion was her resultant weight gain of 10 pounds. She looked healthy and was within weight norms for her age and height. She did not appear obese. Her lament of "Me fat" was countered with suggestions about exercise and diet. Kim's comment to this was a smiling "Me lazy." After the initial weight gain of 10 pounds, her weight stabilized at 115 pounds. Kim's self-image perception of her slight body size and formerly attractive self as an Oriental adolescent complicated her overall present low self-concept. The mores and cultural norms of her youth needed to moderate, not change. Diversity in modes of living and life-style and her extended life-age development called for internal and external self-image adjustments, realignment, and maturation. Alteration and substitution are dynamic parts of the life cycle of human beings. Developmental arrest fostered by emotional deprivation and cultural adjustment shock were static variables that needed therapy intervention to begin a stabilizing dynamic process in Kim's life.

PROCESS IMPLEMENTATION

1—Evaluation

N.D. *Low self-concept*
S   "Me fat." "Me lazy." "Me feel better." "Do better work now."
O   Increased ability to speak in the English language. Better literal language application. Weight gain of 10 pounds.

N.D. *Perceptual disturbance*
S   "Me fat." "Me lazy." "Me feel better." "Do better work now."
O   Increased ability to speak in the English language. Better literal language application. Weight gain of 10 pounds.

N.D. *Interpersonal relationship disturbance*
S   "Me fat." "Me lazy." "Me feel better." "Do better work now."
O   Minimal dosage level of fluphenazine hydrochloride given by intramuscular injection every 3 weeks with minimal discomfort. Antiparkinsonism drug taken daily. Overall attention span, availability to therapy, and functional living status were increased. Thought process appeared more contained as demonstrated by decreasing flight of ideas and associative disturbance and increased communication ability as sender and receiver. Only client complaint, a 10-pound weight gain.

N.D. *Emotional deprivation*
S   "Me fat." "Me lazy." "Me feel better." "Do better work now."
O   Increased ability to speak in the English language. Better literal language application. Weight gain of 10 pounds.

N.D. *Psychotropic medication side effects*
S   "Me fat." "Me lazy." "Me feel better." "Do better work now."
O   Increased ability to speak in the English language. Better literal language application. Weight gain of 10 pounds.

N.D. *Psychotropic medication side effects*
S   "Me fat." "Me lazy." "Me feel better." "Do better work now."
O   Minimal dosage level of fluphenazine hydrochloride given by intramuscular injection every 3 weeks with minimal discomfort. Antiparkinsonism drug taken daily. Overall attention span, availability to therapy, and functional living status were increased. Thought process appeared more contained as demonstrated by decreasing flight of ideas and associative disturbance and increased communication ability as sender and receiver. Only client complaint, a 10-pound weight gain.

Actual outcome
Increased self-disclosure and release from inner tensions. Drug regimen adapted to life-style demands.

2A—Assessment

N.D. *Perceptual disturbance*
S   "Me fat." "Can't tell them." "They no like me anymore." "We go back to stay soon." "Me not good."
O   In her youth, she had accepted that to marry an American and come to the United States signified security, wealth, and happiness. Refused to relinquish old, deeply implanted ideas. Sam promised a trip to her native land.

N.D. *Faulty support system*
S   "Me cry." "Me fat." "Can't tell them." "They no like me anymore." "We go back to stay soon."
O   Lacked human stroking from within family and friendship relationship. Sam perpetuated a promised trip to her native land.

N.D. *Separation anxiety*
S   "Me cry." "Me too tired." "Me fat." "Can't tell them." "They no like me anymore."
O   Unwilling to grieve or give up absent family of origin. Shame related to present life intensified feelings of sadness and loss.

N.D. *Unresolved grief*
  S "Me cry." "Me too tired." "Me fat." "Can't tell them." "They no like me anymore."
  O Unwilling to grieve or give up absent family of origin. Shame related to present life intensified feelings of sadness and loss.
N.D. *Low self-concept*
  S "Me can't." "Me too tired." "Me be good." "Can't tell them." "They no like me." "Me crabby." "Me not good."
  O Cultural subservient frame of reference increased her denial, rejection, and sublimation mechanism. Lack of fulfillment and need gratification increased hostility, conflict within the marriage, and overall fatigue from unsatisfactory life experiences.

3 — Additional nursing diagnosis
None

4A — Variables

Reality timing	+2
Relationships	−2
Stressors and/or crisis	0
Coping resources	0
Significant emotional strength	−2
Significant emotional limitations	−2
Therapy relationship	+4
Physical health status	0
Physical and emotional readiness dimension	+2
Available support system	−2
Meaning significance	+4
Values and belief impact	+4
Other	
BALANCE	+

Additional specific knowledge
See case material.

Analysis and synthesis
N.D. *Perceptual disturbance.* Immediately willing to integrate any possible negative message from significant and nonsignificant others, distorting self-perception and maintaining a low or nonfunctional, reliant person.
N.D. *Faulty support system.* Unwilling or unable to sustain or develop a support system within or outside her nuclear family. Encouragement to renew the bonds with her family of origin in an open, honest manner can release energy for present-centered tasks.
N.D. *Separation anxiety.* Inability to experience a new culture, unexpected reality, and life related to the loss of a security base. No trust is felt or perceived by the client in her marriage relationship.

N.D. *Unresolved grief.* Expectations and reality conflict prevent grief related to loss of the security provided by the family of origin to proceed beyond the stage of shock.
N.D. *Low self-concept.* Inner conflict between reality, expectations, and cultural values decreases self-esteem. The conflict itself consumes energy needed for growth and conflict resolution.

4B — Design of action
N.D. Perceptual disturbance, faulty support system, separation anxiety, unresolved grief, low self-concept.
  1. Plan
    a. Continue to encourage self-disclosure and provide validation for reality perception.
    b. Encourage a renewed and open relationship with family of origin.
  2. Strategy
    a. Active listening.
    b. Validate reality.
    c. Urge renewed and open communication by letter with family of origin.
    d. Support positive behaviors and coping mechanisms.
    e. Introduce persons of similar cultural background.
  3. Expected outcomes
    a. Relinquishment of fantasy and acceptance of authentic life position.
    b. Renewed honest relationship with family of origin via mail.
    c. Developing friendship with a person of similar background.
  4. Criteria
    a. Beginning acceptance of reality of life position.
    b. Mutual communication within family of origin.
    c. Beginning involvement in friendship with a person of similar background.

Dialogue became an essential component of therapy, providing a medium to free energy for positive, new directions. Once secure in the professional relationship, finding that trust, confidentiality, and honesty were constant components, this client, formerly labeled mute, unburdened many intense feelings. The fragility of her English speaking skills did not block her thought process expression. One had to reserve clinical judgment regarding the actual fragmentation of her thoughts, since pursuit of word clarification often validated only the presence of fractured and fragmented speech in the identified language, not in the thinking form itself. Increased emotional sharing for Kim and partial discernment of the burdensome feelings by the therapist produced in Kim an increased calm and self-assurance.

Expectation and reality needed a more vivid focus and a definition and comprehension of the point of departure from actuality. In her youth, Kim had accepted that to marry an American and come to the United States would be the epitome of security, wealth, and happiness. This fantasy had been shattered through the acquisition of the desired imagery. Kim's life was marked by insecurity, economic stressors, and absence of happy or pleasant relationships or experiences. She had not relinquished the fantasies impeding her ability to cope with the realities of her present existence. A stated therapy goal became the abandonment of her fantasy and the acknowledgment of her authentic life, both intellectually and emotionally. Then restorative modification and alteration in her life-style could culminate. Kim had living choices that she did not comprehend, which were blocked by her adamant refusal to relinquish old, deeply implanted notions. Freedom from these beliefs would further free her psychic energy for healthy decision making and positive growth.

In addition, Sam had perpetuated the false expectation by promising Kim that she could return to her native land for a visit, and he even talked at length of the family returning to Kim's native country as permanent residents. Promises, dreams, and visions of the future seemed destined to be no more than fantasy. These continued false assurances perpetuated Kim's fantasy life and further disillusioned her in regard to her marriage and the fulfillment of her desired American dream. Kim lacked human stroking from within family and friend relationships and experienced fatigue from long hours

in monotonous, routine factory work and the even longer hours caring for her husband, daughter, and the total housekeeping management responsibility. Sam drifted from one goal to another, from one educational program to another, and from one interest pursuit to another, rarely completing a task. Kim's Oriental cultural subservient frame of reference increased her denial, rejection, and sublimation mechanisms. Lack of fulfillment and need gratification increased Kim's hostility, conflict within her marriage, and overall fatigue from unsatisfactory life experiences.

Separation from a cohesive family of origin along with an unwillingness to grieve for or give up the absent persons only increased Kim's instability. Separation anxiety was always prominent. Feelings of shame related to her life situation also intensified her sadness and loss response. Kim did not want to acknowledge to her mother the perceived failure of her new life-style. Letters to her family were infrequent and avoided the sensitive issues. They omitted acknowledgment of any adjustment dilemmas.

As therapy encounters unfolded the extent of this problem, Kim was urged to write to her family of origin on a constant and regular basis. She was encouraged to disclose the previously concealed, painful problems to her mother. Weeks passed before Kim taxingly set down her written confession. The weeks before the response from her mother arrived were distressing and laced with erratic behaviors. On some days she was quiet and withdrawn; on other days she experienced pressure of speech, transient states of excitement, and increased, more noticeable clarity efforts in diction.

The long-awaited letter arrived after a month's time. The therapist believed that the communication as interpreted by Kim was harsh in tone and condemning in nature. Kim, aware of the underlying blaming tone, was nonetheless renewed and affirmed by the response. The correspondence offered a supportiveness, acceptance, and fondness from the mother's scolding manner. A sense of being cared for was perceived by Kim in the written emotions expressed to her. These affectionate emotions were fortifying, even though they were expressed on the level of a "naughty child" message. Ongoing correspondence provided a link to her past and to her cultural, familial roots, lending a renewed sense of meaning to Kim's life. Energy expended in covert life measures was freed to generate positive healthy life transformations and adjustment.

Attempts to find other people in the community who spoke Kim's language and dialect were unsuccessful. A liaison relationship in which there existed a common vernacular bond could have promoted an exchange of ideas and means of communication.

The therapist focused on Kim's family of origin, now mandating a frequent exchange of letters and encouraging a continual honest expression of feelings. "Sister no like me," she complained. Further conversation elicited feelings of sibling rivalry. It seemed that her sister had two maids and a husband with a position of prominence and power in the small fishing village where most of Kim's family lived. Her sister's good fortune generated in Kim a false self-message of "I am no good." Her life stance and accepted role of low self-esteem, self-degradation, and shallow self-concept fostered fabrication, misinterpretation, and distortion of truth and factual information.

The therapist and client examined available data within an atmosphere of positive assurance. The therapist's expressions of affirmation created a climate of uneasiness, and such true assurances were often verbally rejected by Kim. A message of "You are OK." was frequently countered with "Me not good." Such dialogue was exchanged without the client's acceptance at first. Resolution began after months of declarative dialogue with the therapist giving positive personal feedback and messages of affirmation. Slowly elicited and unsure "Me did?" and "Me can?" statements were countered by the

therapist with "It is better to hear you say that you are good. You really are a valuable person, Kim." And later "Yes, Kim you are a good person." Client and nurse could smile together in recognition of this accomplishment and growth toward self-affirmation. Kim began to understand that her sister's life accomplishments need not demean her and could even be reason for happiness for another person. Intellectual belief of this fact was present, although emotional lack of acceptance remained prominent.

PROCESS IMPLEMENTATION

1—Evaluation

N.D. *Perceptual disturbance*
- S "Sister no like me." "Me not good." "Me did?" "Me can?"
- O Correspondence unfolded sibling rivalry. Beginning intellectual understanding that her sister's life accomplishments need not demean her. Exchange of smile between client and nurse.

N.D. *Faulty support system*
- S "Sister no like me." "Me not good." "Me did?" "Me can?"
- O Taxingly disclosed life situation in letter to mother. Response offered supportiveness, acceptance, and fondness. Ongoing correspondence provided a link to her past and cultural, familial roots.

N.D. *Separation anxiety*
- S "Sister no like me." "Me not good." "Me did?" "Me can?"
- O Taxingly disclosed life situation in letter to mother. Response offered supportiveness, acceptance, and fondness. Ongoing correspondence provided a link to her past and cultural, familial roots.

N.D. *Unresolved grief*
- S "Sister no like me." "Me not good." "Me did?" "Me can?"
- O Taxingly disclosed life situation in letter to mother. Response offered supportiveness, acceptance, and fondness. Ongoing correspondence provided a link to her past and cultural, familial roots.

N.D. *Low self-concept*
- S "Sister no like me." "Me not good." "Me did?" "Me can?"
- O Taxingly disclosed life situation in letter to

mother. Response offered supportiveness, acceptance, and fondness. Ongoing correspondence provided a link to her past and cultural, familial roots. Correspondence unfolded sibling rivalry. Beginning intellectual understanding that her sister's life accomplishments need not demean her. Exchange of smile between client and nurse.

Actual outcome

Beginning acceptance of authentic life position. Renewed, open, mutual relationship with mother by correspondence. Unable to locate a person of similar origin in the client's immediate locale.

2A — Assessment

N.D.   *Low self-concept*

S   "She smarter than mother." "No talk to mother." "Can't understand." "Me no able." "Too hard."

O   Ann's focus outside of home. Absent parental control, self-restraint, and parental interaction. Ann assumed parent role and spoke for Kim in Sam's absence. Observation of mother-child fondness bond but also child nurturing mother.

N.D.   *Interpersonal relationship disturbance*

S   "She smarter than mother." "No talk to mother."

O   Ann's focus outside of home. Absent parental control, self-restraint, and parental interaction. Ann assumed parent role and spoke for Kim in Sam's absence. Observation of mother-child fondness bond but also child nurturing mother.

N.D.   *Emotional deprivation*

S   "She smarter than mother." "No talk to mother."

O   Ann's focus outside of home. Absent parental control, self-restraint, and parental interaction. Ann assumed parent role and spoke for Kim in Sam's absence. Observation of mother-child fondness bond but also child nurturing mother.

N.D.   *Language barrier*

S   "She smarter than mother." "No talk to mother." "Can't understand." "Me no able."

O   Ann's focus outside of home. Absent parental control, self-restraint, and parental interaction. Ann assumed parent role and spoke for Kim in Sam's absence. Observation of mother-child fondness bond but also child nurturing mother.

N.D.   *Short concentration span*

S   "Can't understand." "Me no able." "Too hard."

O   Absent parental control, self-restraint, and parental interaction. Ann assumed parental role and spoke for Kim in Sam's absence. Short

concentration span observed when anxiety most prominent.

3 — Additional nursing diagnosis

None

4A — Variables

Reality timing	+3
Relationships	+1
Stressors and/or crisis	0
Coping resources	+1
Significant emotional strength	+1
Significant emotional limitations	−2
Therapy relationship	+4
Physical health status	0
Physical and emotional readiness dimension	+3
Available support system	+1
Meaning significance	+4
Values and belief impact	+4
Other	
BALANCE	+

Additional specific knowledge

See case material.

Analysis and synthesis

N.D.   *Low self-concept.* "Good mother" is often an important part of a woman's self-worth. Mothering needs to be flexible to the child's growth needs and abilities. Often personal strengths can be an outgrowth of positive role feelings.

N.D.   *Interpersonal relationship disturbance.* An increased bond and intensity in the mother-child interaction can add strength to client's perception of her overall self-concept and abilities.

N.D.   *Emotional deprivation.* Growth demonstrated through client's reaching out to develop mother-child relationship. Client needs and wants to feel an emotional closeness in her life.

N.D.   *Language barrier.* Task exercises in which client understands the game rules and can receive immediate feedback provide experience for learning language skills and thus decreasing the language barrier. Language skills are significant to client as she compares herself to her daughter in relation to command of the English language.

N.D.   *Short concentration span.* Task involvement is usually a good medium to increase length of attention span, particularly when client demonstrates readiness and both intellectual and emotional commitment to the task.

4B—Design of action

N.D. Low self-concept, interpersonal relationship disturbance, emotional deprivation, language barrier, short concentration span.

1. Plan
   a. Involve mother and child in mutually enjoyable pastime tasks.
2. Strategy
   a. Persuade both parties to become involved in task.
   b. Allot a given time to task.
   c. Establish mutually agreed-on task rules.
   d. Monitor task.
3. Expected outcomes
   a. Mutual enjoyment and dialogue of sharing.
   b. Increased self-discipline, intellectual concentration, and language development for both parties.
   c. Task mastery.
4. Criteria
   a. Adherence to established time and rules and task direction.
   b. Observed increased sharing and enjoyable interaction, increased self-discipline, intellectual concentration, language development, and task mastery.
   c. Expressions of task and relationship satisfaction by client and child.

Kim expressed a feeling of distance between herself and her daughter. "She smarter than mother." Ann's language skill and peer involvement took her to commitments outside the small family circle. Assessment concluded that Ann fell comfortably within the norms of accepted physical and emotional growth and development scales. She had experienced little parental control, and her own lack of self-restraint and self-discipline were evident. Ann assumed the parent role and spoke for Kim in Sam's absence. On occasion, the therapist had observed Ann nurturing Kim. Touch, fondling, and voice tone did validate that mother and child shared a love and a fondness bond, but they were experiencing communication, role, and relationship stressors.

To expand and develop this mother-child relationship positively while focusing on Kim's concern and Ann's observed need, the therapist received the consent of both mother and daughter to begin a mutual and enjoyable task. The couple would participate in an activity each evening for 1 hour without the interference of the television or other distracting activity. Ann chose the game and had the responsibility for teaching the exercise to her mother. The chosen game must have defined rules. This activity could not be changed until Kim had mastered it through demonstrating that she understood the rules. The task itself would increase the daily time contact of mother-child encounters in a positive atmosphere with an emotionally safe and defined activity. Both individuals would have an exercise in self-discipline, intellectual concentration, and language development. A mutual time of enjoyment produced a climate for Ann to begin a dialogue of sharing, confiding, and exchange with her mother. This experience of openness within the mother-child relationship would be more important to Ann as she reached adolescence. Kim perceived less distance between herself and her daughter. The important value of her positive self-image as a good mother was affirmed through these action-oriented experiences, from which emotional interchange was a by-product.

The task itself began under the therapist's tutelage, her presence guiding the tone and progress of the procedure. Occasional monitoring of the interaction and task was accomplished by monthly participation and observations by the therapist. Ann needed to be reminded of the defined limits and was not allowed to deviate from or change the stated rules. Kim needed encouragement to continue in the task attempts when she faltered. Furthermore, she needed the approval and overruling of the therapist through verbal advocacy. Sam was invited to join the group. He had neither the patience nor the interest to become involved and refused the invitation, stating he had other, more interesting things to do with his time. Kim and Ann learned several games, Monopoly being their favorite. This shared involvement continued throughout the therapy, although leveling off to a routine of three or four times a week and gradually acquiring a more spontaneous nature. These hours of contented exchange helped to fill Kim's empty feeling, enhanced the mother-daughter relationship, and provided the lacking intellectual and emotional stimulus for growth at the demand level of each person. Pleasure and intimacy experiences were rare occurrences in Kim's life. Pleasurable allotment of time among people can have a relieving, corrective, and restorative effect to the emotionally depleted individual.

The mother-daughter task did not alter the amount of dialogue time between Kim and the therapist. This helpful assistance from the therapist, yielding a renewed and intensified mother-child relationship, broadened Kim's reality perception, trust in the therapist, and commitment to her health work. Involvement with people and tasks decreased the amount of time Kim could give to fantasy and autistic thinking while increasing her reality orientation to the intricacy of her present required corrective adaptations.

PROCESS IMPLEMENTATION

1—Evaluation

N.D.   *Low self-concept*

S   "She tell me about school." "Me like Monopoly." "We talk long time." "Me feel . . . good."

O   Demonstration of game rule mastery. Adherence to scheduled times for pastime activity. Expression of new words, used in correct manner. Climate of open sharing and enjoyment between mother and child. Sam refused to become involved. Increased appropriate affect. Smiling and laughing during pastime.

N.D.   *Interpersonal relationship disturbance*

S   "She tell me about school." "Me like Monopoly." "We talk long time."

O   Demonstration of game rule mastery. Adherence to scheduled times for pastime activity. Expression of new words, used in correct manner. Climate of open sharing and enjoyment between mother and child. Sam refused to become involved.

N.D.   *Emotional deprivation*

S   "She tell me about school." "Me like Monopoly." "We talk long time."

O   Climate of open sharing and enjoyment between mother and child. Sam refused to become involved.

N.D.   *Language barrier*

S   "She tell me about school." "Me like Monopoly." "We talk long time."

O   Demonstration of game rule mastery. Adherence to scheduled times for pastime activity. Expression of new words used in correct manner.

N.D.   *Short concentration span*

S   "She tell me about school." "Me like Monopoly." "We talk long time."

O   Demonstration of game rule mastery. Adherence to scheduled times for pastime activity.

Actual outcome

General adherence to established time, rules, and task direction. Expressions of decreased emotional distance between mother and child. Observed increase in self-discipline, intellectual concentration, and language development by both parties.

2A—Assessment

N.D.   *Communication disturbance within the marital relationship*

S   "Me no talk." "He no want me but in bed."

O   Relationship founded on withheld truths, reserved mutual trust, and suppressed emotional sharing. Both withheld crucial information and actual expectations. A sense of emptiness and coldness pervaded the marriage for Kim. Sam acknowledged satisfaction and no need for change.

N.D.   *Dependence/independence struggle*

S   "Me no talk."

O   Client portrayed a docile, compliant, and accommodating nature during courtship.

N.D.   *Passive resistance*

S   "Me no talk."

O   Magnifying language barrier to coerce dependence. Reliance gave limited control through a mute stance.

N.D.   *Language barrier*

S   "Me no talk."

O   Magnifying language barrier to coerce dependence. Reliance gave limited control through a mute stance.

N.D.   *Emotional deprivation*

S   "He no want me but in bed."

O   A sense of emptiness and coldness pervaded the marriage for Kim. Sam acknowledged satisfaction and no need for change.

3—Additional nursing diagnosis

None

4A—Variables*

Reality timing	+2
Relationships	−4
Stressors and/or crisis	0
Coping resources	−1
Significant emotional strength	−3
Significant emotional limitations	−3
Therapy relationship	+4
Physical health status	0
Physical and emotional readiness dimension	0
Available support system	−2
Meaning significance	+2
Values and belief impact	+2
Other	
BALANCE	−

Additional specific knowledge

See case material.

Analysis and synthesis

N.D. *Communication disturbance within the marital relationship.* Mutual basic stance of dishonesty in relation to one another predicts failure in a marriage.

N.D. *Dependence/independence struggle.* The dilemma perceived by the client is monumental, and although reliance is uncomfortable she seems to feel that self-reliance may produce a situation in which she will be unable to cope effectively.

N.D. *Passive resistance.* Confrontation could be disruptive. The problems may intensify or not resolve to the client's satisfaction. Despite the discomfort, there is some predictability in the helpless stance.

N.D. *Language barrier.* This functional impediment creates a falsely secure foundation for retreat and dependence and for reliance on her husband. The coercion of this stance traps both parties in an unstable relationship. It is necessary to assess the "game" of each party and its payoffs.

N.D. *Emotional deprivation.* The insatiable need to fill this void of positive feeling experiences creates an energy to suppress needs or to reach out to uncertain encounters. Therapy focus

---

*Note variables apply only to client. To facilitate adaptation or change in a marriage, the two parties involved must demonstrate a willingness and readiness to become open to and involved in the process.

should strengthen the client to choose and to engage in positive growth pursuit.

4B—Design of action

N.D. Communication disturbance within the marital relationship, dependence/independence struggle, passive resistance, language barrier, emotional deprivation.

1. Plan
   a. Encourage client self-disclosure and release of angry and hostile feeling.
   b. Facilitate couple therapy.
2. Strategy
   a. Active listening.
   b. Explore feelings.
   c. Validate perception.
   d. Facilitate couple communication.
3. Expected outcomes
   a. Release of inner feelings of hostility and fear.
   b. Open couple communication.
4. Criteria
   a. Open self-disclosure in therapy.
   b. Initiation of couple therapy.

The interpersonal relationship of Sam and Kim had begun with a false foundation of withheld truths, reserved mutual trust, and suppressed emotional sharing. Kim had not expressed her fantasies and expectations related to marriage and Americanization. She had portrayed a docile, compliant, and accommodating nature to win her man. Sam, too, had withheld crucial information and his actual expectations. It was several years after their marriage before Kim discovered that Sam had two previous marriages which ended in divorce. He did not maintain a relationship with or support the children from these unions. His lack of industry, responsibility, and goal completion were a life pattern not obvious to Kim until the obligations of marriage and the duties of child rearing became her sole charge along with the accountability for family financial earnings. These stressors and the absence of a readily available support system unmasked previously hidden pathology.

One passive measure that Kim used to cope with her situation was to magnify her language barrier, thus demanding action from her husband. Sam was coerced to accept this dependence. Kim's passive resistance gave her some needed control in the marriage but isolated her person to an autistic thinking level. Compliance with accepted communication norms would open the healthy world of new relationships to Kim, but it also presented the threat of tipping the delicate balance in this marriage. Kim's underlying fear was that she would lose Sam, not be capable of maintaining herself and Ann, and would have to return to her native land in poverty, disgrace, and shame. This fright and dread were deeply rooted in her psyche and believed as an actual truth.

Sam was apparently happy in the marriage relationship. The couple shared a mutually satisfactory sexual intimacy, but the absence of emotional intimacy created a strained alliance. Kim's troubled self was reaching for security and integrity. This needed sense of closeness was felt in the mother-daughter relationship and the nurse-client relationship, but for Kim, a sense of hostile coldness pervaded the marriage relationship. Sam expressed satisfaction with the marriage per se and acknowledged no need for change. He allowed the therapist to continue visits because their involvement altered Kim's level of dependence and reliance that at times were perceived as cumbersome by this happy-go-lucky husband.

PROCESS IMPLEMENTATION

1—Evaluation

N.D.   *Communication disturbance within the marital relationship*
   S   "Me no talk." "He no want me but in bed." "Kim angry." "No, me can't tell him." "He get mad." "He send Kim home."
   O   Relationship founded on withheld truths, reserved mutual trust, and suppressed emotional sharing. Both withheld crucial information and actual expectations. A sense of emptiness and coldness pervaded the marriage for Kim. Sam acknowledged satisfaction and no need for change. Obligations of marriage, duties of child rearing, and family finances became client's sole charge. Unwilling to confront problem with husband.

N.D.   *Dependence/independence struggle*
   S   "Me no talk." "Kim angry." "No, me can't

tell him." "He get mad." "He send Kim home."
   O   Client portrayed a docile, compliant, and accommodating nature during courtship. Obligations of marriage, duties of child rearing, and family finances became client's sole charge. Unwilling to confront problem with husband.

N.D.   *Passive resistance*
   S   "Me no talk."
   O   Magnifying language barrier to coerce dependence. Reliance gave limited control through a mute stance. Obligations of marriage, duties of child rearing, and family finances become client's sole charge. Unwilling to confront problem with husband.

N.D.   *Language barrier*
   S   "Me no talk."
   O   Magnifying language barrier to coerce dependence. Reliance gave limited control through a mute stance. Unwilling to confront problem with husband.

N.D.   *Emotional deprivation*
   S   "He no want me but in bed." "Kim angry." "No, me can't tell him." "He get mad."
   O   A sense of emptiness and coldness pervaded the marriage for Kim. Sam acknowledged satisfaction and no need for change.

Actual outcome
   Client released uncomfortable emotions in therapy but was unwilling to discuss identified problems openly with husband. Husband perceived no problem. Behavior dynamics between husband and wife unchanged.

2A—Assessment

N.D.   *Anxiety*
   S   "Me too tired." "Me too busy." "Me lazy."
   O   No interest or activity outside family home and job.

N.D.   *Dependence/independence struggle*
   S   "Me painted at home." "Me can draw . . . see." "Me too tired." "Me too busy." "Me lazy."
   O   No interest or activity outside family home and job.

N.D.   *Low self-concept*
   O   "Me painted at home." "Me can draw . . . see." "Me too tired." "Me too busy." "Me lazy."
   O   No interest or activity outside family home and job.

N.D.   *Interpersonal relationship disturbance*
   S   "Me painted at home." "Me can draw . . . see." "Me too tired." "Me too busy." "Me lazy."

O No interest or activity outside family home and job.

N.D. *Language barrier*

　S "Me painted at home." "Me can draw . . . see." "Me too tired." "Me too busy." "Me lazy."

　O No interest or activity outside family home and job.

N.D. *Passive resistance*

　S "Me painted at home." "Me can draw . . . see." "Me too tired." "Me too busy." "Me lazy."

　O No interest or activity outside family home and job.

3—Additional nursing diagnosis
None

4A—Variables

Reality timing	0
Relationship	−3
Stressors and/or crisis	0
Coping resources	−3
Significant emotional strength	−3
Significant emotional limitations	−3
Therapy relationship	+4
Physical health status	0
Physical and emotional readiness dimension	−1
Available support system	−4
Meaning significance	−1
Values and belief impact	−1
Other	
BALANCE	−

Additional specific knowledge
See case material.

Analysis and synthesis

N.D. *Anxiety.* New situations create intense fear of the unknown, exaggerated by past negative experiences. A sense of loss of control further agitates the client's unstable position.

N.D. *Dependence/independence struggle.* The known or predictable safety from a dependent, reliant stance is chosen to decrease anxiety and alleviate uncertain emotions. The client's covert assumption is a return or partial semblance of an inner feeling of control and safety.

N.D. *Low self-concept.* Client intensely believes she cannot relate in an acceptable fashion; furthermore, she views herself as unacceptable in the American culture.

N.D. *Interpersonal relationship disturbance.* Lack of positive reinforcement and multiple negative reinforcement for inabilities to relate on a person-to-person level lead to chronic relationship withdrawal and feelings of inadequacy. Client needs to view professional relationship experiences as transferable.

N.D. *Language barrier.* This reliable, acceptable protective device is chosen when the nature of the experience or encounter is uncertain.

N.D. *Passive resistance.* Direct confrontation of issues, uncertain encounters, or new experiences are perceived as impossible; thus are rejected and action deferred to the reliable mute stance.

4B—Design of action

N.D. Anxiety, dependence/independence struggle, low self-concept, interpersonal relationship disturbance, language barrier, passive resistance.

1. Plan
   a. Involve client in task to develop her artistic talent and encourage associations with others.
2. Strategy
   a. Persuade participation in art class.
   b. Support artistic development.
   c. Encourage and support communication with other art students.
3. Expected outcomes
   a. Demonstration of artistic talent.
   b. Initial relationship with peers.
4. Criteria
   a. Demonstration of completed art task.
   b. Dialogue relating to new person associations in therapy.

Kim needed to develop an interest or activity outside her home. She possessed an artistic talent, displaying for the nurse paintings that she had done in previous years. Persuaded by the therapist, Kim began an evening art class. This involvement expanded her creative talents and unfolded a previously closed avenue of self-expression. During therapy hours, she proudly demonstrated her work. Two pictures were framed and hung on the living room walls, adding color and warmth to the previously drab room.

Kim would not mingle with the other art students, retreating in a stance of withdrawal and the protective cover of her communication barrier. All therapy efforts to commence relationships or other-person encounters were met with "Me can't," "Me can't talk," "Me don't know how," or "Them don't like me." The therapist cultivated "I can" ideas and elaborated on Kim's ability to relate to Ann and the therapist. Kim staunchly and continually rejected the fact that she could communicate with other people and the nurse's mandate to attempt new encounters. The nurse believed that Kim had the potential to relate to another human being successfully as validated by the professional relationship. The readiness, motivational, and interpersonal strength factors required to execute this behavior were absent. Other intervention attempts to foster relationship encounters would be delayed until ongoing assessment proved a new availability to the defined task. Therapy intervention was again centered on release of the client's inner emotions, both positive and negative. A new thrust of intense person affirmation and feedback with a focus on improved behavior and true task achievement was also instituted.

Several weeks after this intensive plunge into psychotherapy, Kim experienced renewed catharsis from the unburdening of painful emotions. Assessment of the relationship strength and cohesion dictated a more confrontive and directive nursing approach and response. The client wavered between resistance and cooperation with this fresh therapy tack, but a new level of adult interaction and verbal exchange was attained. This strengthened alignment of nurse and client was marked by Kim's ambivalence, incipient insight, and initial verbalization of desire for changes in her life.

PROCESS IMPLEMENTATION

1—Evaluation

N.D.   *Anxiety*
   S   "Me can't." "Me can't talk." "Me don't know them." "Them don't like me."
   O   Became involved in art class, producing two pictures. During therapy hour, proudly demonstrated her work. Refused to mingle with peers and withdrew to protective cover of communication barrier.

N.D.   *Dependence/independence struggle*
   S   "Me can't." "Me can't talk." "Me don't know them." "Them don't like me."

   O   Became involved in art class, producing two pictures. During therapy hour, proudly demonstrated her work. Refused to mingle with peers and withdrew to protective cover of communication barrier.

N.D.   *Low self-concept*
   S   "Me can't." "Me can't talk." "Me don't know them." "Them don't like me."
   O   Became involved in art class, producing two pictures. During therapy hour, proudly demonstrated her work. Refused to mingle with peers and withdrew to protective cover of communication barrier.

N.D.   *Interpersonal relationship disturbance*
   S   "Me can't." "Me can't talk." "Me don't know them." "Them don't like me."
   O   Became involved in art class, producing two pictures. During therapy hour, proudly demonstrated her work. Refused to mingle with peers and withdrew to protective cover of communication barrier.

N.D.   *Language barrier*
   S   "Me can't." "Me can't talk." "Me don't know them." "Them don't like me."
   O   Became involved in art class, producing two pictures. During therapy hour, proudly demonstrated her work. Refused to mingle with peers and withdrew to protective cover of communication barrier.

N.D.   *Passive resistance*
   S   "Me can't." "Me can't talk." "Me don't know them." "Them don't like me."
   O   Became involved in art class, producing two pictures. During therapy hour, proudly demonstrated her work. Refused to mingle with peers and withdrew to protective cover of communication barrier.

Actual outcome
   Painted, framed, and hung two pictures on living room wall. Withdrew from peers and rejected the intellectual concept that she could communicate with others.

2A—Assessment

N.D.   *Anxiety*
   S   "Me mad."*
   O   Husband decided to make an abrupt family and job move. Refused to allow couple therapy sessions even for the sole purpose of clarification. Transitional data vague. Pacing. Restless body

---

*Absence of subjective data indicate limited verbal exchange, extended periods of silence in therapy, or lack of comment to the clinician's queries.

gestures. Silence. Eye-to-eye contact decreased.

N.D. *Dependence/independence struggle*
S *
O Retreated to a nonverbal English stance or the use of her native tongue. Silence.

N.D. *Communication disturbance within the marital relationship*
S "Me mad."*
O Husband decided to make an abrupt family and job move. Refused to allow couple therapy session even for the sole purpose of clarification. Transitional data vague. Retreated to a nonverbal English stance or the use of her native tongue. Silence.

N.D. *Language barrier*
S *
O Retreated to a nonverbal English stance or the use of her native tongue. Silence.

N.D. *Passive resistance*
S *
O Retreated to a nonverbal English stance or the use of her native tongue. Silence.

N.D. *Thought disorder*
S *
O Retreated to a nonverbal English stance or the use of her native tongue. Silence. Pacing. Restless body gestures. Eye-to-eye contact decreased. Inappropriate affect. Maintained person distance.

N.D. *Autism*
S *
O Retreated to a nonverbal English stance or the use of her native tongue. Silence. Pacing. Restless body gestures. Eye-to-eye contact decreased. Inappropriate affect. Maintained person distance.

3—Additional nursing diagnosis
None

4A—Variables

Reality timing	−5
Relationships	−5
Stressors and/or crisis	−5
Coping resources	−5
Significant emotional strength	−5
Significant emotional limitations	−5
Therapy relationship	−1
Physical health status	0
Physical and emotional readiness dimension	−5

*Absence of subjective data indicates limited verbal exchange, extended periods of silence in therapy, or lack of comment to the clinican's queries.

Available support system	−5
Meaning significance	−5
Values and belief impact	−5
Other	
BALANCE	−

Additional specific knowledge
See case material.

Analysis and synthesis

N.D. *Anxiety*. Life crisis precipitates intense inner tension and the use of reliable but ineffective coping mechanisms. Withdrawal to an ongoing mute stance profoundly expresses client's negative response and reaction to the uncertain, threatened life position.

N.D. *Dependence/independence struggle*. Unable to cope effectively with the dynamics of the situation. Withdrawal to an extremely dependent state only intensifies client's vulnerability rather than offering control and security.

N.D. *Communication disturbance within the marital relationship*. Patterns of frequent, erratic mobility, insecure job objectives, and changing life direction and overall instability seem impossible to confront. At some point client must confront these issues in her marriage if she is to survive emotionally.

N.D. *Language barrier*. This communication obstacle is a hindrance to movement within therapy and to resolution in the overall life of the client.

N.D. *Passive resistance*. The dynamics of this indifferent form of aggression is highly controlling and destructive in nature. To relinquish this stance is perceived as a giving-up of one's power. The deception of this seeming nonresistant stance is protective to client's pathology. Client cannot conceptualize sincere, open truthfulness.

N.D. *Thought disorder*. The tight entrenchment in the intense passive resistance stance of the client and commitment to its false protection continue to encourage self-absorption to the point of perpetuation of the valued deception as reality.

N.D. *Autism*. Regression to the mute stance decreases and/or blocks stimuli and encourages broad fantasy life development and response as if it were an authentic experience.

4B—Design of action
N.D. Anxiety, dependence/independence struggle, communication disturbance within the marital relationship, language barrier, passive resistance, thought disorder, autism.

1. Plan
   a. Facilitate the imminent move with person support.
   b. Encourage the relationship termination process.
   c. Identify a mental health liaison at the new destination.
2. Strategy
   a. Accept current level of functioning.
   b. Elicit necessary data.
   c. Encourage couple communication.
   d. Structure new professional support system.
   e. Role model termination process.
3. Expected outcomes
   a. Acknowledgement of necessary data by husband.
   b. Limited couple communication.
   c. Acceptance of new professional support system.
   d. Involvement in the experience of the termination process.
4. Criteria
   a. Necessary data offered by husband.
   b. Limited but viable couple communication.
   c. Verbal acceptance and commitment to contact the identified new professional support system.
   d. Limited verbal comment indicating the experiencing of termination emotions.

At this crucial point, therapy was abruptly terminated by Sam's decision to move the family 1000 miles across the country. He had received a job opportunity, the nature of which remained vague even under the clinician's persistent questioning. Sam called the position a "once-in-a-lifetime opportunity." He again aborted the attainment of his educational objective.

Kim was openly angry and hostile in therapy about this life crisis but would not dispute the move with Sam or confront the more important issue of the decision-making format within their marriage. She would not allow a couple-therapy session with the clinician even for the sole defined purpose of clarifying and gathering specified data. The disruptive force of this life modification could have caused less turmoil had some factual information concerning the transition surfaced. The date of the expected move, the exact location, and actual information about

their new place of residence, data about Ann's school, and facts about Sam's new employment position and income level were minimal. Such data would have aided in the transition process. Kim's reaction to the crisis was to withdraw, become increasingly reliant on Sam, oftentimes retreating to a nonverbal English stance and the use of her native tongue in response to the therapist's questions. Her restless body gestures returned, and she could be observed pacing when the nurse arrived at their home.

Silences in therapy involved lengthy intervals, often lasting 15 minutes. Eye-to-eye contact decreased, and it appeared that Kim wished to evade direct eye contact. Severely threatened by the coming environmental change, loss of employment, and abrupt separation from the therapist, Kim attempted to retreat from experiencing the emotional trauma of the impending crisis. As in previous separations and loss, she felt the shock effect and mentally directed the pain into her unconscious mind to avoid the anguish of coping with the ensuing grief feelings.

Limited understandable verbal communication was present between Kim and the therapist. Encounters were lengthy and resembled the initial contact period. After receiving Kim's verbal consent, the nurse made a telephone call to the community mental health center located in the broadly defined area where Sam intended to settle his family. This initial communication was supported by a detailed written report containing extensive factual data, a therapy progress summary, and recommendations of intervention measures to facilitate the implementation of continued therapy for Kim. Drug maintenance information and a drug evaluation were detailed in this report. Additional medical information and supportive findings were supplemented by the physician. Kim was handed a card with the address, telephone number, and name of a contact person at this community mental health center. She was directed to telephone the center to schedule an appointment with this liaison person the first week she was located in the new area. Kim hesitantly agreed to the plan. She placed the information card in her purse, but one had to question her ability to follow the directions in her present state of intense distress and reliance. Sam received the same verbal and written orientation to the agreed-on plan, and he further consented to assume responsibility for the completion of the task. Implications from past patterns of behavior led one to hypothesize that contact with a new source of help for Kim would not be completed until her behavior became uncomfortable or intolerable for Sam.

Time restriction was a negative variable to the successful termination of this professional relationship. The recently acquired depth and renewed emotional involvement by the client now became a deterrent to the task at hand. The linkage with a new caring person was important to the therapy transition and to the psychological restabilization of Kim. Aware that Kim actually heard more than she wished others to be aware she had heard, and in spite of her withdrawal maneuvers, the therapist expressed mutual separation feelings. "Our time together has been good. Today you don't feel very well, but you have felt better and you will feel good again. I believe your new therapist will help you. He wants to try to help." In addition, honestly, caringly, slowly, and distinctly, the clinician expressed her own feeling of loss related to Kim's departure. "I will miss you, Kim. We have shared many feelings," she said, pointing to head and heart.

Emotions were expressed simply. Information on how to find new employment was given. When the actual time for a last parting arrived, the therapist spontaneously hugged Kim, whose response was one of emotional restraint but not of physical resistance or withdrawal. She had tears in her eyes. "It's good to cry when you hurt, Kim. I will really miss you, too," were the therapist's departing comments.

Tears visible for the first time in 2 years and at an appropriate time signified healthy but painful emotions and also an expression of meaning. Consequent emotional well-being

could depend on the commitment to and the actual involvement in a new therapy relationship as well as in the emotional strength attained in this terminating relationship.

There are many uncontrolled variables in any therapist-client relationship. Final severance of a meaningful, helpful, progressing relationship presents a dilemma that can be perplexing for client and therapist alike. The clinician is tempted to reason, "If only I had more time" and find it paradoxical to begin the cessation of carefully chosen objectives and goals. The quandary is further complicated by procedures and critical performance inauguration already begun. The recent emergence of rudimentary behaviors, sources of stress, and origin variance data make this laboriously earned knowledge seem inconsequential. Toilsome progress is lost for the moment. Retreat to previous stumbling blocks and pathological behaviors perplexingly hinder the critical situation for the client and present new challenges for the nurse. Knowledgeable application of nursing process and objective evaluation bring to focus the existence of growth and concrete progress through therapy. Finally, the positive learning experience from an inescapable termination of a relationship through the true living of the feelings involved creates a medium to foster growth and health and establishes a basis for future interpersonal relationships.

Further assessment and evaluation demonstrate the ease of transition and change of focus by the therapist when a tool such as nursing process is applied, lending a theoretically proved sound approach and objectivity to the problem. A threat to such a circumstance exists when emotionally charged material perpetuates pathology rather than alleviates the stress and improves the pathological behaviors. A basic method of approach or framework of thought underlying a professional stance and a knowledgeable conceptual base give the nurse clinician a logical and reliable foundation to provide the competence, flexibility, and judgment aptitude needed in both crisis and noncrisis client situations. Sound, skilled nursing intervention for a nurse generalist or for a clinical specialist is guided to completion by the choice of a valid nursing process methodology and the proficient application of the framework to nursing practice.

SUMMARY PERSONAL PROFILE*

Social adjustment

S   †
O   Openly angry and hostile in therapy about life circumstance but would not confront issues with husband. Withdrew, became increasingly reliant on husband, and most often retreated to nonverbal English stance and use of her native tongue. Pacing. Restless body gestures. Decreased eye-to-eye contact. Limited, understandable verbal communication between client and therapist. Tears at time of actual termination. Did not physically withdraw from therapist.

Emotional health status

S   †
O   Openly angry and hostile in therapy about life circumstance but would not confront issues with husband. Withdrew, became increasingly reliant on husband, and most often retreated to nonverbal English stance and use of her native tongue. Pacing. Restless body gestures. Decreased eye-to-eye contact. Limited, understandable verbal communication between client and

therapist. Tears at time of actual termination. Did not physically withdraw from therapist.

Physical health status

S   †
O   Height 5 feet. Weight 115 pounds. Fluphenazine hydrochloride in lowest minimal dosage by intramuscular injection every 3 weeks, accompanied by an antiparkinsonism drug daily. Continued to follow eating pattern of her family of origin.

Spiritual dimension

S ⎫
O ⎭ No acknowledged or observable change.

Daily living skill performance

S   †
O   Withdrew, became increasingly reliant on husband, and most often retreated to nonverbal English stance and use of her native tongue.

Coping skill repertoire

S   †
O   Openly angry and hostile in therapy about life circumstance but would not confront issues with husband. Withdrew, became increasingly reliant on husband, and most often retreated to nonverbal English stance and use of her native tongue. Pacing. Restless body gestures. Decreased eye-to-eye contact. Limited, understandable verbal communication between client and therapist. Tears at time of actual termination. Did not physically withdraw from therapist.

Maturational struggle according to Erikson's developmental stages

S   †
O   Basic trust vs. basic mistrust—limited minimal drive and hope.

---

*It should be noted that client summary profile is a description of client's coping style, interaction manner, and behavior during a crisis period. It is hypothesized that previous growth through therapy is *temporarily* reversed because of situational variables and stress.

†Absence of subjective data indicates limited verbal exchange, extended periods of silence in therapy, or lack of comment to the clinician's queries.

Autonomy vs. shame and doubt—struggle intensified under stress.

Identity vs. role confusion—struggle intensified under stress.

Self-integration

S †

O Openly angry and hostile in therapy about life circumstance but would not confront issues with husband. Withdrew, became increasingly reliant on husband, and most often retreated to nonverbal English stance and use of her native tongue. Pacing. Restless body gestures. Decreased eye-to-eye contact. Limited, understandable verbal communication between client and therapist. Tears at time of actual termination. Did not physically withdraw from therapist.

Quality of life

S †

O Openly angry and hostile in therapy about life circumstance but would not confront isssues with husband. Withdrew, became increasingly reliant on husband, and most often retreated to non-verbal English stance and usc of her native tongue. Pacing. Restless body gestures. Decreased eye-to-eye contact. Limited, understandable verbal communication between client and therapist. Tears at time of actual termination. Did not physically withdraw from therapist.

SUGGESTED READINGS

Adams, G.: Human sexuality, recognizing the range of human sexual needs and behavior, American Journal of Maternal-Child Nursing **1**:165-169, May/June, 1976.

American Nurses' Association: Standards of psychiatric mental-health nursing practice, Kansas City, 1973, The Association.

Baker, C., and Huff, B., editors: Physicians' desk reference, ed. 30, Oradell, N.J., 1976, Medical Economics, Inc.

Berne, E.: Transactional analysis in psychotherapy, New York, 1961, Grove Press, Inc.

Bullmer, K.: The art of empathy, New York, 1975, Human Sciences Press, Inc.

Dixon, B.: Interviewing when the patient is delusional, Journal of Psychiatric Nursing **69**:25-34, Jan., 1973.

Doller, J.: Tardive dyskinesia and changing concepts of antipsychotic drug use: a nursing prospective, Journal of Psychiatric Nursing **15**:23-26, Nov., 1977.

Hall, E.: The hidden dimension, Garden City, N.Y. 1966, Doubleday & Co., Inc.

Harris, T.: I'm OK—you're OK, New York, 1967, Harper & Row, Publishers.

Hitchens, E.: Helping psychiatric outpatients accept drug therapy, American Journal of Nursing **77**:1144-1148, July, 1977.

Hopper, J.: Effective therapy with antipsychotic medications, Nurse Practitioner **2**:32-33, Sept./Oct., 1976.

Kelly, H.: The sense of an ending, American Journal of Nursing **69**:2378-2381, Nov., 1969.

Kline, N., and Davis, J.: Psychotropic drugs, American Journal of Nursing **73**:54-63, Jan., 1973.

Knapp, M.: Nonverbal communication in human interaction, New York, 1972, Holt, Rinehart & Winston, Inc.

Kolb, L.: Modern clinical psychiatry, Philadelphia, 1977, W. B. Saunders Co.

Krieger, D.: Therapeutic touch, the imprimatur of nursing, American Journal of Nursing **75**:784-787, May, 1975.

Leininger, M.: Transcultural nursing, New York, 1978, John Wiley & Sons, Inc.

Ray, O.: Drugs, society, and human behavior, ed. 2, St. Louis, 1978, The C. V. Mosby Co.

Roberts, S. L.: Territoriality: space and the schizophrenic patient, Perspectives in Psychiatric Care **7**(1):28-33, 1969.

Rubin, T.: The angry book, New York, 1969, Collier Books.

Sencide, L.: Taking the labels off, Nursing Times **74**:52, Jan. 12, 1978.

Walker, R.: Developing cultural awareness, AORN Journal **27**:1302-1304, June, 1978.

Yoder, J.: Alienation as a way of life, Perspectives in Psychiatric Care **15**(2):66-71, 1977.

Zahourek, R., and Crawford, C.: Forced termination of psychotherapy, Perspectives in Psychiatric Care **16**:193-199, July-Aug., 1978.

---

†Absence of subjective data indicates limited verbal exchange, extended periods of silence in therapy, or lack of comment to the clinician's queries.

CHAPTER 11

ON ACHIEVING A FELICITOUS NURSE-CLINICIAN STANCE

Since the inception of the community mental health movement in the 1960s, psychiatric hospital populations have decreased drastically. At the same time sufficient support systems for this group of clients have not evolved with comparable or necessary remedial programs to facilitate the autonomous adjustment or life-style adaptations of the long-term client. This new population of clients receiving short-term treatment and immediate return to community life who would formerly have received extended and/or custodial care in a hospital setting are in need of maintenance therapy. They need adequate treatment to facilitate growth and adjustment to allow them to become functioning members of the community. Their self-reliance is essential to community adaptation, but it is most often absent because of the nonautonomous life stance, resulting from chronic illness and extended hospitalizations. Nursing offers a broad-based means to relate to and interact with this unique group, helping to develop their daily living skills and cultivate their self-esteem and self-sufficiency.

The nurse-clinician can be the elementary force for health modification in the lives of these clients. Their chronic psychiatric status demands intervention to prevent further disruption of living and skillful guidance to initiate or reinitiate a basic life stance of new and increased effective coping styles, improved interacting manner, and positive behavior patterns. The relationship and interactions affiliation combine with an excellent nursing process design to achieve this end. The dynamics of each encounter will be unique to the particular client and the particular nurse involved.

The person of the nurse is the germane component of the relationship and the therapy. Authenticity is a person quality that the nurse engaged in long-term client care must possess. The extended time the client has spent under the tutelage of psychiatric personnel endows him with a keen sense of judgment regarding the nurse's trust and sincerity. The characteristic of authenticity lends an authoritative stance to the nurse that no amount of knowledge or skill can compensate. Rapport and a climate of trust are established through this basic person component of an effective therapy program.

Honesty is a basic component of both the authentic clinician and the authentic nurse-client relationship. No baseline for confidence, reliance, and secureness in any relationship is built on deception. Hope is undermined by dishonesty. Therapy messages must be truthful, sincere, and trustworthy. Communication perceived as dishonest by clients increases ambivalence, a deterring quality already prevalent in their disrupted lives. There is a kindness and protectiveness in truth that one cannot appreciate until one becomes intensely committed to it. Defensive reactions from clients to reality-based truth can only validate the need to confront and cope with the issues at hand. Candor and directness can be tempered by the therapist's care, concern, support, and realistic expectations.

It is not uncommon that dishonesty is first portrayed nonverbally in a covert clinician attempt to avoid confrontive interactions that may be perceived as difficult or uncomfortable. Deception, no matter how masterful, can discredit one's effectiveness. The clinician becomes for the client one more person whose likelihood of offering effective guidance has become decreased through deceit. There is margin for error within the relationship if one makes an honest mistake. There is no margin for error when fraudulence and untruthfulness are basic ingredients in the encounter. Not only is mockery made of the relationship but this professional fraudulence spills over to one's peers, decreasing credibility to the body of knowledge one espouses. The integrity of the relationship rests with the clinician. Role modeling an open, honest style of interacting and calmly, kindly confronting client messages that evidence ambivalence, ambiguity, dissimilarity, incompatibility, or disparity of thought or feeling facilitate truth and the credibility of the interpersonal relationship.

Self-reliance is alien to the long-term, psychiatrically disturbed client. The accountability for the relationship rests with the nurse-clinician. Nursing process provides the adaptable, sound methodology to implement a goal-directed, structured, relevant nurse-client affiliation. The scope of the interpersonal relationship creates the means for the client to learn and to experience dependable, responsible behavior.

There is no shame for the clinician in apology or admission of error. The force of nursing process mandates frequent evaluation and ongoing assessment to prevent misunderstanding, to examine possible misconception, and to allow space to correct error. The human quality of the nurse permits mistake and oversight, but it also grants warmth, care, concern, and nurturing. No body of knowledge or process can provide these components to support personal growth. A solid person-to-person relationship uniquely combines the human strength and limitation of one individual to foster the human potential of another individual.

A mature and cultivated other-person sensitivity is required of the nurse to pierce the often indifferent, stoic, apathetic, and inert-appearing client. Insensitivity and self-absorption are defensive maneuvers that a client employs to shield the fragile psyche from pain and the uncertainty of life. Discernment of the true emotional self of the client is unfolded by the perceptive, compassionate, empathetic feelings of the therapist. The client experiences new sensations of comfort and security, which slowly allow for the revealing of inner concerns and fragile susceptibilities. Experiencing a relationship with a truly sensitive therapist permits emptiness and superficiality to begin to give way to the inception of other-person awareness. Role modeling of this deeply human, impressionable quality of sensitivity often allows the client to risk emulating a sense of other-person awareness and sensitivity without feeling vulnerable.

Chronicity often contains negative messages of an end point in itself. The dependence and lack of self-esteem perpetuate an aura of hopelessness and helplessness for both client and caregiver. A sense of objective nurse involvement and commitment both to the client and to the health tasks is elementary to the nurse-client relationship. Few significant persons have believed in the client's potential for improvement, however limited, that is essential for him to sense before beginning any health-directed program. The clinician's positive attitude perpetuates a sense of self-confidence foreign to the client. Objectivity creates a realism for the nurse, keeping a sense of perspective for both parties, allowing the quality of humanness to emerge with its unique strengths, limitations, and potentials.

A therapist's feeling of hope lends new meaning to the client's existence. The vulnerable, dependent position of the client evidences pervading attitudes of futility, desperation, dejection, and pessimism, finalizing in an overall sense of despair. Self-disappointment only breeds increased vulnerability and helplessness. Dynamically, the client's vague perceptions of self are erased with a new life meaning, involving potential, dormant strength, latent growth, and delayed capabilities. A sense of hope can unharness energy, abilities, experimentation, and renewed endeavor. A permeating, continuing sense of hope gives power to the therapist to fortify the vulnerable client while penetrating the previously ineffectual life position.

Self-awareness, self-discernment, and self-discipline are qualities in a therapist that combine with flexibility to enhance the knowledge and skill of the individual nurse-clinician. Awareness is an acknowledgment of one's behavior, emotions, and behavioral impact. Self-discernment is an accurate insight and integration of one's behavior, emotions, and motivation. Self-discipline is the ability to restrain, control, and order one's intellectual and emotional behavior and direction. Flexibility is a person quality that allows one to adapt and modify one's behavior according to the demands of a situation or to the needs of another person.

Awareness and insight should underlie the professional person of the nurse. Keen self-judgment and accurate self-knowledge encourage correct and precise perception, promoting credibility, integrity, and accountability. These self-development qualities are not easily acquired. A certain amount of painstaking, diligent striving is required to bring the true self into focus and to further integrate and distinguish the self and the ethos of the professional self. The projected image of the self should be in accurate alignment with the real self. For the professional nurse to function proficiently as an accomplished therapist, there must be no sense of conflict within the personhood and the professional stance.

The professional ethos has a more ordered existence and contains specific ethics, beliefs, and values. The rules of conduct are usually overt in nature. The professional discipline itself partially defines the role. The prescribed structure creates a degree of safety and a margin for error. Education defines practice, correct course of action, usual policy, and accepted process and methods of transaction as well as defining a knowledge base. Some learned professional tactics are covert in nature, and some game rules change according to the politics of the players and the dominating institution. The accepted professional ethos frequently sanctions the nurse-client relationship, rapidly surpassing social and personal boundaries and allowing for an unhesitating sense of emotional intimacy.

The person ethos is a broad sense of self acquired through the total life developmental process and the experience of living. Many persons choose a professional discipline because it easily meshes with the accepted values and beliefs of their inner self or because of the protective nature of the profession. Areas of internal disagreement and antagonism must be resolved as the professional person is educated in the science and art of the chosen vocation. There is less pretense for the person, fewer protective structures, and defined courses of action. One stands autonomously in the life decision-making process, schooled by previous life experience, knowledge, and emotional strength and resilience. Integrated individuals have developed a self-assurance of who they are (identity), where they are going (goals), and what their life is about (purpose). They also possess a compatible professional identity, goals, and purpose. Harmony of life principle lends itself to personal satisfaction from professional endeavors.

Self-discipline is a person quality and professional characteristic that allows the clinician to use knowledge from awareness and insight to mold or adjust his ethos as the situation demands. Flexibility lends individuality and durability to the client's situation. The clinician's flexibility promotes constancy and intensity in the therapy relationship. Furthermore, this adaptability encourages needed patience for the nurse in the long process of uncovering and validating clouded data from a complicated and perplexing network of self-perpetuating, disorganized client behaviors. The judgments mandated by the psychosocial client interaction are intense requirements, constantly calling for reassessment and realignment of the clinician's core values and beliefs basic to the cohesive stance of person and nurse.

John Powell, in his book *Unconditional Love,* describes the personhood of the individual espousing a life principle (identity, goal, purpose) of unconditional love:

More specifically, loving you does not mean that I cease to love myself. On the contrary, the idea that I cannot love you unless I love myself is universally accepted by psychologists. Those who do not love themselves are sad, plagued by a constant sense of emptiness which they are always trying to fill. Like a person with a painful toothache, they can think only of themselves and they are constantly in search of a dentist, someone to make them feel better. If I do not love myself, I can only use others; I cannot love them.

My loving you can never be an abdication of my own self. I could possibly give my life for you out of love, but I could never deny my identity as a person. I will try to be what you need me to be, to do what you need done, to say whatever you need to hear. At the same time I am committed to an honest and open relationship. As a part of my gift of love, I will always offer my thoughts, preferences, and all my feelings, even when I think they may be unpleasant or even hurtful to your feelings. If we are committed to total honesty and total openness, our relationship will never be a sticky one, marked by hidden agenda, repressed resentments, displaced emotions, acting out in adolescent ways what we do not have the courage to speak out. Unless we agree to honor honesty and openness, we will never be sure of each other. Our relationship will seem more like a charade than a real life drama.

Finally, in my commitment of unconditional love I promise you a person, not a piece of putty. A ''person'' means that I have rights, as well as responsibilities. I have a right, for example, to express my own thoughts and feelings, to have my own preferences and the liberty to follow them. I also have an area of personal choice which is mine, and I must insist on keeping this area for myself. Making my own decisions and taking responsibility for them is an essential part of the human maturation process. Of course, I will never make decisions which involve both of us, but there are decisions that I must make for myself. These are some of the rights implied in being a person, and I intend to assert these rights and to insist that you respect them. Be ready to find in me a person you can bump into. Of course, you have a corresponding set of rights, and I will try to be very careful in respecting them. I will not only respect your rights, but I will expect you to exercise your own personhood in asserting these rights and in insisting on my respect for them.

And please have the courage to tell me at all times what you are thinking and feeling. I have no X-ray eyes to know your hidden thoughts or feelings. I cannot guess your preferences. You must tell me. Making assumptions is a dangerous game. Do not think you are loving me by playing chameleon or by twisting yourself into a pretzel shape trying to please me. If you do, I will probably tire of you or become bored with you. I will certainly feel unchallenged by you and by our relationship.

Lastly, I cannot ever let you use or manipulate me. We must love persons and use things. I am a person, not a thing. To let you use me would be no act of love, either for you or for myself. Please understand that I will never set myself up as your judge. I cannot now nor will I ever be able to read your intentions. I can know your intentions only by asking you. But I will never allow your temper tantrums or your tears to compromise my communication. If I feel suspicious of you, I will confront you with my feelings. If I feel hurt by something you have said or done, I will say "Ouch!" When you affirm or console or congratulate me, I will forever be visibly grateful to you. The me that shall be yours will be the unabridged and unedited version. In the words of the poet Richard Lovelace: "I could not love thee, dear, so much/ Lov'd I not honor more."

I am an actor, not a reactor. This means that I must always decide how I am going to act. I cannot put this responsibility in your hands. I will try to combine as much tact and kindness as I can with my honesty and openness, but I can never allow myself to be manipulated into a compromise, either in my conduct or in communication. My thoughts and my feelings are not for hire. I will not be used.

Whatever else love may ask of us, it does not ask us to be doormats or compulsive pleasers or peace-at-any price persons. The primary gift of love is the offering of one's most honest self through one's most honest self-disclosure.*

The personification of a life principle of unconditional love in one's private life and personal relationships is a core element in the establishment of true regard for a moral value of intense respect for human dignity or a professional caring ethic.

It can be said that a caregiver to the chronically distressed client would be well fortified with a personal life principle of unconditional love. This life principle would strengthen and sustain one's professional endeavors. Many encounters with clients call for answering the question: What is the loving thing to do? or What is the caring thing to do? One can be tempted also to ask what is the easiest or simplest thing to do? or What is the quickest or least taxing thing to do? These questions in

themselves and the choice of caregiver response can establish the pattern and potential for a healing relationship.

Sameness is not a constant component of a human being; personal growth dynamics change potential. Compatibility is a changing relationship variable. The person dynamics of the long-term client are usually muted. The relationship between client and nurse can be a forceful power, used to create or resist the process of chronicity. An impelling force can result from an integrated personal-professional ethos of the nurse-clinician, opening rapport and a climate of trust through an authentic and knowledgeable stance while demonstrating care, concern, integrity, and hope. This potency can encourage an unfolding and a reaching-out to experience by the client, disengaging a negative position of resignation and retreat from living. Healing begins within such relationship dynamics.

The explanation of the interpersonal factors between client and clinician has a vital quality. In actuality, life is reinstituted through the heart and breath of the relationship. One must be careful in a didactic description and interpretation not to misconstrue the overall picture as a simplistic, rote exercise of skill. Caregiving to the long-term client demands tremendous patience in pacing oneself to the client's functional level. Repetition may become a tedious, although necessary, task. Feedback may be absent or minimal so that the clinician who values productivity may question the intrinsic worth of the association. Work satisfaction must often come from the commitment to the person or the task rather than from goal completion. Basic and elementary goal achievement may not be visible for a year or more. Belief in the possibility of reaching realistic objectives can be difficult to enkindle when visible progress is absent. Personal fortitude must be supported from peer relationships and personal encounters and endeavors. The danger comes when the client-therapist relationship is perceived only as a

---

*Reprinted from Powell, John: Unconditional love, Niles, Ill., 1978, Argus Communications. Used with permission from Argus Communications, Niles, Ill.

routine and tiresome interview, an unpleasant task, or a burdensome encounter rather than an uncertain, often perplexing interaction but one with possibility for health, growth, and healing. The nurse can be strengthened by a conscious awareness of helping, accurate practice guidelines giving direction to nursing action. (See Appendix B.) The spark of challenge to the clinician's potential, skill, proficiency, and commitment must remain alive.

In 1978 the President's Commission On Mental Health issued a report evaluating the quality and availability of mental health care in the United States. This assessment established a national priority to meet the needs of people with chronic mental illness. Present inadequacies of the mental health service delivery system were acknowledged. The report recommends that special programs of change targeted for the long-term client be developed at three levels; (1) the individual level, or the client and his family; (2) the program level, or a prospectus designed to assist the disabled individual; and (3) the organizational level, or the structure that administers and coordinates these programs. This report clearly specifies problems encountered by the severely and chronically ill psychiatric client and proposes a design of action with distinct reference to the perplexing, unsettled life stance of this individual in our present social structure. The possibility of implementation of the recommendations of this report gives new and renewed hope to client and caregiver alike.

SUGGESTED READINGS

Arnold, H.: Four A's: a guide to one-to-one relationships, American Journal of Nursing **76**:941-943, June, 1976.

Collins, M.: Communication in health care, St. Louis, 1977, The C. V. Mosby Co.

Craig, A., and Hyatt, B.: Chronicity in mental illness: a theory on role change, Perspectives in Psychiatric Care **16**:139-154, June, 1978.

Fromm, E.: Art of loving, New York, 1956, Harper & Brothers, Publishers.

Harris, T.: I'm OK—you're OK, New York, 1967, Harper & Row, Publishers.

Joint Commission on Mental Illness and Health: Action for mental health, New York, 1961, Basic Books.

Jourard, S.: Transparent self, Princeton, N.J., 1964, Van Nostrand Co.

Murrary, J.: Failure of the community mental health movement, American Journal of Nursing **75**:2034-2036, Nov., 1975.

O'Brien, M.: Communications and relationships in nursing, St. Louis, 1978, The C. V. Mosby Co.

Powell, J.: Unconditional love, Niles, Ill., 1978, Argus Communications.

Report To the President From The President's Commission On Mental Health, Vol. I, Washington, D.C., 1978, Government Printing Office.

Report To the President From the President's Commission On Mental Health, Vol. II, Washington, D.C., 1978, Government Printing Office.

Rogers, C.: On becoming a person, Boston, 1961, Houghton-Mifflin Co.

Satir, V.: People making, Palo Alto, Calif., 1972, Science & Behavior Books, Inc.

Slovinsky, A., et al.: Back to the community: a dubious blessing, Nursing Outlook **24**:370-374, June, 1976.

Sundeen, S., et al.: Nurse-client interaction, St. Louis, 1976, The C. V. Mosby Co.

Topalis, M., and Aguilera, D.: Psychiatric nursing, ed. 7, St. Louis, 1978, The C. V. Mosby Co.

NURSING DIAGNOSES CATEGORIZED ACCORDING TO THEMES

It is significant to note that the themes are not mutually exclusive. All nursing diagnoses are unique to the specific client and situation and may change in theme, depending on person, place, time, psychopathology, and the dynamics of the nurse-client relationship.

SYMPTOMS OF EMOTIONAL DISTRESS

Absent support systems
Affect disturbance
Anxiety
Communication disturbance within the marital relationship
Controlling (manipulative) behavior
Denial
Dependence/independence struggle
Emotional deprivation
Environmental deprivation
Family disruption
Faulty self-image
Faulty support system
Fear
Financial stress
Inability to perform required tasks of daily living

Inability to solve problems effectively
Intellectualization
Interpersonal relationship disturbance
Intimacy/isolation struggle
Limited physical energy
Loneliness
Low self-concept
Low stress tolerance
Obesity
Passive resistance
Psychophysiological reaction to stress
Rigid life stance
Separation anxiety
Short concentration span
Suicide potential
Suspicious behavior
Transient memory loss
Trust/mistrust struggle
Unrealistic expectations in relationships
Unrealistic self-expectations

DESCRIPTIONS OF PROMINENT CLIENT BEHAVIORS

Acceptance of the illness role
Acceptance of the mental illness role

Affect disturbance
Antisocial and abusive behavior
Anxiety
Apathy
Breathing difficulties
Communication disturbances within the marital
   relationship
Controlling (manipulative) behavior
Denial
Dependence/independence struggle
Difficulty in adjustment to parenting
Difficulty in adjustment after long-term hos-
   pitalization
Edema
Faulty self-image
High blood pressure
Inability to perform required tasks of daily liv-
   ing
Inability to solve problems effectively
Interpersonal relationship disturbance
Intellectualization
Intimacy/isolation struggle
Lack of insight
Language barrier
Limited physical energy
Low self-concept
Low stress tolerance
Obesity
Passive resistance
Pregnancy
Psychophysiological reaction to stress
Psychotropic medication side effects
Rigid life stance
Self-centered life focus
Short concentration span

Suicide potential
Suspicious behavior
Transient memory loss
Trust/mistrust struggle
Unhealthy learned behavior
Unkempt environment
Unrealistic expectations in relationships
Unrealistic self-expectations
Unstructured life-style

SIMPLISTIC DESCRIPTIONS OF CORE PATHOLOGY

Anxiety
Affect disturbance
Apathy
Autism
Controlling (manipulative) behavior
Decompensation episode
Denial
Dependence/independence struggle
Depression
Fear
Inability to complete the grieving process
Intellectualization
Interpersonal relationship disturbance
Intimacy/isolation struggle
Loneliness
Low self-concept
Passive resistance
Perceptual disturbance
Psychophysiological reaction to stress
Suspicious behavior
Thought disorder
Trust/mistrust struggle
Unresolved grief

GUIDELINES FOR PSYCHOSOCIAL INTERVENTION

The nurse-clinician should remain cognizant of the need to do the following:

1. Accept the client in his current state of functioning.
2. Accept the reality of the client's situation.
3. Accept client setbacks and reversals as an essential component of growth.
4. Allow initial dependency; it may facilitate overall autonomy.
5. Allow negative, as well as positive, client feelings.
6. Assess and validate personal space parameters, using care and precision in the selection of physical space maneuvers. Distance and touch choices are critical relationship decisions.
7. Assess and examine the congruence of a client's feelings, thoughts, and actions.
8. Assess body language of both client and nurse. Be alert to the impact of body language on the interaction process and interpersonal relationship dynamics.
9. Assess physical health status and intervene when necessary to prevent or ameliorate the identified symptomatic behaviors.
10. Assess and evaluate daily living skill capabilities. Intervene when change or adaptation is demanded by life position, client choice, psychopathology, and/or the helping-healing growth process.
11. Comment on factual data without personal judgment.
12. Confront recurrent client messages that evidence ambivalence, ambiguity, dissimilarity, incompatibility, or disparity of thought, feeling, or action.
13. Confront with an assured, calm, kind stance and sufficient authentic objective data to support the issue or issues in question.
14. Demonstrate integrity, credibility, and accountability as a person and a professional.
15. Develop the qualities of sensitivity and other centeredness.
16. Elicit self-disclosure only for the purpose of intervention. Unfolding intimate client data necessitates helping with resolution of revealed issues.
17. Elicit feedback whenever possible from the client for establishing goals and evaluating progress.
18. Encourage experiencing or "trying on" new behaviors within the secure confines of the nurse-client relationship.
19. Establish the boundaries of the professional relationship, especially in the areas of

confidentiality, role of the nurse, and client expectations.

20. Establish and modify treatment plans and goals to fit the assessed needs of the client.
21. Evaluate communication context, being alert to the client's meaning.
22. Examine both the strengths and limitations of the client, allowing for ongoing change of the human condition.
23. Expect client growth and involvement, adjusted to client reality.
24. Express personal affirmation and supportive and corrective feedback for the client's positive actions and interactions.
25. Help the client to develop, maintain, and increase an authentic positive sense of self.
26. Honor the essential need for a meaningful and/or useful relationship in the client's life.
27. Honor the client's values and beliefs and life choices not related to psychopathology.
28. Honor the client's perception of a sense of risk, danger, or uncertainty as he approaches new situations, interpersonal encounters, and change. Serve as a guide, facilitator, and source of sustenance to the client's efforts toward clarifying reality.
29. Interact honestly with the client, presenting reality and truth.
30. Interact clearly and concisely, using care and precision in language choice and application.
31. Interact by employing positive statements and open-ended questions. Avoid blaming statements.
32. Interact on an adult-to-adult level with congruence of thought, word, and action.
33. Involve the client in goal setting whenever possible. Verbal and written contracts often facilitate the client's involvement.
34. Involve the client in appropriate task-centered life activities.
35. Listen actively for both manifest and latent communication messages.
36. Portray a sense of hope.

37. Present a knowledgeable, proficient nurse-clinician stance.
38. Respect the client's humanness.
39. Respect the client's uniqueness and individuality.
40. Remain open to nontraditional client-nurse experiences.
41. Remain knowledgeable of and alert to the psychopathology of the client and its impact on the client's life-style.
42. Remember that when in doubt, assessing for additional data and validating data through observation, collaboration, and theory will help to clarify the correct course of action.
43. Remember that the responsibility and accountability for the course of the helping relationship rest with the nurse. A structured, goal-directed approach can create a sense of trust and foster growth.
44. Remember that the "thereness" or presence of support is often an effective form of sustenance or maintenance for the client.
45. Remember that ongoing assessment of the everchanging human condition is necessary.
46. Remember that personal awareness, self-discipline, and flexibility are essential characteristics of the nurse.
47. Remember that role modeling is an effective method of teaching new life adaptation skills.
48. Remember that the experiencing of a feeling or action may be necessary to the client's growth.
49. Remember that the vital quality of the interpersonal relationship combined with excellence of nursing process design can be the elementary force for health modification.
50. Remember that the dynamics of each encounter will be unique to the particular client and the particular nurse involved in the specific interpersonal relationship and the specific interview.

Index

(